Affective Computing in Healthcare

Applications based on biosignals and artificial intelligence

Online at: https://doi.org/10.1088/978-0-7503-5182-9

IPEM–IOP Series in Physics and Engineering in Medicine and Biology

About the Series

The series in Physics and Engineering in Medicine and Biology will allow the Institute of Physics and Engineering in Medicine (IPEM) to enhance its mission to 'advance physics and engineering applied to medicine and biology for the public good'.

It is focused on key areas including, but not limited to:

- clinical engineering
- diagnostic radiology
- informatics and computing
- magnetic resonance imaging
- nuclear medicine
- physiological measurement
- radiation protection
- radiotherapy
- rehabilitation engineering
- ultrasound and non-ionising radiation.

A number of IPEM–IOP titles are being published as part of the EUTEMPE Network Series for Medical Physics Experts.

A full list of titles published in this series can be found here: https://iopscience.iop.org/bookListInfo/physics-engineering-medicine-biology-series.

Affective Computing in Healthcare

Applications based on biosignals and artificial intelligence

Edited by
M Murugappan
Department of Electronics and Communication Engineering, Kuwait College of Science and Technology, Kuwait, Kuwait

IOP Publishing, Bristol, UK

ISBN 978-0-7503-5182-9 (ebook)
ISBN 978-0-7503-5180-5 (print)
ISBN 978-0-7503-5183-6 (myPrint)
ISBN 978-0-7503-5181-2 (mobi)

DOI 10.1088/978-0-7503-5182-9

Version: 20230801

IOP ebooks

British Library Cataloguing-in-Publication Data: A catalogue record for this book is available from the British Library.

Published by IOP Publishing, wholly owned by The Institute of Physics, London

IOP Publishing, No.2 The Distillery, Glassfields, Avon Street, Bristol, BS2 0GR, UK

US Office: IOP Publishing, Inc., 190 North Independence Mall West, Suite 601, Philadelphia, PA 19106, USA

To my parents, my wife Subbu, and my Children Sakthi and Harish.

Contents

Preface

The field of affective computing has progressed tremendously in the past few years and has gained wide acceptance in various applications that involve e-learning, marketing, customer service, smart transportation, healthcare, and many more. Affective computing takes advantage of different modalities such as facial expressions, biosignals, gestures, and speech in order to develop technology that can detect different emotions (happiness, anger, sadness, fear, disgust, and surprise) of users. Over the past few years, it has become increasingly common in healthcare to employ this technology for clinical diagnosis. An affective computing system has also been developed for attempting to identify emotional disturbances or impairments in patients using an automated diagnosis system. In the past, it has been primarily used as a tool for diagnosing emotional disturbances associated with a variety of diseases, including depression, stress, emotional stress, anxiety, bipolar disorder, attention deficit disorder, strokes, Parkinson's disease (PD), autism spectrum disorders (ASD), mood disorders, etc. The majority of existing emotional computing applications rely on facial expressions and physiological signals such as Electrocardiograms (ECGs), Electromyograms (EMGs), Electroencephalograms (EEGs), Electrooculograms (EoGs), Skin Temperature (ST), Galvanic Skin Response (GSR), Photoplethsymogram (PPG), etc to assess the emotional state changes on the subjects. There have been numerous methods and algorithms proposed by researchers to extract meaningful information from biosignals and facial images so that they can extract meaningful information related to different emotions. In order to make decisions, artificial intelligence (AI) methods have been based on machine learning algorithms and deep learning algorithms. In spite of the fact that facial expression-based emotion recognition is a simple, cost-effective, and computationally efficient means of assessing emotions, the researchers have primarily chosen to use biosignals to assess the subject's emotions because they are highly robust and have the ability to capture highly refined information from physiological changes in an uncontrolled manner.

Researchers from a variety of countries have been involved in the development of the book, Affective Computing in Healthcare: Applications based on Biosignals and Artificial Intelligence. A total of eleven papers were selected for publication after the papers were reviewed by 31 reviewers in a double-blind fashion. There were several topics covered in the book, including the anxiety recognition using a new EEG signal analysis approach based on samples density in Chebyshev chaotic map, Evaluating the cognitive load during Lexical Decision Task for Monolinguals and Bilinguals using EEG, Detection of psychological stress using Principal Component Analysis of Phonocardiography signals, Affective Computational Advertising based on Perceptual Metrics, Machine Learning Based Emotions Recognition in Arousal-Valence Space using Photoplethysmogram Signals, EEG-Based Human Emotion Classification from Single-Channel Feature Extraction Methods Using Entropy Features and mRMR for Feature Selection, Detection of Physiological Body Movements by the Analysis of EEG Signals using Deep Neural Networks, Voice-enabled real-time affective framework for negative emotion monitoring, Differential Diagnosis Tool in health care application using Respiratory sounds under Emotion and Convolutional Neural Network, Gender and Emotion Recognition from Implicit User Behavior Signals, and Affective Computing and the Impact of VR/AR in the Healthcare Industry and Medical Domain.

As the editor of this book, I would like to thank the authors for revising and correcting their papers based on the feedback they received from our reviewers. I would also like to thank the reviewers for arranging a time slot within their schedules to review the papers. This will enable them to provide constructive feedback on their content with suggestions for improvement. I am delighted to be the editor of this book. It is with sincere gratitude that I acknowledge the authors and reviewers who have dedicated their time to the creation of this book.

M. Murugappan
Editor

Editor biography

M Murugappan

Professor Dr M Murugappan has been working at Kuwait College of Science and Technology (KCST), Kuwait as a Full Professor in Electronics, Department of Electronics and Communication Engineering since 2016. It is also his pleasure to serve as a Visiting Professor at the School of Engineering at Vels Institute of Science, Technology, and Advanced Studies in India. He is also an International Visiting Fellow at the Center of Excellence in Unmanned Aerial Systems at Universiti Malaysia Perlis in Malaysia. In 2006, he graduated from Anna University, India with an ME degree in Applied Electronics. He received his PhD from Universiti Malaysia Perlis, Malaysia in 2010 for his contribution to the field of mechatronic engineering. Between 2010 and 2016, he worked as a Senior Lecturer at the School of Mechatronics Engineering, Universiti Malaysia Perlis, Malaysia. In this role, he taught a variety of courses related to biomedical and mechatronics engineering. As a result of his excellent publications and research, he has been awarded several research awards, medals, and certificates. In a study by Stanford University, he was recently ranked among the top 2% of scientists working in experimental psychology and artificial intelligence for three consecutive years (2020–22). His research into affective computing has received more than $750,000 in grants from Malaysia, Kuwait, and the UK. His publications include more than 140 peer-reviewed conference proceedings papers, journal articles, and book chapters. Several of his journal articles have been recognised as best papers, best papers of the fiscal year, etc. Prof. Murugappan is a member of the editorial boards of *PLoS One*, *Human Centric Information Sciences*, the *Journal of Medical Imaging and Health Informatics*, and the *International Journal of Cognitive Informatics*. In addition to being the Chair of the IEEE Kuwait Section's Educational Activities Committee, he is an active reviewer for *IEEE Transactions on Multimedia*, *IEEE Transactions on Affective Computing*, *IEEE Transactions on Health Informatics*, and *IEEE Transactions on Biomedical Signal Processing*. He is interested in affective computing, affective neuroscience, the Internet of Things (IoT), the Internet of Medical Things (IoMT), cognitive neuroscience, brain–computer interfaces, neuromarketing, neuroeconomics, medical image processing, machine learning, and artificial intelligence. Throughout his career, he had a strong collaborative relationship with leading researchers in the fields of biosignal/image processing, artificial intelligence, IoT, and cognitive neuroscience. He is a member of several international professional societies including IEEE, IET, IACSIT, IAENG, and IEI.

List of contributors

RaamaNarayanan AnanthaNarayanan
Department of Bio-Medical Engineering, Sri Sivasubramaniya Nadar College of Engineering, Kalavakkam, Tamil Nadu, India

R Balasubramani
NMAM Institute of Technology, (Visvesvaraya Technological University, Belagavi), Nitte, Karnataka, India

Amandeep Cheema
Thapar Institute of Engineering and Technology, Patiala, Punjab, India

Moajjem Hossain Chowdhury
Universiti Kebangsan Malaysia, Malaysia

Muhammad E H Chowdhury
Qatar University, Doha 2713, Qatar

Faezeh Daneshmand-Bahman
Department of Biomedical Engineering, Imam Reza International University, Mashhad, Razavi Khorasan, Iran
Health Technology Research Center, Imam Reza International University, Mashhad, Razavi Khorasan, Iran

Suma Dawn
Jaypee Institute of Information Technology, Noida, India

B Geethanjali
Department of Bio-Medical Engineering, Sri Sivasubramaniya Nadar College of Engineering, Kalavakkam, Tamil Nadu, India

Fizza Ghulam Nabi
University of the Punjab, Lahore, Pakistan

Roland Goecke
University of Canberra, Australia

Ateke Goshvarpour
Department of Biomedical Engineering, Imam Reza International University, Mashhad, Razavi Khorasan, Iran
Health Technology Research Center, Imam Reza International University, Mashhad, Razavi Khorasan, Iran

Md Sakib Abrar Hossain
University of Dhaka, Dhaka, Bangladesh

Md. Shafayet Hossain
Qatar University, Doha 2713, Qatar

Shweta Jain
Indian Institute of Technology, Ropar, India

Rodrigo Jamisola Jr
Botswana International University of Science and Technology, Palapye, Botswana

Harish Katti
Indian Institute of Science, Bengaluru, India

Jason Elroy Martis
NMAM Institute of Technology (Visvesvaraya Technological University, Belagavi), Nitte, Karnataka, India

Lucky Odirile Mohutsiwa
Botswana International University of Science and Technology, Palapye, Botswana

Soujanya Narayana
University of Canberra, Australia

Rajkumar Palaniappan
University of Technology Bahrain, Salmabad, Kingdom of Bahrain

Sukeerthi Sakthivel
Department of Bio-Medical Engineering, Sri Sivasubramaniya Nadar College of Engineering, Kalavakkam, Tamil Nadu, India

M S Sannidhan
NMAM Institute of Technology (Visvesvaraya Technological University, Belagavi), Nitte, Karnataka, India

Md. Nazmul Islam Shuzan
Universiti Kebangsan Malaysia, Malaysia

Mandeep Singh
Thapar Institute of Engineering and Technology, Patiala, Punjab, India

Ramanathan Subramanian
University of Canberra, Australia

K B Sudeepa
NMAM Institute of Technology (Visvesvaraya Technological University, Belagavi), Nitte, Karnataka, India

Kenneth Sundaraj
Universiti Teknikal Malaysia Melaka (UTeM), Melaka, Malaysia

Prabha Sundaravadivel
Department of Electrical and Computer Engineering, The University of Texas at Tyler, Texas, USA

Aithal Sunil Kumar
NMAM Institute of Technology (Visvesvaraya Technological University, Belagavi), Nitte, Karnataka, India

Mahesh Veezhinathan
Department of Bio-Medical Engineering, Sri Sivasubramaniya Nadar College of Engineering, Kalavakkam, Tamil Nadu, India

Vikneswaran Vijean
Universiti Malaysia Perlis, Malaysia

Parker Wilmoth
Department of Electrical and Computer Engineering, The University of Texas at Tyler, Texas, USA

IOP Publishing

Affective Computing in Healthcare
Applications based on biosignals and artificial intelligence
M Murugappan

Chapter 1

Anxiety recognition using a new EEG signal analysis approach based on sample density in a Chebyshev chaotic map

Faezeh Daneshmand-Bahman and Ateke Goshvarpour

Anxiety is an unpleasant and stressful feeling experienced in different situations. Interfering with the normal functioning of the person, it can become a disorder. Anxiety disorder is associated with many physical and psychological effects. However, despite its high prevalence, an accurate diagnosis is only possible when the symptoms are sufficient and severe. Traditional diagnosis, a time-consuming process, depends on how the patient responds to self-reported questions. Alternatively, the electroencephalogram (EEG), a non-invasive clinical tool for screening brain activity, has attracted the attention of many researchers in the last few decades. This chapter proposes a novel computer-aided technique for detecting anxiety levels using EEG. Accordingly, the DASPS database was used to classify 19-channel EEGs into two and four anxiety levels. A two-dimensional phase space, called a Chebyshev chaotic map, was reconstructed. To the best of our knowledge, a Chebyshev chaotic map has not been utilised in biosignal analysis previously. The shape of the resulting trajectory depends on a variable that determines the degree of chaos. Multiple positive numbers were assigned to this variable to analyse its effect on the results. Innovative indicators were used for quantifying the map, including maximum density and the sample where the maximum density occurred. Then, minimum-redundancy maximum-relevance approach was implemented to reduce the feature number. *K*-fold cross-validation with a *k* of 2, 5, and 10 was applied to divide the data into training and testing groups. Finally, a decision tree and a *k*-nearest neighbour classifier with a *K* value of 2–8 were applied. The features were input into the module in four ways, including 5, 10, and 15 top-ranked against all measures to examine the impact of the number of selected attributes on anxiety detection rates. A maximum accuracy of 93.75% and 100% was obtained when detecting two and four anxiety levels, respectively. Compared to state-of-the-art EEG anxiety-detection systems, the proposed scheme is superior from a performance perspective.

1.1 Introduction

Affective computing is an active field of research that tries to identify, analyse, interpret, and simulate human emotional states using recent emerging technologies. Another goal of these methods is to provide efficient healthcare tools and systems for objective assessment, monitoring, and recognition of psychological disorders such as anxiety.

Anxiety, the most prevalent mental health problem worldwide [1–3], covers a wide range of mental disorders. The Fifth Edition of the Diagnostic and Statistical Manual of Mental Disorders (DSM-5) includes a broad spectrum of syndromes in the category of anxiety, including selective mutism, panic attack/disorder, specific phobia, agoraphobia, substance/medication-induced anxiety disorder, separation anxiety disorder, generalised anxiety disorder, social anxiety disorder (social phobia), and anxiety disorder due to another medical condition [4]. Gender-dependent prevalence, with anxiety being 1.5 to 2 times more likely among women, has been documented formerly [5]. Some previous studies have itemised trait and state as the two main anxiety groups [6]. The former designates personality traits and is measured while the individual is in a resting condition [7]. Conversely, the responses of the human body, either psychological or physiological, to the introduction of mental strain are measured in the latter [8]. Anxiety has many side effects [9], and it can also arise with other maladies, including major depressive disorder, personality disorders, and substance abuse. In addition, it constitutes an economic burden and causes significant deficiency in individual life quality [10].

Currently, anxiety diagnosis relies on self-reporting questionnaires, including the Diagnostic Interview Schedule [9], the Spielberg State and Trait Anxiety Inventory, Structured Clinical Interview for DSM-IV Disorders [11], the Composite International Diagnostic Interview, the aforementioned DSM-5, the Hospital Anxiety and Depression Scale, and the like [4]. An expert healthcare practitioner is required to interpret these tests. However, anxiety is only correctly diagnosed in this way when the symptoms are sufficient and severe [11]. Thus, developing efficacious clinical-diagnosis-aided tools or healthcare monitoring arrangements is of great importance to reduce healthcare expenditures and facilitate practitioners' work. To this end, physiological anxiety-based affective computing has been developed. Among methods of measuring physiological responses, the electroencephalogram (EEG) is held in special esteem due to its low cost, non-invasive nature, and high time resolution benefits [12].

EEG analysis in affect recognition has been considered in prior research [13–18]. Some efforts have also been made to detect anxiety as an affective computing application in health promotion systems by analysing EEG signals [19–25].

In a study conducted by Giannakakis *et al* [19], EEG signals were collected from 18 volunteers over 40 sessions while watching a 1 min video. Several features were implemented, including alpha-band asymmetry, coherence, brain load index, spectral centroid frequency, temporal properties of Hjorth parameters, and correlation dimensions. Early feature evaluation was performed using the Wilcoxon test. Next, sequential backward selection (SBS) and sequential forward selection (SFS) were implemented to select the feature. A higher alpha-band asymmetry for resting rather than anxious conditions was reported. On the contrary, the brain load index was higher for anxiety than the resting condition [19]. Klados *et al* [20] collected EEGs from 32 students in three circumstances, including (i) pre-test rest, (ii) three working memory tasks and four arithmetic tasks, and (iii) post-test rest. Event-related potentials with simple graph-theoretical parameters of functional connectivity were extracted from the corresponding signal. The optimum features were then selected using CfsSubsetEval and applied to a naïve Bayesian tree (NBTree) classifier. Math anxiety was diagnosed with 93.75% precision [20]. Baghdadi *et al* [8] provided an EEG database, namely DASPS, of 23 healthy participants and characterised them with several spectral, temporal, and time–frequency attributes. The features were applied to a support vector machine (SVM), stacked sparse auto-encoder (SSAE), and *k*-nearest neighbour (*K*-NN) classifier to detect two and four anxiety levels. The SSAE outperformed the other classifiers with a maximum accuracy of 83.5% and 74.60% for two and four anxiety levels, respectively [8]. Daneshmand-Bahman and Goshvarpour [21] analysed EEGs from the DASPS database using a Lyapunov exponent, different fractal dimensions, and approximate entropy. An accuracy, precision, F1 score, and sensitivity of 80%, 92.75%, 84.15%, and 80.58%, respectively, were obtained using a minimum-redundancy maximum-relevance (mRMR) feature-selection approach and multilayer perceptron (MLP) neural network [21]. Xie *et al* [22] analysed the EEGs of 10 individuals with depression and anxiety and 10 healthy controls in a resting state and Stroop tasks. Then, the phase lag index (PLI) was utilised to obtain the functional connectivity of the brain networks. Additionally, a convolutional neural network (CNN) was used for classification. The maximum achieved accuracy was 67.67% for anxiety and depression diagnoses [22]. Recently, Muhammad and Al-Ahmadi attempted to provide an objective human anxiety assessment agenda utilising the DASPS database [23]. First, electrode selection was accomplished using statistical analysis. Next, frequency domain attributes were calculated. Following EEG frequency band and feature selection, classification was implemented using multiple machine-learning procedures. Use of a random forest (RF) classifier resulted in an accuracy of 94.90% and 92.74% using nine and 10 features, respectively [23]. Li *et al* [24] collected EEG data from 12 participants. They quantified the signals utilising linear and non-linear characteristics. Specifically, spectral measures, such as total power, maximum power spectral density (max), and the frequency at maximum power density (f0), as well as Hjorth parameter, hemispherical asymmetry (HA), mean absolute amplitude (Ppmean), mean square, and variance were calculated as linear attributes, and approximate entropy (ApEn), complexity (C0) and correlation dimension (D2) were extracted as non-linear features. The correlation analysis was applied for feature selection. Then, two classifiers, SVM and *K*-NN, were used to classify the data into four anxiety levels. A maximum accuracy of 62.56% was obtained by the SVM [24]. Al-Ezzi *et al* [25] collected EEG data from 88 participants. The data were then processed using fuzzy entropy. Five machine-learning algorithms, including a naïve Bayes classifier (NBC), *K*-NN, linear discriminant analysis (LDA), a decision tree (DT), and a SVM, were examined to detect four anxiety levels. Their classification results showed a maximum accuracy of 86.93%, sensitivity of 92.46%, and specificity of 95.32% using the NBC [25].

This brief literature review shows that some of the proposed approaches have been implemented based on conventional frequency and statistical analyses [8, 19, 23]. Owing to the non-stationary and chaotic nature of EEG signals, however, these procedures do not have the potential to provide sufficient information about the signal behaviour. On the other hand, some researchers have utilised non-linear methods, which involve high computational complexity [20, 22]. Further, there is still a need to provide more accurate methods with better performance in diagnosing anxiety. The present chapter aims to provide a reliable system for classifying anxiety into two and four levels to address these challenges.

The main contribution of the proposed anxiety-detection scheme is by proposing innovative non-linear measures based on a Chebyshev chaotic map, which is consistent with the non-linear nature of EEGs. To the best of the authors' knowledge, Chebyshev chaotic maps have not yet been used to analyse biological signals. To quantify the map, we present an inventive technique based on the density of points. Additionally, a bulky feature vector length can be an influencing factor on classification rates. Consequently, we also examine the effect of the number of optimal features on anxiety recognition rates.

1.2 Material and methods

1.2.1 EEG DASPS database

This chapter makes use of the pre-processed EEG time series available in the DASPS database [8]. The database includes 14 standard EEG channels, according to the international 10–20 system. The chosen positions of the EEG electrodes were AF3, F7, F3, FC5, T7, P7, O1, O2, P8, T8, FC6, F4, F8, and AF4, while two mastoid sensors were considered as a ground point and indirect references. A wireless EEG headset, the Emotiv EPOC, was used to acquire the EEG signals. All EEG signals were recorded in an isolated room. The sampling frequency was 128 Hz. Then, ocular/muscular artifacts and EEG baseline were removed using a 4–45 Hz finite impulse response pass-band filter [8]. Twenty-three healthy subjects (13 female and 10 male) with an average age of 30 years participated in the study; all were without any psychological diseases.

The DASPS database applied flooding to induce anxiety. The recitation of real-life conditions was applied to motivate the participant. After performing a survey, six situations were selected where volunteers acknowledged the highest anxiety levels, including loss, family issues, financial issues, deadlines, witnessing a deadly accident, and mistreatment.

A consent form was asked to be signed before starting the experiment. Additionally, participants were enquired to fill out a Hamilton Anxiety Rating Scale (HAM-A) to calculate the initial severity of their anxiety level. Following the preparation period, in which the participants were required to maintain minimal movement and to close their eyes, the reciting/imagining of the aforementioned situations commenced. During this period, the psychotherapist recited the scenarios for 15 s, one-to-one. In each recitation, the volunteers had to recall the state of affairs and rate their valence and arousal by a nine-scale Self-Assessment Manikin (SAM) within 15 s. The valence was scored negative to positive, and arousal was ranked from calm to exciting. Using the SAM scores, the

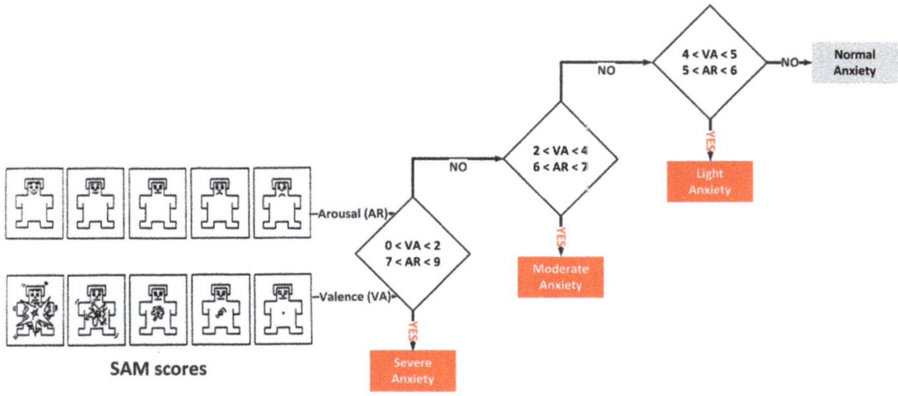

Figure 1.1. The process of labelling different anxiety levels.

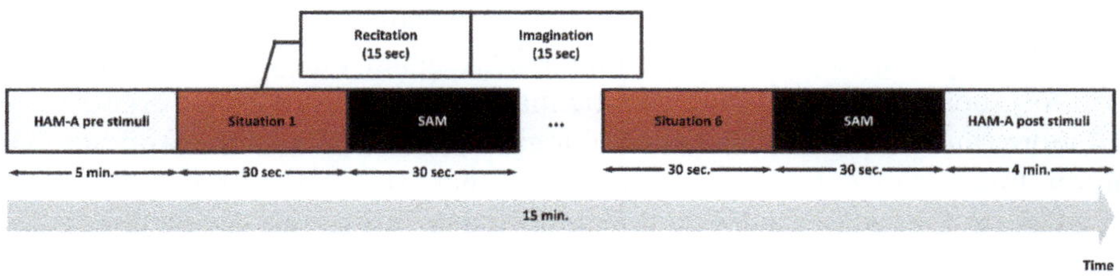

Figure 1.2. Protocol of anxiety stimulation.

labelling of four anxiety levels was performed. For arousal scores between 7 and 9 and valence scores between 0 and 2, the anxiety was labelled as 'severe'. Arousal scores from 6 to 7 and valence scores from 2 to 4, the anxiety was marked as 'moderate'. Arousal scores of 5 to 6 and valence scores of 4 to 5 indicated 'light' anxiety; otherwise, they were tagged as 'normal' anxiety (figure 1.1). Two-level anxiety classes were defined as normal and mild anxiety in one group and moderate and high anxiety in the other one. At the end of the trial, the psychoanalyst reassessed some items from the HAM-A rating to adjust the subject's anxiety level. Figure 1.2 shows all steps of the protocol. In conclusion, 136 'Normal' trials, 26 'Light' trials, 26 'Moderate' trials, and 88 'Severe' trials were labelled [8].

1.2.2 Normalisation

Since the database has already made the pre-processed EEG signals available to the public, only normalisation was performed here. Normalisation, a linear transformation to standardise the data in [0, 1], is calculated by equation (1.1):

$$\hat{x}_1 = \frac{x_i - \min(x_i)}{\max(x_t) - \min(x_t)}, \tag{1.1}$$

where the lower and upper values of EEG data (x_i) are shown by min(x_i) and max (x_i), respectively. This is a particular type of min–max normalisation with

$\max(\hat{x}_i) = 1$ and $\min(\hat{x}_i) = 1 = 0$ [26]. The following equation transfers data to [−1, 1], a preferred range for a Chebyshev chaotic map:

$$x_{\text{new}}\ \hat{x}_i \times 2 - 1. \tag{1.2}$$

Using equation (1.2), the max (x_{new}) = +1 and the min (x_{new}) = −1.

1.2.3 Chebyshev chaotic map

It has already been shown that chaotic maps have a non-linear structure [27]. A Chebyshev chaotic map, a one-dimensional chaotic plot [28], is recommended to elude trapping in local optima and to benefit the rummage [29]. It fulfills vital qualifications, comprising semi-group and chaotic characteristics [30, 31]. Chebyshev chaotic maps have been applied in a wide range of studies in various fields of science, including wireless body area networks [30], secure biometric-based authentication schemes [32], public-key cryptography [31], and authentication protocols [27]. However, to the best of our knowledge, a Chebyshev chaotic map has not been previously utilised in biomedical signal analysis. Furthermore, the reason for applying a Chebyshev chaotic map is to provide a better ergodic system and a more random output compared to logistic, Hénon, and sine mappings [33]. In addition, unlike conventional Poincaré plots, where signal amplitude information is used to draw the map, Chebyshev chaotic maps utilise the signal phase (cosine transformation). These features encouraged the use of a Chebyshev chaotic map for EEG signal processing and classification.

Chebyshev's polynomial, $T_n(y)$, as a polynomial in the type of y with degree n [31], that is, $n \in Z$, $y \in [-1, 1]$ and $T_n(y)$:$[-1, 1] \rightarrow [-1, 1]$, is defined by equation (1.3):

$$T_n(y) = \cos(n.\ \arccos(x)), \tag{1.3}$$

where n shows the degree of chaos and x is the normalised EEG samples. Additionally, the trigonometric functions $\cos(x)$ and $\arccos(x)$ are defined as cos (x): $R \rightarrow [0,\pi]$ and $\arccos(x)$: $[-1,1] \rightarrow [0,\pi]$ [30].

The Chebyshev polynomial has significant characteristics like Parseval's identity and orthogonality. Recent findings [34] have highlighted a more precise approximation of polynomial functions in interpolation using the Chebyshev polynomial as compared to Fourier series.

1.2.3.1 Chebyshev chaotic map data density quantifiers

Two data density quantifiers have been proposed to quantify Chebyshev chaotic maps. One hundred and twenty-eight strips parallel to the vertical axis of the map were formed. Next, the data density at each strip was calculated [35]. The maximum data density of all stripes was the first indicator. The sample where the maximum density occurred was the second quantifier of the map. Consequently, the total number of features was 28 (2 × 14; Chebyshev chaotic map data density indices × number of EEG channels). Figure 1.3 shows a sample of a Chebyshev chaotic map displaying how the map is divided into 128 ribbons. Also, the ribbon with the highest density of points has been specified on the plot.

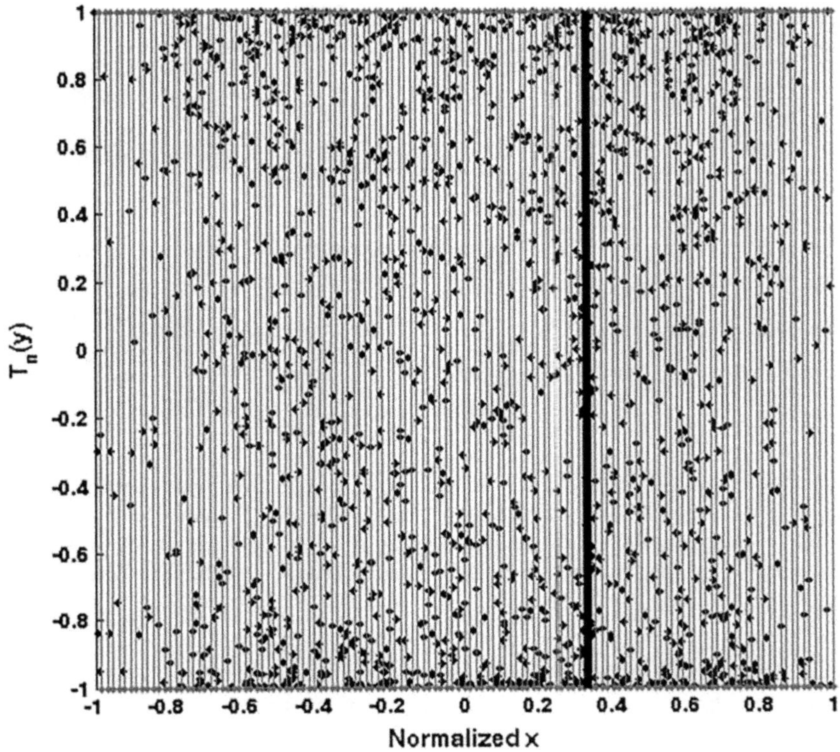

Figure 1.3. Schematic representation of how to segment and extract attributes from a Chebyshev chaotic map. The grey lines show 128 ribbons on the map. The density of points is calculated for each ribbon. A filled black line indicates the ribbon with the highest density of points.

Figure 1.4 demonstrates a sample EEG signal for normal/anxious states, their Chebyshev chaotic maps, and the corresponding colour density contours. As can be seen in the figure, dissimilar Chebyshev chaotic maps, with different positions for the distribution of higher-density points, are obtained for the different anxiety levels.

1.2.4 Feature selection

Feature-selection methods are divided into the filter [36], wrapper [37], and embedded [38] approaches. Unlike wrapper- and embedded-based methods, which are combined with the learning process to select the optimal subset of features, filter-based techniques are performed independently of the learning process. The learning process of the wrapper and embedded procedures usually entails a nested cross-validation (CV) strategy, which may cause augmented computational costs or overfitting, especially with few available observations. Therefore, a filter-based feature-selection approach was considered. The mRMR approach belongs to the family of filter-based algorithms. It effectively selects features by keeping the most relevant features (i.e., holding the most correlation with a class by calculating the

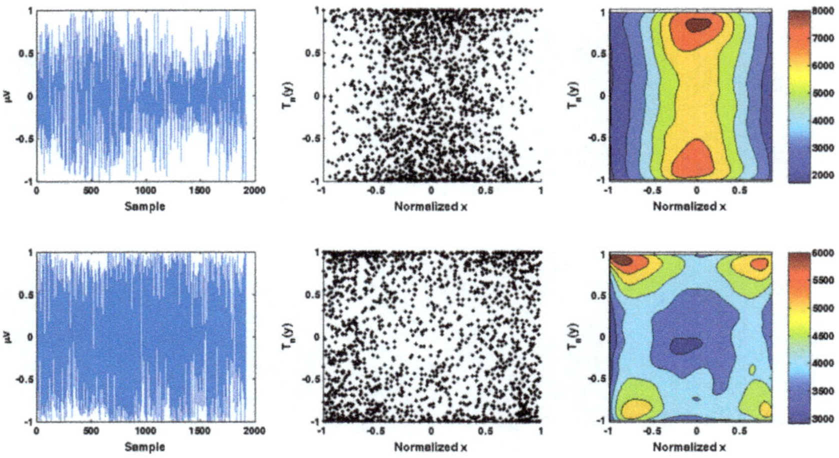

Figure 1.4. Top: Normalised brain signal, Chebyshev chaotic map, and colour density contour of the Chebyshev map for a person in a normal state (from left to right). Bottom: Normalised brain signal, Chebyshev chaotic map, and colour density contour of the Chebyshev map for an anxious person (from left to right). For the density contour, the cold colours show lower data density, and the warm colours show a higher density of data points.

F-statistic or mutual information, MI) and omitting the redundant features (by calculating the Pearson correlation coefficient or mutual information).

In this chapter, mRMR was implemented using MI. Here, the minimal-redundancy maximum-relevance criteria rank the features. mRMR is designed to find the maximum dependence between a feature set, *X*, and class, *c*, using MI. The MI is obtained using equation (1.4) when the marginal probabilities *p*(*a*) and *p*(*b*) and the joint probability *p*(*a*,*b*) between these two characteristics are determined:

$$I(A;\, B) = \sum\nolimits_{b\in B}\sum\nolimits_{a\in A} p(a,\, b)\log\left(\frac{p(a,\, b)}{p(a)\,p(b)}\right). \tag{1.4}$$

Maximum relevance includes features that apply to equation (1.5):

$$\max D(X,\, c);\, D = \frac{1}{|\,X\,|}\sum\nolimits_{X_i\in X} I(X_i;\, c). \tag{1.5}$$

Given that feature selection only creates redundancy using the maximum relevance, the minimum-redundancy criterion is added to it, which is obtained using equation (1.6):

$$\min R(X);\, R = \frac{1}{|\,X\,|}\sum\nolimits_{X_i,\, X_j\in X} I\left(X_i,\, X_j\right). \tag{1.6}$$

The combination and optimisation of the two formulas, equations (1.5) and (1.6), lead to the creation of the mRMR [39].

To examine the impact of the number of selected features on the anxiety-detection rates, they were input into the classification module in four ways, including all attributes, the five top-ranked features, the 10 top-ranked features, and the 15 top-ranked features.

1.2.5 Classification

The *K*-NN algorithm belongs to a class of supervised, distance-based machine-learning methods [40]. The distance from all samples in the vicinity of the indefinite data is calculated. Then, the ones with the shortest distances to them are filtered out.

The *K*-NN regards the *k*-nearest training data samples (neighbours) adjacent to the query it is testing. Then, a majority voting rule is performed to inspect which classification to produce. Consider that *K*-NN(d) is the set of *k*-nearest neighbours for the test data (d). The score of each nearest-neighbour data in the training set with the most similarity to the test data is used as the class weight of the neighbour data (equation 1.7):

$$\text{score}(d,\ t_i) = \sum\nolimits_{d_j=KNN(d)} \text{sim}\left(d,\ d_j\right)\delta\left(d_j,\ c_i\right). \tag{1.7}$$

If d_j fits c_i, $\delta(d_j,c_i)$ could be equal to 1 or 0 [41].

The shortest distance from the test sample to the training one is calculated using different algorithms, including Euclidean, Manhattan, Minkowski, and Hamming distances [8, 42]. Through trial and error, the user sets an integer as the k parameter for optimal classification results. Here, we examined different k values varying between 2 and 8.

A DT is a machine-learning technique [43]. Such DTs represent one of the most outstanding methods known for data classification [44]. A DT is a tree where each node indicates an attribute, each branch represents a decision (rule), and each leaf shows an outcome (class labels). The tree is placed reverse down, so the roots are at the highest, and the leaves represent many results at the lowest. The root shows the original dataset. The tree then arrives at the first node, where a definite variable feature is used to divide the population into classes [43]. Since the DT is based on human thinking, it is suitable for interpreting data [45]. This classifier is widely used because it is easy, without ambiguity, and strong, even in the presence of lost values [46]. Also, this model does not rely on hierarchical features but on hierarchical decisions [47].

A *K*-fold CV strategy was adopted to divide the data into training and validation. This strategy splits the data into k subsets [48], with the $k-1$ subsets as training and the remaining subset as a validation set. By repeating the process k times, all subsets are included in the validation set [49]. We set k as different values, including 2, 5, and 10.

In a multi-class strategy, the classifier performance was appraised using accuracy, sensitivity, and F1 score (equations (1.8)–(1.10)):

$$\text{Accuracy} = \frac{\text{TP} + \text{TN}}{\text{TP} + \text{TN} + \text{FP} + \text{FN}}, \tag{1.8}$$

$$\text{Sensitivity} = \frac{\text{TP}}{\text{TP} + \text{FN}}, \tag{1.9}$$

$$\text{F1 score} = \frac{2 \cdot \text{TP}}{2 \cdot \text{TP} + \text{FP} + \text{FN}}, \tag{1.10}$$

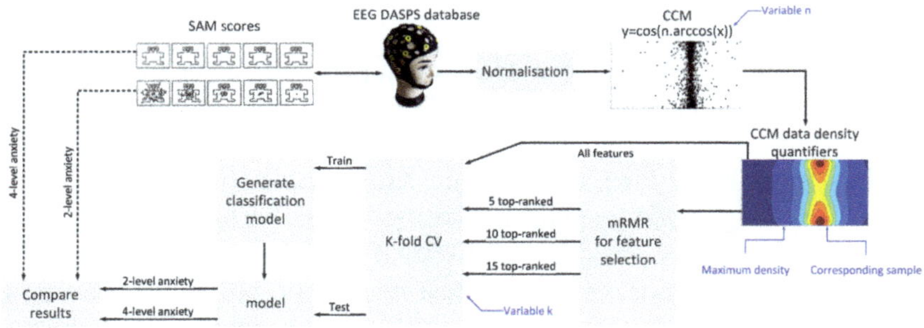

Figure 1.5. Block diagram of the proposed methodology for anxiety recognition.

where TP (True Positive)/TN (True Negative) refers to positive/negative data correctly identified, and FP (False Positive)/FN (False Negative) indicates negative/positive data incorrectly diagnosed.

Figure 1.5 shows an overview of the proposed approach.

1.3 Results

Chebyshev's chaotic map formula (equation (1.3)) incorporates a variable that indicates the degree of chaos (n). First, the effect of changing this variable on the shape of the Chebyshev chaotic map's trajectory was investigated. For this purpose, different positive integers were ascribed to n (figure 1.6).

As the figure shows, increasing the value of n causes the location of the maximum density of points to be determined more precisely. As such, for higher n values ($n = 500$ and 1000), the position of the maximum density has not changed significantly.

Table 1.1 shows the best results for the K-NN classifier. The best classifier performance for distinguishing two and four anxiety levels with varying values of n in a Chebyshev chaotic map is shown in two modes, for all features and the number of features that had the best result. Table 1.2 highlights the selected indices.

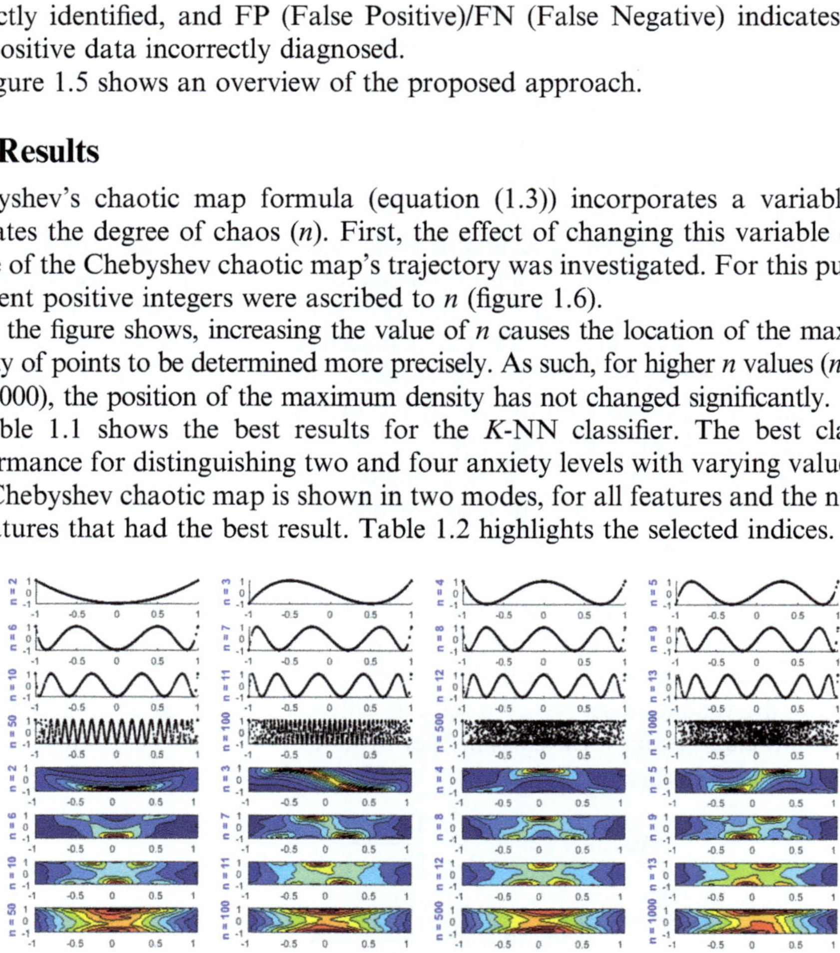

Figure 1.6. The effect of 'n' values on a Chebyshev chaotic map's trajectory and the density distribution of the trajectory points. The first four rows show the reconstruction of a Chebyshev chaotic map for n = 2–13, 50, 100, 500, and 1000. The corresponding colour density of the Chebyshev chaotic map's points is shown in the last four rows of the figure.

Table 1.1. The best results of the *K*-NN classification.

		Two-level anxiety detection					Four-level anxiety detection				
n for Chebyshev chaotic map	Feature vector	NF	*K* for *K*-NN, *K* for *K*-fold	AC	SN	F1	NF	*K* for *K*-NN, *K* for *K*-fold	Accuracy	Sensitivity	F1
2	All	—	(8, 2)	78.75	70	66.66	—	(8, 10)	100	100	74.07
	Selected	15	(8, 2)	90	82.25	66.31	5*	(8, 2)	100	100	67.62
3	All	—	(8, 2)	82.5	77.5	67.01	—	(8, 5)	100	100	75.47
	Selected	5	(8, 5)	90.62	71.05	70.88	10	(8, 2)	100	100	68.18
4	All	—	(8, 2)	83.75	72.5	69.89	—	(8, 2)	100	98.03	63.82
	Selected	10	(8, 2)	92.5	78.75	67.35	5	(8, 5)	100	100	69.84
5	All	—	(8, 2)	85	73.75	67.01	—	(8, 2)	100	100	72.05
	Selected	10	(8, 2)	91.25	78.75	68.62	10#	(8, 2)	100	100	68.02
6	All	—	(8, 5)	90.62	81.25	66.66	—	(8, 5)	100	100	73.07
	Selected	15	(8, 2)	88.75	72.5	70.35	15	(8, 2)	100	100	68.65
7	All	—	(8, 5)	90.62	81.25	73.68	—	(8, 5)	100	100	70.17
	Selected	10	(8, 2)	81.25	78.75	67.70	5	(8, 2†)	100	100	72.72
8	All	—	(8, 5)	87.5	78.12	69.33	—	(8, 2)	100	100	67.85
	Selected	15	(8, 5)	87.5	81.25	71.6	15	(8, 2)	100	98.03	64.23
9	All	—	(8, 2)	92.5	75	68.88	—	(8, 10)	100	100	78.78
	Selected	5	(8, 2)	87.5	78.75	68.47	15	(8, 2)	100	100	71.14
10	All	—	(8, 5)	84.37	81.25	72.72	—	(8, 5)	100	100	75.86
	Selected	15	(8, 2)	87.5	81.25	69.38	5	(8, 5)	100	100	74.19
11	All	—	(8, 2)	88.75	77.5	69.89	—	(7, 5)	100	100	100
	Selected	10	(8, 2)	93.75	85	69.95	10	(8, 2)	100	100	63.7
12	All	—	(8, 5)	87.5	78.12	74.07	—	(8, 2†)	100	100	72
	Selected	10	(8, 2)	86.25	78.75	69.74	15	(8, 2)	100	100	72.22
13	All	—	(8, 2)	85	75	66.32	—	(8, 2)	100	98.3	74.82
	Selected	10	(8, 5)	87.5	75	65.85	15&	(8, 5)	100	100	73.33
50	All	—	(8, 2)	81.25	76.25	68.44	—	(8, 2)	100	100	64.78
	Selected	10	(8, 2)	93.75	83.75	67.01	15	(8, 5)	100	100	76.66
100	All	—	(8, 2)	85	73.75	69.03	—	(8, 5)	100	100	70.58
	Selected	15	(8, 5)	87.5	81.25	67.53	15‡	(8, 5)	100	100	73.33
500	All	—	(8, 5)	87.5	75	70	—	(8, 10)	100	100	74.07
	Selected	10	(8, 2)	88.75	76.25	66	10♠	(8, 2)	100	100	65.24
1000	All	—	(8, 2)	85	76.25	69.74	—	(8, 2)	100	100	67.58
	Selected	15	(8, 5)	93.75	84.37	72.5	5	(8, 5)	100	100	66.66

Notes: NF: number of selected features; AC: accuracy; SN: sensitivity.
* In addition to the number of features mentioned, the maximum accuracy was also 100% for 10 features and twofold CV.
# In addition to the number of features mentioned, the maximum accuracy was also 100% for 15 features and fivefold CV.
† In addition to twofold CV, the maximum accuracy was also 100% for fivefold CV.
& In addition to twofold CV, the maximum accuracy was also 100% for tenfold CV.
& In addition to the number of features mentioned, the maximum accuracy was also 100% for five features and twofold CV, five features and tenfold CV, and 10 features and fivefold CV.
‡ In addition to the number of features mentioned, the maximum accuracy was also 100% for five features and fivefold CV.
♠ In addition to the number of features mentioned, the maximum accuracy was also 100% for five features and five/twofold CV.

Table 1.2. The selected features for the *K*-NN classifier.

	Two-level anxiety detection		Four-level anxiety detection	
n for Chebyshev chaotic map	Number of features selected	Feature-selected channel	Number of features selected	Feature-selected channel
2	15	A2, B9, B14, B6, B5, B12, B13, B7, B10, B2, B3, B8, B4, B1, B11	5	A2, B9, B14, B6, A3
3	5	A1, B12, B9, B14, B7	10	A1, B12, B9, B14, B7, B1, A2, B11, B4, B6
4	10	A1, B9, B14, B4, B6, B10, B12, B5, B7, B2	5	A1, B9, B14, B4, B6
5	10	A1, B12, B9, B14, B6, B1, B11, B7, B5, B4	10	A1, B12, B9, B14, B1, B6, A4, B11, B5, B7
6	15	A1, B14, B9, B4, B12, B6, B5, B11, B7, B1, B10, B13, B8, B2, B3	15	A1, B14, B9, B4, B12, B6, A2, B11, B7, B1, B10, B5, B13, A8, B8
7	10	A1, B12, B9, B14, B6, B1, B11, B5, B4, B13	5	A1, B12, B9, B14, B1
8	15	A1, B14, B9, B4, B12, B6, B10, B1, B5, B11, B7, B8, B2, B13, B3	15	A1, B14, B9, B4, B12, B6, A3, B10, B1, B8, B5, B11, B7, A4, B13
9	5	A1, B12, B9, B14, B7	15	A1, B9, B12, B14, B7, B11, A2, B1, B6, B13, B4, B3, A13, B5, B10
10	15	A1, B12, B9, B14, B1, B6, B4, B5, B11, B13, B10, B7, B3, B8, B2	5	A1, B12, B9, B14, B1
11	10	A1, B9, B12, B14, B1, B6, B4, B11, B7, B5	10	A1, B9, B12, B14, B1, B7, A2, B6, B4, B11
12	10	A1, B12, B9, B14, B11, B5, B6, B1, B4, B13	15	A1, B12, B9, B14, B11, B5, A3, B6, B1, B4, B13, B10, A2, B7, B8
13	10	A1, B9, B12, B14, B1, B6, B11, B4, B5, B7	15	A1, B9, B14, B12, B1, B6, A2, B11, B4, B5, B13, B7, A3, B10, B3
50	10	A1, B9, B12, B14, B6, B4, B11, B5, B1, B13	15	A1, B9, B12, B14, B6, B1, A2, B11, B4, B5, B13, B10, A3, B7, B8
100	15	A1, B9, B12, B14, B6, B1, B11, B5, B4, B13, B7, B10, B3, B2, B8	15	A1, B9, B12, B14, B6, B1, A2, B11, B4, B5, B13, B10, A3, B7, B8
500	10	A1, B9, B12, B14, B6, B4, B11, B5, B1, B13	10	A1, B9, B12, B14, B6, B1, A12, B11, B4, B5
1000	15	A1, B9, B12, B14, B6, B4, B11, B5, B1, B13, B7, B10, B3, B2, B8	5	A1, B9, B12, B14, B6

Notes: A: maximum density; B: the sample where the maximum density occurred; channel numbers from 1 to 14 in the following order: 1: AF3, 2: F7, 3: F3, 4: FC5, 5: T7, 6: P7, 7: O1, 8: O2, 9: P8, 10: T8, 11: FC6, 12: F4, 13: F8, 14: AF4.

As table 1.1 shows, generally the best results were obtained by 8-NN. The maximum accuracy was 93.75% for $n = 1000$, 15 features, and fivefold CV in two anxiety levels. In this case, the sensitivity was 84.37%, and the F1 score was 72.5%. The maximum accuracy was 93.75% for 10 selected features, and $n = 11$ or 50. However, the other classification performance criteria were slightly lower compared to the previous case. On the contrary, the lowest accuracy rate was 78.75% for all the features, $n = 2$, and twofold CV.

All n values yielded the maximum accuracy of 100% for four-level anxiety detection. The maximum sensitivity was 100% for all n values, except for $n = 4$, 8, and 13, where its value dropped to 98.3%. A maximum F1 score of 100% was attained for $n = 11$, all the features, 7-NN, and fivefold CV.

Table 1.2 reveals that the best attribute is the sample in which the maximum density occurred. Also, according to the results, the best channel concerning the most repetitions in selected features is channel 1.

Table 1.3 shows the maximum results using the DT for varying n values in a Chebyshev chaotic map. The best performances for distinguishing two and four anxiety levels are calculated in two modes, including all features and the selected features. Table 1.4 illustrates the selected attributes.

Table 1.3. The best results of the DT classifier.

		Two-level anxiety detection					Four-level anxiety detection				
n for Chebyshev chaotic map	Feature vector	NF	*K* for *K*-fold	AC	SN	F1	NF	*K* for *K*-fold	Accuracy	Sensitivity	F1
2	All	—	10	74.07	76.47	78.78	—	5	77.77	87.5	62.22
	Selected	10	10	74.07	73.68	80	5	2	81.81	84.90	68.70
3	All	—	10	70.37	80	73.33	—	5	82.35	93.75	66.66
	Selected	10	10	67.85	71.42	74.28	5	5	86.36	92.85	75
4	All	—	2	53.62	61.11	57.89	—	2	75.55	85.10	66.11
	Selected	5*	2	59.42	65.78	64.10	5	5	86.66	92.85	83.33
5	All	—	2	52.89	60.86	62.92	—	2	75.51	87.09	60.65
	Selected	10	2	56.52	61.62	63.85	10	5	100	100	70.58
6	All	—	10	70.37	75	75	—	2	86.04	88.09	62.18
	Selected	5	10	67.85	76.92	72.72	10	10	100	100	83.33
7	All	—	2	53.62	58.88	62.35	—	10	100	100	69.56
	Selected	10	10	70.37	78.57	73.33	10	10	100	100	66.66
8	All	—	2	54.34	61.97	58.38	—	2	84.78	94.73	63.15
	Selected	15	2	54.34	60.24	61.34	10	5	100	100	67.92
9	All	—	2	52.89	61.90	56.96	—	2	83.67	86.95	62.99
	Selected	5	10	78.57	81.25	81.25	5	10	100	100	81.48
10	All	—	5	65.45	65.11	74.66	—	5	100	100	74.07
	Selected	5	5	64.28	65.78	71.42	5	5	93.75	93.33	56
11	All	—	2	55.79	62.33	61.14	—	5	88.23	92.85	66.66
	Selected	5	10	71.42	75	77.77	5	2	82.92	91.42	66.12

(*Continued*)

Table 1.3. (*Continued*)

		Two-level anxiety detection					Four-level anxiety detection				
n for Chebyshev chaotic map	Feature vector	NF	*K* for *K*-fold	AC	SN	F1	NF	*K* for *K*-fold	Accuracy	Sensitivity	F1
12	All	—	5	61.81	72	70.27	—	2	79.24	86.66	66.66
	Selected	15	2	55.07	60.46	62.65	15	2	85.36	87.5	58.33
13	All	—	10	78.57	85.71	80	—	5	88.23	100	68
	Selected	5	10	71.42	72.22	76.47	5	2	88.37	88.37	60.31
50	All	—	10	66.66	73.33	70.96	—	5	86.36	89.47	76
	Selected	15	5	65.45	72.41	69.69	10	2	83.92	90.24	64.38
100	All	—	2	56.52	62.5	65.53	—	5	94.11	100	61.90
	Selected	5	2	58.69	65.75	65.88	15	5	93.75	100	64.15
500	All	—	10	67.85	68.42	74.28	—	5	87.5	94.11	64
	Selected	5	2	60.14	63.44	68.20	10	2	85.10	90.24	63.24
1000	All	—	2	54.34	60	61.81	—	5	87.5	92.30	66.66
	Selected	5	2	55.07	61.25	61.25	15	5	95	94.73	67.92

Notes: NF: number of selected features; AC: accuracy; SN: sensitivity.
*In addition to the stated result, the maximum accuracy was obtained utilising 10 features.

According to table 1.2, utilising a DT, the maximum accuracy for two-level anxiety diagnosis was 78.57% for n = 13, all the features, and 10-fold CV. In this case, the sensitivity was 85.71%, and the F1 score was 80%. The maximum accuracy was 78.57% for n = 9 and five selected features.

For four-level anxiety detection, the best results were obtained for n = 6, 10 features, and 10-fold CV, where the accuracy and sensitivity were 100%, and the F1 score was 83.33%. The maximum accuracy was also 100% for n = 7–10. However, compared to the previous condition, the other performance criteria were lower. On the contrary, the lowest accuracy rate was 71.51% for all the features and twofold CV.

The results of table 1.4 show that channel 1 has the most repetitions compared to other EEG electrodes. In addition, from the two indicators of the Chebyshev chaotic map, the characteristic of the sample in which the maximum density occurred has the highest selection rate.

Table 1.4. The selected features for DT classifier.

	Two-level anxiety detection		Four-level anxiety detection	
n for Chebyshev chaotic map	Number of features selected	Feature-selected channel	Number of features selected	Feature-selected channel
2	10	A2, B9, B14, B6, B5, B12, B13, B7, B10, B2	5	A2, B9, B14, B6, B5
3	10	A1, B12, B9, B14, B7, B1, B11, B4, B6, B13	5	A1, B12, B9, B14, B7

4	5	A1, B9, B14, B4, B6	5	A1, B9, B14, B4, B6
5	10	A1, B12, B9, B14, B6, B1, B11, B7, B5, B4	10	A1, B12, B9, B14, B1, B6, A4, B11, B5, B7
6	5	A1, B14, B9, B4, B12	10	A1, B12, B9, B4, B12, B6, A2, B11, B7, B1
7	10	A1, B12, B9, B14, B6, B1, B11, B5, B4, B13	10	A1, B12, B9, B14, B1, B6, A2, B11, B13, B5
8	15	A1, B14, B9, B4, B12, B6, B10, B1, B5, B11, B7, B8, B2, B13, B3	10	A1, B12, B9, B4, B12, B6, A3, B10, B1, B8
9	5	A1, B12, B9, B14, B7	5	A1, B9, B12, B14, B7
10	5	A1, B12, B9, B14, B1	5	A1, B12, B9, B14, B1
11	5	A1, B9, B12, B14, B1	5	A1, B9, B12, B14, B1
12	15	A1, B12, B9, B14, B11, B5, B6, B1, B4, B13, B10, B7, B2, B3, B8	15	A1, B12, B9, B14, B11, B5, A3, B6, B1, B4, B13, B10, A2, B7, B8
13	5	A1, B9, B12, B14, B1	5	A1, B9, B14, B12, B1
50	15	A1, B9, B12, B14, B6, B4, B11, B5, B1, B13, B7, B10, B3, B2, B8	10	A1, B9, B12, B14, B6, B1, A2, B11, B4, B5
100	5	A1, B9, B12, B14, B6	15	A1, B9, B12, B14, B6, B1, A2, B11, B4, B5, B13, B10, A3, B7, B8
500	5	A1, B9, B12, B14, B6	10	A1, B9, B12, B14, B6, B1, A12, B11, B4, B5
1000	5	A1, B9, B12, B14, B6	15	A1, B9, B12, B14, B6, B1, A3, B11, B4, B5, B13, B10, A4, B7, B8

Notes: A: maximum density; B: the sample where the maximum density occurred; channel numbers from 1 to 14 in the following order: 1: AF3, 2: F7, 3: F3, 4: FC5, 5: T7, 6: P7, 7: O1, 8: O2, 9: P8, 10: T8, 11: FC6, 12: F4, 13: F8, 14: AF4.

Figure 1.7 shows the highest performance of the two classifiers. Comparing the results (tables 1.1 and 1.3, and figure 1.7), it is revealed that the *K*-NN outperformed the DT.

1.4 Discussions

Anxiety is an affective disorder that any person may experience at some situation in life. With the prevalence of COVID-19, this disorder is increasing. With timely diagnosis and treatment of anxiety, its exacerbation and complications can be prevented. This chapter presented an innovative anxiety-detection system using a Chebyshev chaotic map (with a variable value of n). The map was characterised using new density-based indicators. The mRMR algorithm was also used for feature selection. The attributes were applied to DT and *K*-NN classifiers using four

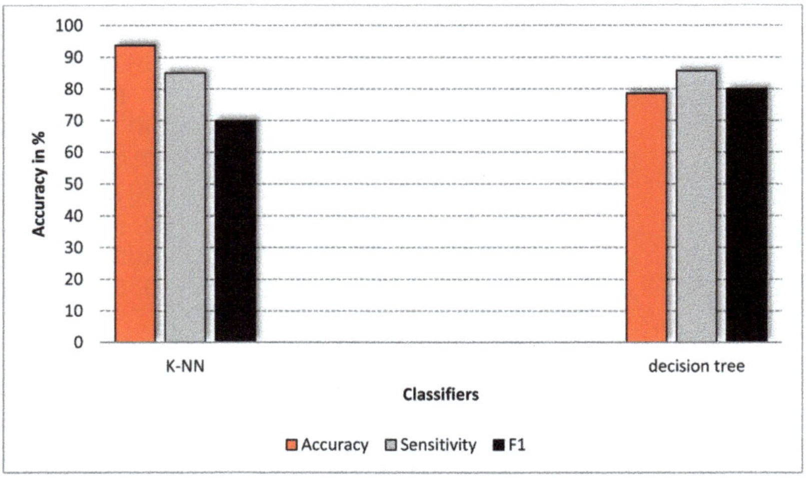

(a)

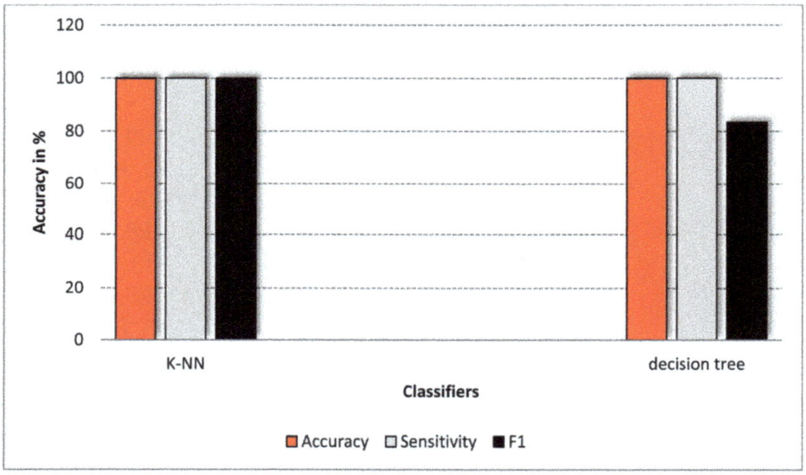

(b)

Figure 1.7. The maximum *K*-NN and DT classification results for separating (a) two anxiety levels, and (b) four anxiety levels.

different input strategies, including all features, the five top-ranked features, the 10 top-ranked features, and the 15 top-ranked features. Our results showed that the *K*-NN's performance was superior to that of the DT. The maximum recognition rate was 93.75% for two-level anxiety detection and 100% for four-level anxiety detection. The selected value of n (in Chebyshev's chaotic map formula) significantly affected the recognition of two anxiety levels, but not in the four anxiety levels case. The number of top-ranked features obtained by the feature-selection algorithm and the adjustment of the amount of k in the k-fold CV had a significant effect on recognition rates. Extracting thet Chebyshev chaotic map's measures took about

70 s for each person in each n value and all EEG channels. The shorter the calculation time, the lower the computational complexity.

A comparison of this new anxiety-detection algorithm with other studies is provided in table 1.5. Differences in approaches and the heterogeneity of systems can be seen from different aspects.

Table 1.5. Overview of studies presented in the field of anxiety detection in terms of number of data, number of channels, analysis method, and results.

Study	Number of subjects	Number of electrodes	Method of analysis	Best results
[19]	18	32	Feature extraction: alpha-band asymmetry, coherence, brain load index, spectral centroid frequency, Hjorth parameter, and correlation dimensions. Feature selection: SBS and SFS. Statistical analysis: ANOVA.	– Asymmetry in the anxiety group is lower than the control group. – Brain index in the control group is lower than the anxiety group.
[20]	32	57	Feature extraction: evoked related potential, simple graph-theoretical parameters extracted from functional connectivity. Feature selection: CfsSubsetEval. Classification: NBTree.	Precision: 93.75%
[8]	23	14	Feature extraction: fractal dimension, Hjorth parameter, band power, Hilbert–Huang spectrum, band power, and root. Root mean square (RMS) using discrete wavelet transform, differential asymmetry, and quantitative features. Classifications: *K*-NN, SVM, SSAE.	Accuracy: 83.50% (two-level anxiety) 74.60% (four-level anxiety) using SSAE
[21]	23	14	Feature extraction: Higuchi–Petrosian–Katz fractal dimensions, Lyapanov exponent, approximate entropy. Feature selection: mRMR.	Precision: 92.75% (two-level anxiety)

(*Continued*)

Table 1.5. (*Continued*)

Study	Number of subjects	Number of electrodes	Method of analysis	Best results
			Classification: MLP.	
[22]	20	31	Feature extraction: proximity matrix obtained by PLI. Classification: CNN.	Accuracy: 67.67%
[23]	23	14	Feature extraction: asymmetry index, rational index, and mean power. EEG frequency band and feature selection: leave-one-out CV and wrapper method. Classifications: MLP, SVM, *K*-NN, RF, DT.	Accuracy: 94.90% (two-level anxiety) 92.74% (four-level anxiety)
[24]	12	128	Feature extraction: Hjorth parameter, total power, max, f0, HA, Ppmean, mean square, variance, ApEn, C0, and D2. Feature selection: correlation. Classifications: SVM and *K*-NN.	Accuracy: 62.56%
[25]	88	32	Feature extraction: fuzzy entropy. Classifications: *K*-NN, LDA, NBC, DT, and SVM.	Accuracy: 86.93% Sensitivity: 92.46% Specificity: 95.32%
Present work	23	14	Feature extraction: innovative Chebyshev chaotic map-based features. Feature selection: mRMR. Classifications: DT and *K*-NN.	Accuracy: 93.75% (two-level anxiety) 100% (four-level anxiety)

The present chapter evaluates the DASPS database [8]. However, since there is no standard database, most of the previous literature has collected data themselves. Consequently, the data are different in terms of the number of electrodes, recording devices, sample number, demographic information (such as gender and age ranges), and anxiety induction protocol. In particular, the sample number varied from 12 [24] to 88 [25]. Also, the number of electrodes differed from 14 [8] to 128 [24].

The innovative features of a Chebyshev chaotic map, which belongs to non-linear approaches and, as yet, has not been evaluated in biosignal analysis, have been suggested in this chapter. Former experiments in EEG anxiety detection have usually focused on the conventional time domain [8, 19, 24] and frequency domain [8, 19, 24], and time–frequency measures [8] and statistical features [24]. However, due to the non-stationary and chaotic nature of EEG signals, insufficient information is obtained from these methods. Dealing with the problem of signal instability can be solved with non-linear analysis approaches. However, as mentioned, these approaches have been considered in few previous studies [19, 21].

The proposed scheme evaluated *K*-NN with different structures and DT. Additionally, the role of adjusting *k* values for the *k*-fold CV and input vectors (in terms of feature number) was tested on anxiety-detection rates. Some studies have focused on the statistical differences between EEG measurements of control and anxious groups [19]. Alternatively, others have attempted to categorise anxiety [8, 20–25]. *K*-NN has been suggested in several studies as a classifier [8, 23–25]. Usually, a method has been dedicated for feature selection [19–21, 23, 24]; however, these methods have not always been the same.

The chosen framework achieved a maximum accuracy of 93.75% for diagnosing two-level anxiety and 100% for detecting four-level anxiety. A lower detection rate has been previously reported on the same database [8]. In [23], a slightly higher rate (by about 1%) was reported in the detection of two anxiety levels, which is negligible. Others achieved classification rates of 62.56% [24] to 94.90% [23]. Compared to state-of-the-art EEG anxiety-detection systems, the proposed scheme is superior from a performance perspective.

1.5 Conclusion

In recent years, providing an automatic anxiety diagnostic tool has become a challenging issue due to the increasing prevalence of anxiety. Consequently, researchers are looking for new methods with a higher recognition rate. In this chapter, it was attempted to provide new biomarkers based on a Chebyshev chaotic map to classify anxiety into two and four levels. Innovative indicators were proposed based on sample density for map quantification, including (i) maximum density, and (ii) the sample where the maximum density occurred. Then, the extracted features were applied to the mRMR algorithm to select the top-ranked features. Finally, the features were applied to the DT and *K*-NN. The DASPS dataset was used for system evaluation. The proposed algorithm achieved a maximum accuracy of 93.75% and 100% for two- and four-level anxiety detection, respectively. In addition, the potential of the variable *n* in Chebyshev's chaotic map equation and the classifier structure were emphasised in the detection of anxiety levels.

The present study had limitations. One such was the limited number of signals provided by the database. The evaluation of mass data makes it possible to infer an algorithm's generalisability, which is not accessible currently. Here, a Chebyshev chaotic map was used for the first time in biological data analysis, and only two parameters were introduced for the quantification. The map's characteristics could be revealed by a more detailed evaluation utilising slightly different tools. The present research evaluated a filter-based feature-selection approach for channel/feature selection. Despite obtaining fascinating results, changing the algorithm may affect the results. Furthermore, anxiety, induced by different cues, includes a wide range of abnormalities. The causes and consequences of anxiety can yield the occurrence of a range of other neurological disorders. This study only examined cases that used flooding to drive anxiety.

Regarding the study's limitations, the following suggestions are provided for future research: (i) to evaluate large-scale datasets to ensure the effectiveness of the proposed algorithm; (ii) here, point-density-based indicators were proposed for the Chebyshev chaotic map's quantification, whereas in future studies, the map should be described by other measures; (iii) the suggested system implemented mRMR for selecting top-ranked attributes, but other feature-selection approaches should be tested; and (iv) the proposed algorithm should be assessed by diagnosing other neurological disorders.

Acknowledgments

This article uses the DASPS database [8]. The authors would like to thank Ms Baghdadi and her colleagues for making the data available for free.

Compliance with ethical standards

Funding

This research did not receive any specific grant from funding agencies in the public, commercial, or not-for-profit sectors.

Conflict of interest

The authors declare that they have no conflict of interest.

Statements of ethical approval

This article does not contain any studies with human participants performed by any of the authors.

References

[1] Liu Y, Chen H, Zhang N, Wang X, Fan Q, Zhang Y and Li M 2021 Anxiety and depression symptoms of medical staff under COVID-19 epidemic in China *J. Affect. Disord.* **278** 144–8

[2] McElroy E, Fearon P, Belsky J, Fonagy P and Patalay P 2018 Networks of depression and anxiety symptoms across development *J. Am. Acad. Child Adolesc. Psychiatry* **57** 964–73

[3] Schäfer J Ö, Naumann E, Holmes E A, Tuschen-Caffier B and Samson A C 2017 Emotion regulation strategies in depressive and anxiety symptoms in youth: a meta-analytic review *J. Youth Adolesc.* **46** 261–76

[4] Millet N, Longworth J and Arcelus J 2017 Prevalence of anxiety symptoms and disorders in the transgender population: a systematic review of the literature *Int. J. Transgend.* **18** 27–38

[5] Bandelow B, Michaelis S and Wedekind D 2017 Treatment of anxiety disorders *Dialogues Clin. Neurosci.* **19** 93

[6] Saviola F, Pappaianni E, Monti A, Grecucci A, Jovicich J and De Pisapia N 2020 Trait and state anxiety are mapped differently in the human brain *Sci. Rep.* **10** 1–11

[7] Arsalan A and Majid M 2022 A study on multi-class anxiety detection using wearable EEG headband *J. Ambient Intell. Humaniz. Comput.* **13** 5739–49

[8] Baghdadi A, Aribi Y, Fourati R, Halouani N, Siarry P and Alimi A M 2019 DASPS: a database for anxious states based on a psychological stimulation arXiv preprint arXiv:1901.02942

[9] Bandelow B and Michaelis S 2015 Epidemiology of anxiety disorders in the 21st century *Dialogues Clin. Neurosci.* **17** 327

[10] Michael J A, Wang M, Kaur M, Fitzgerald P B, Fitzgibbon B M and Hoy K E 2021 EEG correlates of attentional control in anxiety disorders: a systematic review of error-related negativity and correct-response negativity findings *J. Affect. Disord.* **291** 140–53

[11] McKnight P E, Monfort S S, Kashdan T B, Blalock D V and Calton J M 2016 Anxiety symptoms and functional impairment: a systematic review of the correlation between the two measures *Clin. Psychol. Rev.* **45** 115–30

[12] Mannan M M N, Kamran M A and Jeong M Y 2018 Identification and removal of physiological artifacts from electroencephalogram signals: a review *IEEE Access* **6** 30630–52

[13] Dar M N, Akram M U, Yuvaraj R, Khawaja S G and Murugappan M 2022 EEG-based emotion charting for Parkinson's disease patients using convolutional recurrent neural networks and cross dataset learning *Comput. Biol. Med.* **144** 105327

[14] Goshvarpour A and Goshvarpour A 2019 EEG spectral powers and source localization in depressing, sad, and fun music videos focusing on gender differences *Cogn. Neurodyn.* **13** 161–73

[15] Goshvarpour A and Goshvarpour A 2020 A novel approach for EEG electrode selection in automated emotion recognition based on lagged Poincare's indices and sLORETA *Cogn. Comput.* **12** 602–18

[16] Goshvarpour A and Goshvarpour A 2023 Novel high-dimensional phase space features for EEG emotion recognition *SIViP* **17** 417–25

[17] Bong S Z and Khairunizam W *et al* 2017 Implementation of wavelet packet transform and nonlinear analysis for emotion classification in stroke patients using brain signals *Biomed. Signal Process. Control* **36** 102–12

[18] Anandhi B and Jerritta S *et al* 2020 Performance analysis of wavelet transform in the removal of baseline wandering from ECG signals in children with autism spectrum disorder (ASD) *Advances in Electrical and Computer Technologies Lecture Notes in Electrical Engineering* vol 672 (Singapore: Springer)

[19] Giannakakis G, Grigoriadis D and Tsiknakis M 2015 Detection of stress/anxiety state from EEG features during video watching *2015 37th Annual Int. Conf. of the IEEE Engineering in Medicine and Biology Society (EMBC) (August 2015) (Piscataway, NJ)* (IEEE) pp 6034–7

[20] Klados M A, Pandria N, Athanasiou A and Bamidis P D 2017 An automatic EEG based system for the recognition of math anxiety *2017 IEEE 30th Int. Symp. on Computer-Based Medical Systems (CBMS)(June 2017) (Piscataway, NJ)* (IEEE) pp 409–12

[21] Daneshmand-Bahman F and Goshvarpour A 2021 Classification of EEG signals in two levels of normal and anxious using nonlinear features *J. Cogn. Psychol.* **9** 54–69 (in Persian)

[22] Xie Y, Yang B, Lu X, Zheng M, Fan C, Bi X and Li Y 2020 Anxiety and depression diagnosis method based on brain networks and convolutional neural networks *2020 42nd Annual Int. Conf. of the IEEE Engineering in Medicine and Biology Society (EMBC)(July 2020) (Piscataway, NJ)* (IEEE) pp 1503–6

[23] Muhammad F and Al-Ahmadi S 2022 Human state anxiety classification framework using EEG signals in response to exposure therapy *PLoS One* **17** e0265679
[24] Li Z, Wu X, Xu X, Wang H, Guo Z, Zhan Z and Yao L 2022 The recognition of multiple anxiety levels based on electroencephalograph *IEEE Trans. Affect. Comput.* **13** 519–29
[25] Al-Ezzi A, Al-Shargabi A A, Al-Shargie F and Zahary A T 2022 Complexity analysis of EEG in patients with social anxiety disorder using Fuzzy entropy and machine learning techniques *IEEE Access* **10** 39926–38
[26] Singh B K, Verma K and Thoke A S 2015 Investigations on impact of feature normalization techniques on classifier's performance in breast tumor classification *Int. J. Comput. Appl.* **116** 11–15
[27] Dharminder D and Gupta P 2021 Security analysis and application of Chebyshev's chaotic map in the authentication protocols *Int. J. Comput. Appl.* **43** 1095–103
[28] Qi F, Huang S, Li T, Yang H and Kang X 2019 2D Henon-Chebyshev's chaotic map for image encryption *2019 IEEE 21st Int. Conf. on High Performance Computing and Communications; IEEE 17th Int. Conf. on Smart City; IEEE 5th Int. Conf. on Data Science and Systems (HPCC/SmartCity/DSS) (Zhangjiajie, China, August 2019)* (Piscataway, NJ: IEEE) pp 774–81
[29] Kaveh A, Mahdipour Moghanni R and Javadi S M 2021 Chaotic optimization algorithm for performance-based optimization design of composite moment frames *Eng. Comput.* 1–13
[30] Gao G, Peng X, Tian Y and Qin Z 2016 A chaotic maps-based authentication scheme for wireless body area networks *Int. J. Distrib. Sens. Netw.* **12** 2174720
[31] Meshram C, Obaidat M S and Meshram S G 2018 Chebyshev's chaotic map-based ID-based cryptographic model using subtree and fuzzy-entity data sharing for public key cryptography *Security and Privacy* **1** e12
[32] Chatterjee S, Roy S, Das A K, Chattopadhyay S, Kumar N and Vasilakos A V 2016 Secure biometric-based authentication scheme using Chebyshev's chaotic map for multi-server environment *IEEE Trans. Dependable Secure Comput.* **15** 824–39
[33] Shakiba A 2020 Generating dynamical S-boxes using 1D Chebyshev's chaotic maps *J. Comput. Secur.* **7** 1–17
[34] Karjanto N 2020 Properties of Chebyshev polynomials arXiv preprint arXiv:2002.01342
[35] McLean M 2022 Data density plot (https://mathworks.com/matlabcentral/fileexchange/31726-data-density-plot), MATLAB Central File Exchange (accessed 21 March 2022)
[36] Yu L and Liu H 2003 Feature selection for high-dimensional data: a fast correlation-based filter solution *Proc. 20th Int. Conf. on Machine Learning (ICML-03)* ed T Fawcett and N Mishra (Menlo Park, CA: AAAI Press) pp 856–63
[37] Kohavi R and John G H 1997 Relevance wrappers for feature subset selection *Artif. Intell.* **97** 273–324
[38] Lal T N, Chapelle O, Weston J and Elisseeff A 2006 Embedded methods *Feature Extraction: Foundations and Applications* ed I Guyon, M Nikravesh, S Gunn and L A Zadeh (Berlin: Springer) pp 137–65
[39] Ramírez-Gallego S, Lastra I, Martínez-Rego D, Bolón-Canedo V, Benítez J M, Herrera F and Alonso-Betanzos A 2017 Fast-mRMR: fast minimum redundancy maximum relevance algorithm for high-dimensional big data *Int. J. Intell. Syst.* **32** 134–52
[40] Salvador–Meneses J, Ruiz–Chavez Z and Garcia–Rodriguez J 2019 Compressed *K*-NN: *K*-nearest neighbors with data compression *Entropy* **21** 234
[41] Alsaffar A and Omar N 2015 Integrating a lexicon based approach and *k*-nearest neighbour for malay sentiment analysis *J. Comput. Sci.* **11** 639

[42] Lusiandro M A, Nasution S M and Setianingsih C 2020 Implementation of the advanced traffic management system using *k*-nearest neighbor algorithm *2020 Int. Conf. on Information Technology Systems and Innovation (ICITSI) (October 2020) Piscataway, NJ* (IEEE) pp 149–54

[43] Zhang Z 2016 Decision tree modeling using R *Ann. Transl. Med.* **4**

[44] Charbuty B and Abdulazeez A 2021 Classification based on decision tree algorithm for machine learning *J. Appl. Sci. Technol. Trends* **2** 20–8

[45] Patel H H and Prajapati P 2018 Study and analysis of decision tree based classification algorithms *Int. J. Comput. Sci. Eng.* **6** 74–8

[46] Song Y Y and Ying L U 2015 Decision tree methods: applications for classification and prediction *Shanghai Arch. Psychiatry* **27** 130

[47] Frosst N and Hinton G 2017 Distilling a neural network into a soft decision tree arXiv preprint arXiv:1711.09784

[48] Bengio Y and Grandvalet Y 2003 No unbiased estimator of the variance of *k*-fold cross-validation *NIPS'03: Proc. 16th Int. Conf. on Neural Information Processing Systems (December 2003)* pp 513–20

[49] Anguita D, Ghio A, Ridella S and Sterpi D 2009 *K*-fold cross validation for error rate estimate in support vector machines Proc. 2009 Int. Conf. on Data Mining, DMIN 2009 *(Las Vegas, USA, July 13–16 2009)* pp 291–7

IOP Publishing

Affective Computing in Healthcare
Applications based on biosignals and artificial intelligence
M Murugappan

Chapter 2

Evaluating cognitive load during lexical decision tasks for monolinguals and bilinguals using EEG

Mahesh Veezhinathan, B Geethanjali, Sukeerthi Sakthivel and RaamaNarayanan AnanthaNarayanan

Cognitive load plays an important role in the efficient transfer of information. In this, it relies on the processing of information that relates to working memory. In this chapter, a study was designed with two independent groups (monolinguals and bilinguals) to assess information processing and cognitive load during a lexical decision task (LDT) with increasing level of difficulty. The monolinguals are native speakers of Tamil, with their education taking place also in the same language, whereas the bilinguals selected are native Tamil speakers with their medium of instruction instead in English. The bilinguals are proficient in both English and Tamil. The LDT stimulus, with varying robustness in lexical range (650L and 1500L), was employed using a Psytool kit. An electroencephalogram was used to record across 19 electrode locations during the task (i.e., stimuli present) along with in a resting state (i.e., no stimuli). The relative band powers across all the electrode locations were extracted, and this information was used to calculate the event-related changes and the task performance. When comparing the task performances significant changes ($p < 0.05$) were found in accuracy (non-word, related word, and unrelated word) for both monolinguals and bilinguals. The theta synchronisation was significantly different ($p < 0.05$) and noted at the Fp1, Fp2, O1, and P4 electrode positions during 650L for monolinguals; in bilinguals the theta synchronisation was significantly different ($p < 0.05$) at the F3, F4, F8, Fp1, Fp2, O1, and P4 electrode locations during 650L and the Fp1, P3 T3, T4, and T5 electrode locations during 1500L. Well-connected functional connectivity was noted in the left hemisphere electrode locations in bilinguals when compared with monolinguals. Apart from that, this also proves that, even at difficult lexical levels, their decision-making was good and accuracy improved when compared with monolinguals. This helps bilinguals in improvising their learning abilities by inhibiting irrelevant stimuli. Bilingual participants also showed increased connectivity in the brain region associated with attention. The task performance in bilinguals was enhanced when compared to monolinguals.

doi:10.1088/978-0-7503-5182-9ch2

2.1 Introduction

One of the most important characteristic capabilities of the human species is the ability to practice language and carry out effective communication. Almost 50% of the world's population speaks more than one language [1]. Bilingualism is generally explained as when an individual can utilise at least two languages, whereas monolingualism can be simply defined as when an individual can utilise a single language. It has been determined that exposure to a foreign language at a young age, as well as continued utilisation of two languages throughout an individual's lifetime, results in an improvement of cognitive capabilities. Past research work has shown that bilingualism is more advantageous at both ends of the age spectrum. Bilingual children show better task switching, attention, and other cognitive capabilities, whereas elsewhere it has been shown that bilingual adults afflicted with Alzheimer's take twice as long to progress in the symptoms of the disease as their monolingual counterparts. A study conducted by Meyer and Schvaneveldt found that individuals reply very rapidly to words that are related to each other in comparison to non-related words [2]. This illustrates the concept of 'priming', in which participants can be made to respond to subsequent words immediately, once after the exposure of a word, typically displayed on a screen.

In addition to this, cognitive load also plays a major role in information storage and retrieval. Cognitive load should thus be measured for efficient transfer of information, as it is a well-known index of perceptive activity [3]. Exposure to multiple languages assumes a significant part in the efficacious achievement of intellectual activities while performing executive control [4]. Cognitive load can be characterised into three various types: intrinsic load, extrinsic load, and germane cognitive load. These can be used to analyse the load on working memory during the execution of tasks [5, 6]. Usually, cognitive load varies from person to person based on age and intelligence. Lower lexile measures are easy to read. The selected bilinguals are participants who have a medium level of instruction in English. Electroencephalogram (EEG) measurements are the best method to estimate cognitive load, and offer a high degree of sensitivity [7].

The authors of a previous study state that the right hemisphere will be more dominant during second-language processing than first-language processing [8]. Since bilinguals demonstrated less adaptation, which may also be due to interference from the elicited other language, Friesen *et al* [9] chose a monolingual population that can speak English as their native language but who have the least exposure to a second language. As a result, when compared to monolinguals, bilinguals' simple lexical selection caused greater disagreement. Baumgart *et al* pointed out that executive control is related to intellectual performance and acquires an advantage if inhibitory control and attention attain a higher extent [10]. Cognitive control can be used to measure problem-solving skills, planning, working memory, inhibitory control, and attention, which are derived from the executive function. Bialystok *et al* proposes a *picture selection task*, wherein a fixation cross is initially displayed on a screen, displayed for 500 or 1500 ms, and then images are shown on both sides for 500 or 1500 ms. At the same time, participants will hear any one of the picture's associated words and are instructed to press the key relevant to the corresponding image and sound. The stimuli are arbitrarily produced by the program. After, the completion time taken to respond will be evaluated by a program. They also utilised a *Peabody Picture Vocabulary Test-III*, in which participants had to identify a picture corresponding to a spoken word. This is one of the commonly employed English vocabulary knowledge tests [1].

The authors also employed non-linguistic tasks, where the participants had to press a button as a response to measure congruent and incongruent trials. In this non-linguistic task, a blue or red square appears on any one side of the screen (i.e., either left or right). The participant has to concentrate on the display and respond by pressing the key depending on the coloured square, irrespective of the display location on the screen. Bialystok *et al* pointed out that executive control comprises language retrieval and its training [11]. This will usually be associated with the frontal lobe, which is responsible for switching attention unconsciously from one task to the other, planning, and deciding skills performed in the short-term memory [1, 8, 12]. Using the Stroop and Simon task, we can examine the executive control [13]; likewise, by utilising the Flanker test, which is a non-semantic task [14]. It has been shown that language switching and mixing can happen when there is an expansion in the perfusion of the left caudate nucleus and the left side of the frontal lobe [15].

Monolinguals and bilinguals have differences in cognitive processing. Bilinguals have more activation brain areas, and it has been shown that, in bilingualism, sub-networks by which the functions of the brain have been damaged can be restructured and reconnect with other undamaged areas. Also, bilinguals exhibit stronger executive functioning than monolinguals. Bilingualism thus has an impact not only on language but also on cognition and in supporting the networks of the brain [16]. The perisylvian region is responsible for language, which incorporates Wernicke's region and Broca's region. Broca's region is tied to talking, and Wernicke's region is associated with perception [17].

Our study focuses mainly on the effect of lexical tasks, with increasing lexical levels, and their impact on cognitive load as performed by monolinguals and bilinguals. Various aspects of bilingualism have been studied in neurology. Such studies have provided insight into information processing regarding the cognitive functions of individuals possessing bilingualism. To this end, it is hoped that analysing the relationship between the linguistic processing of low-level tasks (650L) and high-level tasks (1500L) for monolinguals and bilinguals will help to understand the brain connectivity pattern across various regions of the brain, and will also help to quantify the effect of cognitive load. The primary motivation behind the study is to decide and analyse the cognitive load and linguistic performance of both monolinguals and bilinguals with regard to etymology. In his work, two different lexile measures were used to quantify the cognitive load and learning abilities of the individuals by providing non-words, related words, and unrelated words for both monolinguals and bilinguals. For this, the task performance for each category was calculated and its associated event-related changes using EEG.

2.2 Methodology

Eligible participants between the stipulated age ranges were selected and divided according to their native language and preferred instructional method. These participants then underwent modified lexical judgment tasks that comprised presenting words as visual task stimuli for a period of 1500 ms. A reaction time of 500 ms was provided to capture their responses. A 10–20 electrode system was used to record the participants' EEG signals at various locations, including the central area (C3, C4, Cz), frontal area (F3, F4, F7, F8, Fz), frontal planar area (Fp1, Fp2), parietal lobe (P3, P4, and Pz), occipital lobe (O1, O2, and Oz), as well as two reference electrodes (A1 and A2). The acquired raw data were first extracted. Data analysis was then carried out using appropriate software tools; to accelerate data processing, the obtained EEG signals were separated into distinct intervals based on the number of seconds of data. Suitable filters with distinct pass bands and stop bands were employed to remove noise and artefacts and to filter out the required signal. The values obtained were inspected to determine any distributional similarities. By optimising all electrode placement points, the relationships between the findings can be revealed. Further, by taking into consideration these event-related changes in the corresponding EEG bands, the interconnectivity between the different regions of the brain will be evidenced.

2.2.1 Block diagram

Monolinguals were presented with stimuli of increasing lexical order 650 L and 1500 L in the Tamil language, whereas bilinguals were presented with both English and Tamil. The low lexical level (650 L) stimuli were presented first for 1500 ms and subjects were asked to respond whether it was a related word or not-related word during the response period (500 ms), then followed by high lexical level (1500L). The workflow of the study and sample stimuli presentation are shown in figures 2.1 and 2.2, respectively.

2.2.2 Participant selection

Twenty healthy participants from ages 18–20 studying in the engineering program were selected, and two independent groups (monolinguals and bilinguals) were segregated based on their mother tongue and their medium of instruction for learning. In the monolingual group, ten healthy adults (nine men, one woman) were selected for this study based on their language preference. They had learnt Tamil as their mother tongue and took it as well as their instructing medium, and had nominal exposure to the english language (i.e., as a second language). For the bilingual group, ten healthy adults (two men, eight women) were employed for this study. The participants were again selected based on their mother tongue, being native Tamil speakers, only this time their medium of took instruction is English. These bilinguals had an equal knowledge of English and Tamil. All the participants are right-handed and have no history of seizure or medication. They were asked to relax and made to sit on a comfortable chair in a sound proof room. The study was carried out in accordance with the guidelines of the Institutional Ethics Committee

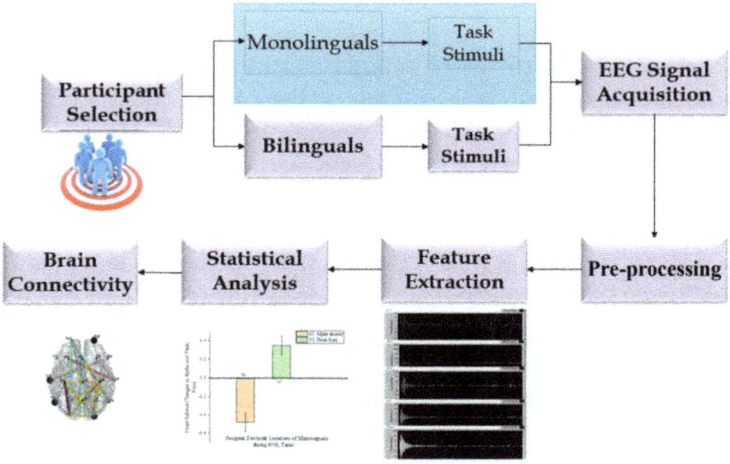

Figure 2.1. Functional flowchart of the evaluation of cognitive load for monolinguals and bilinguals.

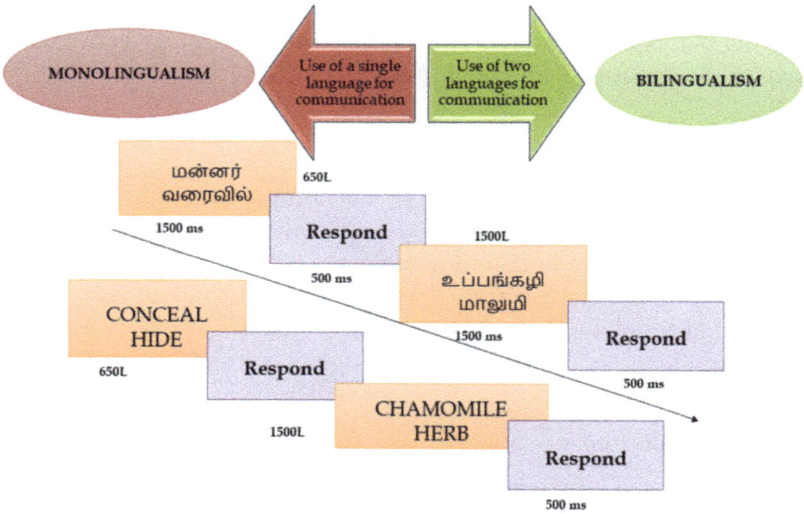

Figure 2.2. Design of task stimuli for Tamil and English for monolinguals and bilinguals.

of the Institute for Human Volunteer Research. The participants signed a document of informed consent after the experiment protocol was discussed.

2.2.3 Lexical decision task

The stimuli were selected for our study from Psytoolkit (psytoolkit.org), a database of psychological tasks, available online. The lexical decision tasks (LDTs; here, in English and Tamil) were modified to suit our studies. The procedure of the task stimuli is shown in figure 2.3. To evaluate the linguistic activity of both the bilingual and monolingual subjects, the LDT chosen was an etymological task. In view of their

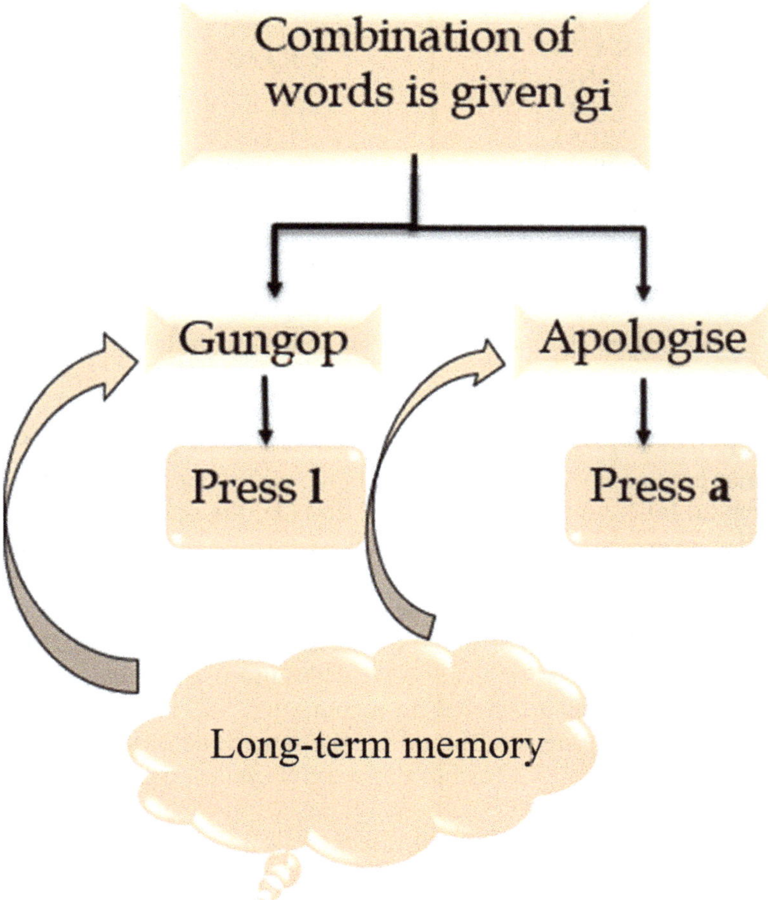

Figure 2.3. Task procedure.

lexical degree of difficulty, English tasks were classified as low (650L) and high (1500L) level. This same task was performed to identify the ability of the second language (L2) in the bilingual subjects, as they are familiar with two languages. The first language (L1), here taken as Tamil, and its LDT was completed by gathering the troublesome words, which were approved by experts. These words are categorized as challenging and easy to determine the degree of proficiency in the monolingual group.

The lexile text ranges for English were taken from standard guidelines [2]. The lexile text ranges for Tamil were prescribed by Tamil linguistics professors based on Tamil textbooks for the 4th and 11th grades, where we can interpret differences in the texts given. The lexile ranges for both the languages are tabulated as per the figure 2.4.

2.2.4 Data acquisition

As mentioned, the chosen modality used in this study was EEG. To record these signals, a standard 10–20 electrode system was utilised. The electrodes were

GRADES	TEXT RANGE (L) - ENGLISH
11-12	1185-1385
9-10	1050-1335
6-8	925-1185
4-5	740-1010
2-3	420-820
1	190-530

(A)

GRADES	TEXT RANGE (L) - TAMIL
11	1500
4	650
2-3	400
1	250

(B)

Figure 2.4. Lexile level charts: (A) English, and (B) Tamil.

positioned on the scalp with respect to the brain lobes [18]. The central area electrodes are denoted as C3, C4, Cz; the frontal area as F3, F4, F7, F8, Fz; the frontal planar area as Fp1, Fp2; the parietal lobe electrodes are given as P3, P4 and Pz; the occipital lobe electrodes are O1, O2 and Oz; the reference electrodes (right and left earlobes) are A1 and A2; and a ground electrode was placed behind the ear. The right side of the brain was denoted by even numbers, whereas the left side of the brain was denoted by odd numbers. Silver/silver chloride (Ag/AgCl) electrodes were used on the scalp with the help of 10–20 EEG paste [19]. To filter the EEG signals, a low-pass filter and high-pass filter are used with cut-off frequencies of 0.1–50 Hz. The acquired EEG signals are stored on a computer, and analysis is executed off-line. The EEG recording devices should set the same time base of 30 mm s^{-1} and sensitivity of 7.5 $\mu V\ mm^{-1}$. The electrodes were placed on the scalp after abrading the skin with surgical spirit. This was done to reduce impedance for better recording. After arranging the electrodes, an impedance check was done to test for open electrodes. EEG was then recorded on a reference montage for all 19 electrodes.

2.2.5 Experiment protocol

The experimental protocol took 22 min for bilingual subjects and 12 min for monolingual subjects, wherein they were subjected to all the tasks, one after the other, and for which EEG recordings were taken. These are displayed in figure 2.5. A period of rest was given between tasks, wherein the participants had to close their eyes. The protocol's tasks were of equal durations of 3 min, and the rest period between each of the tasks lasted for 2 min; the same experiment protocol here followed is taken from prior studies [19, 20].

2.2.6 EEG data processing

Using the protocol outlined in figure 2.5, the acquired raw data are then separated. The data were processed using LabVIEW 19. The EEG signals were divided into specific epochs based on their seconds of data to make the data processing faster. The signal processing is executed as per figure 2.6. The sampling was done with a frequency of 256 Hz [21], and was averaged with the help of a smoothing filter by means of a triangular window. The above process was performed to improve the signal-to-noise ratio of the signal, and then the band was limited to 4–40 Hz. As the delta band had a slow drift, this

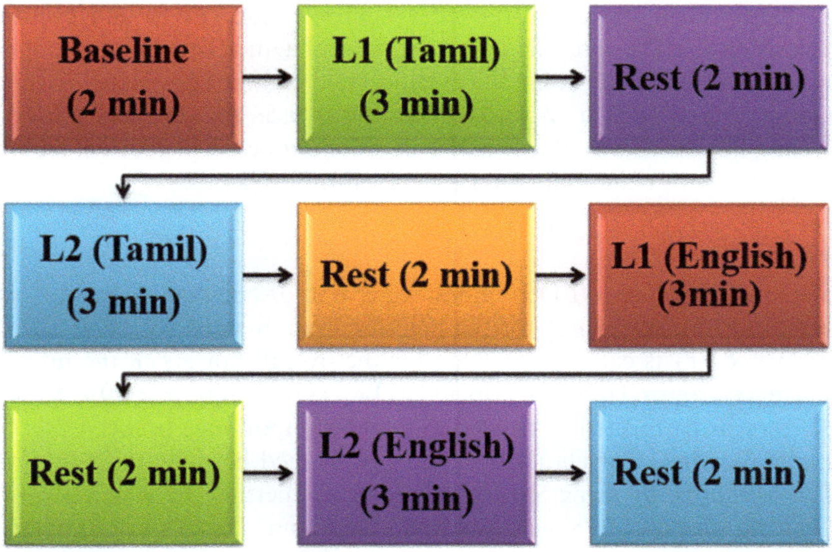

Figure 2.5. Protocol for bilinguals.

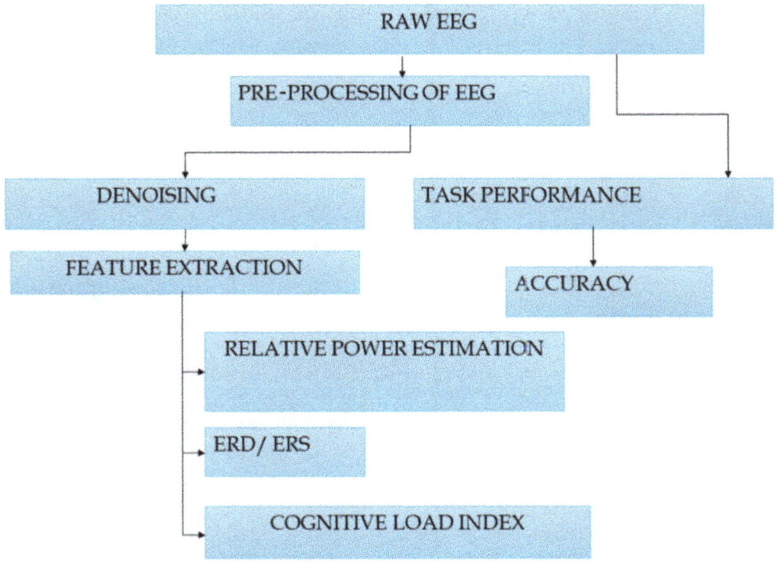

Figure 2.6. Signal processing and feature extraction.

band was ignored. The noise and artefacts were removed by the use of a band-pass filter (BPF), with a pass band of 4 Hz to 40 Hz. As per the different frequency bands, each signal was separated into an alpha band (8 Hz to 13 Hz), beta band (13 Hz to 30 Hz), theta band (4 Hz to 8 Hz), and gamma band (30 Hz to 40 Hz) [21, 22]. A Butterworth filter was chosen as it did not have ripples in the pass band. By ignoring the delta band, eye-movement artefacts were removed. Calculation of the total power and individual power spectral densities was done and, for later analysis, the values were stored.

From these values, the event-related synchronization (ERS) and event-related synchronization (ERD) were calculated for the alpha and theta bands from the task and rest values. ERD/ERS infers the event-related changes associated with cortical information processing [23]. Wavelet denoising is used for characterisation of the signal. Using this transform, the signal gives more frequency resolution, and it serves as a good solution for the time–frequency localisation [24, 25].

2.2.7 Statistical analysis

The calculated ERS and EDS values were not distributed normally, so non-parametric tests are performed for the measured parameters. By using a Friedman test, massive contrasts can be estimated for the overall powers of the multitude of four recurrence groups. Here, the critical level was taken to be $p = 0.05$. A connected example test was performed to gauge the singular importance between every one of the variable matches. Correlation was then performed between tasks and between rests. This was done by using Spearman's rank coefficients, by which a correlation matrix can be plotted for all the electrode locations. The feature extraction and statistical analysis processe are shown in figures 2.7 and 2.8, respectively.

The entire analysis was undertaken using the IBM SPSS Statistics software (v24). For monolinguals, the mean relative part energies of the alpha, beta, theta, and gamma bands are measured while performing the tasks as well as in a resting state

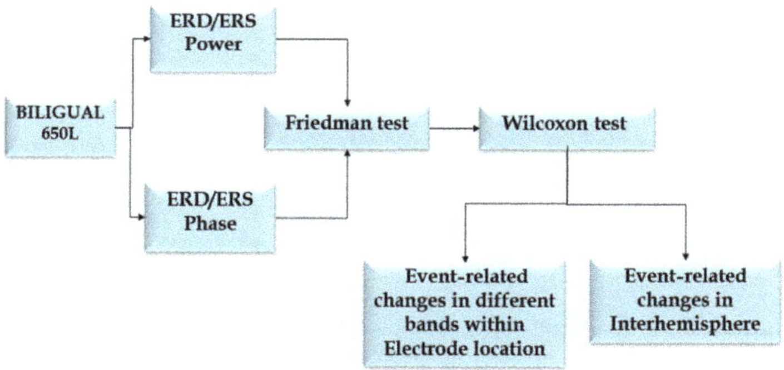

Figure 2.7. Feature extraction for low-level task in bilinguals.

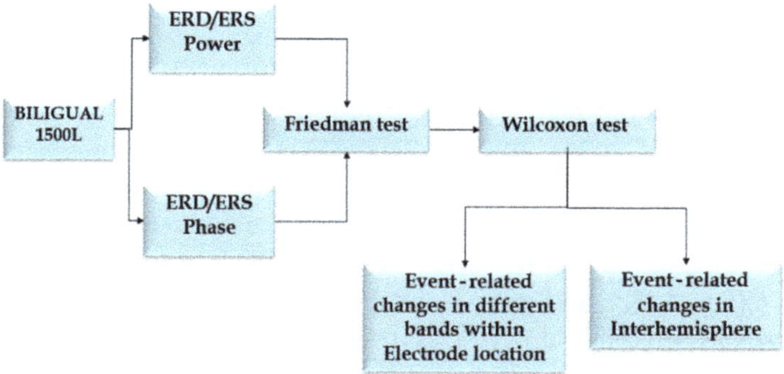

Figure 2.8. Feature extraction for high-level task in bilinguals.

from all 19 electrode locations. The Friedman test is completed for both the mono- and bilingual groups, respectively; from the measured parameters (the relative component energies of the alpha, beta, theta, and gamma bands) a statistically significant difference was noted. Then, a Wilcoxon ranked test is used for the analysis between the left and right hemispheric areas, and also between the frequency bands in each electrode location.

A comparison of the monolingual and bilingual groups can be done statistically using a Mann–Whitney U test. The performance of semantic, long-term memory is related with alpha desynchronization, and the capacity to encode new data is related with theta synchronisation. Subsequently, the event-related changes of the alpha and theta bands were estimated. The results of the acquired signal and signal processing are displayed in figures 2.9–2.12.

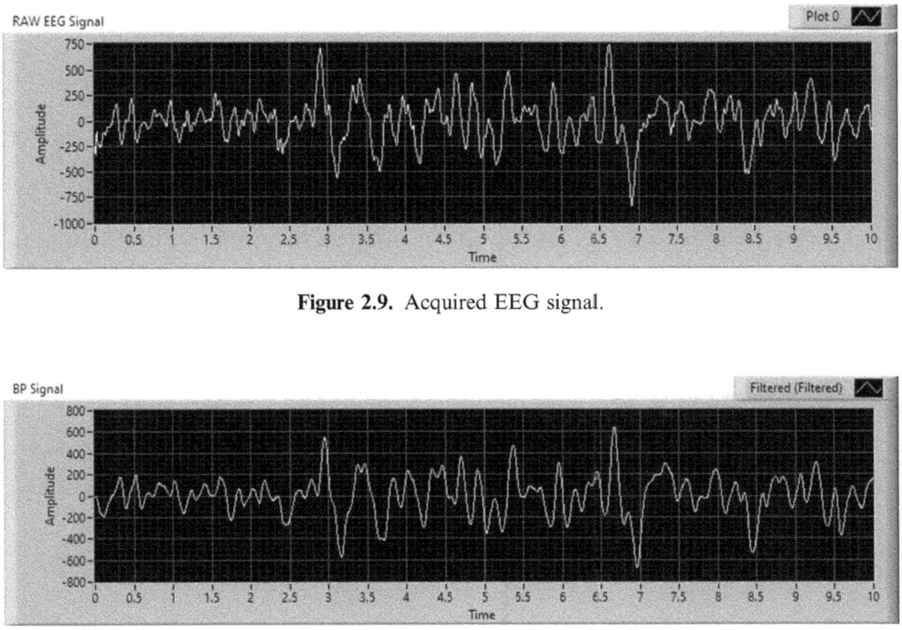

Figure 2.9. Acquired EEG signal.

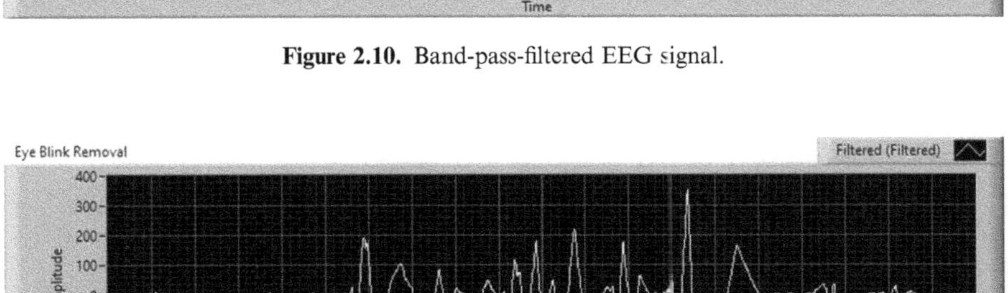

Figure 2.10. Band-pass-filtered EEG signal.

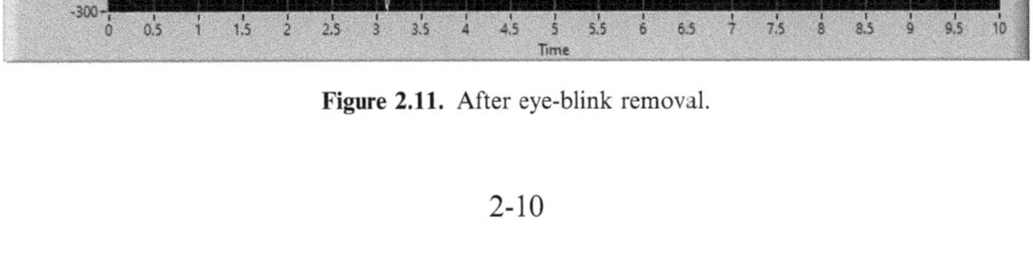

Figure 2.11. After eye-blink removal.

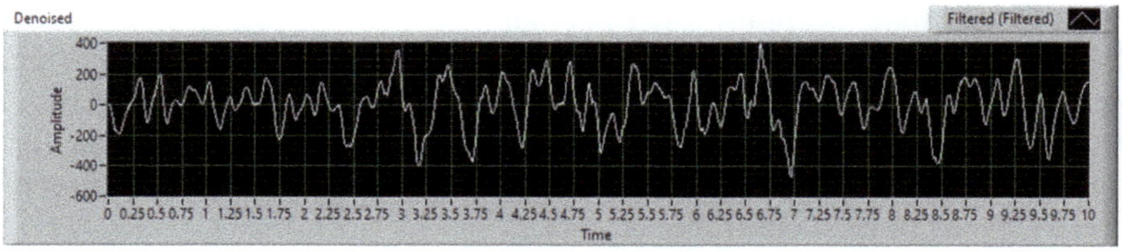

Figure 2.12. Pre-processed EEG signal for analysis.

2.3 Results

2.3.1 Task performance analysis

Accuracy and reaction-time analysis can be used to evaluate the task performance. The reaction time provides the time taken to respond for every stimulus, whereas the accuracy will give the correctness of the response given by the participant.

The accuracy of a task is measured using the following formula:

$$\%\text{Accuracy} = \frac{\text{No. of correct responses}}{\text{Total no. of presented stimuli}} * 100. \tag{2.1}$$

The key finding from this comparative study is that the bilingual group were more accurate compared to the monolingual group in both levels of lexical task (650L and 1500L). From this data, it can be concluded that differences between bilingual groups and monolingual groups are statistically significant. Graphical representations of the task accuracy are given in figures 2.13–2.15.

2.3.2 Reaction-time analysis

The participants made lexical decisions (determining whether or not both the presented strings were words) that were measured in terms of response times.

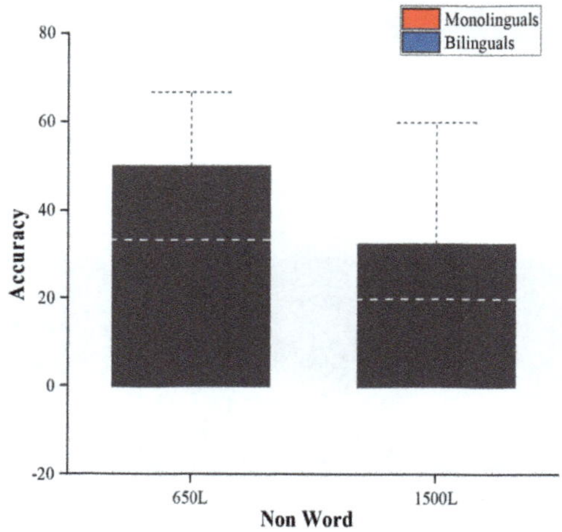

Figure 2.13. Accuracy for non-words.

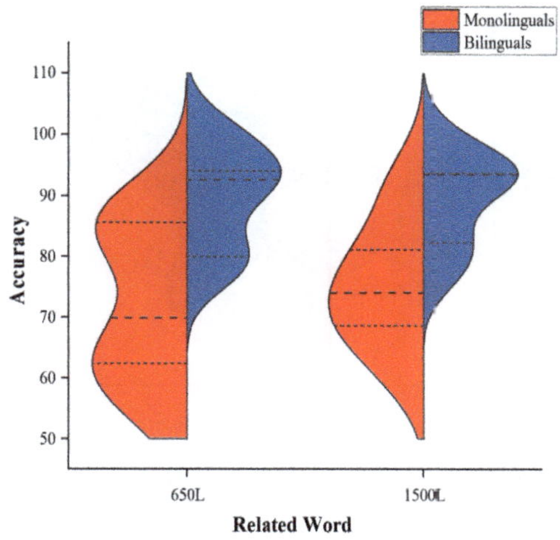

Figure 2.14. Accuracy for related words.

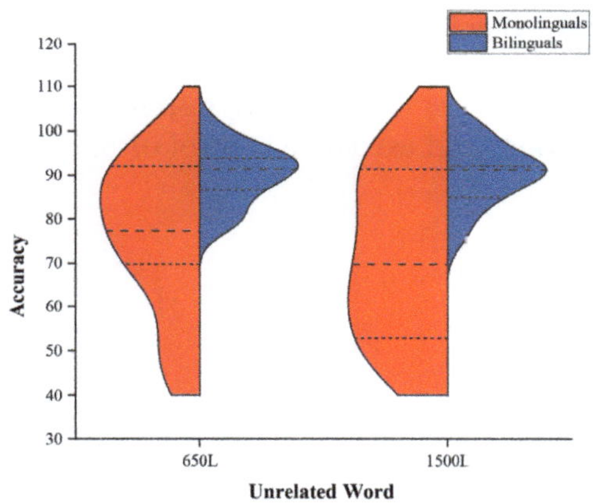

Figure 2.15. Accuracy for unrelated words.

Although the reaction times of the bilinguals were high, they furthermore responded accurately when compared to monolinguals [26]; statistically significant differences found in the bilingual group while performing the 650L non-word task. A graphical representation is shown in figure 2.16.

2.3.3 Event-related changes within frequency bands

The ERD can be measured by using the following steps [22, 27, 28]:

1. Filter the EEG frequency bands using a BPF, then square and average the data.
2. Average the obtained data over the number of epochs.
3. Articulate the changes in the band power as compared to a reference interval by using the below formula:

$$\text{ERD} = \frac{\text{BPR} - \text{BPT}}{\text{BPR}} * 100, \tag{2.2}$$

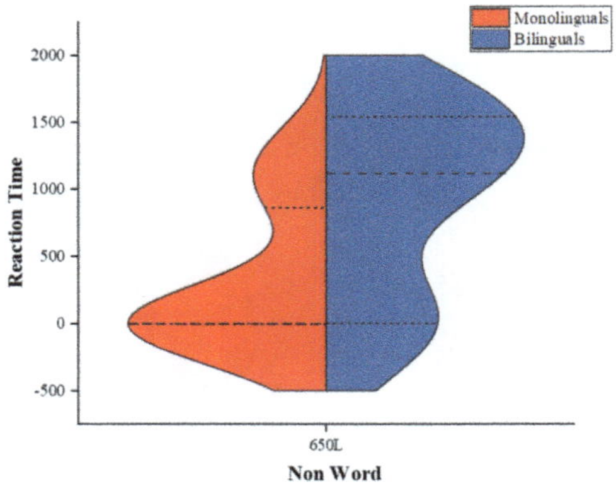

Figure 2.16. Reaction times for non-word task (650L).

where 'BPT' is the band power task and 'BPR' is the band power rest.

Processing in the cortical area will be reflected in the EEG power. EEG power is negatively associated with the theta band, whereas it is positively correlated with the alpha frequency range. Significant differences ($p < 0.05$) were noted in the monolingual group during the 650L task in the Fp1, Fp2, O1, and P4 locations, as depicted in figure 2.17. These locations are responsible for short-term memory, working memory, attention, and executive control of behaviour, respectively.

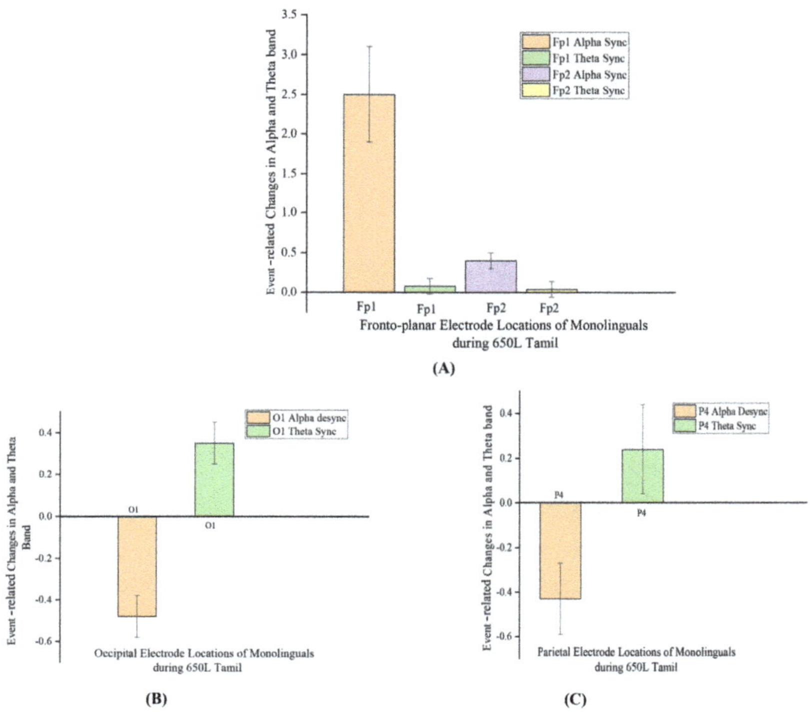

Figure 2.17. Event-related changes in the monolingual group during the 650L task at (A) Fp1 and Fp2, (B) O1, and (C) P4.

Significant differences were noted in the monolingual group during the 1500L task in the F8, Fp1, T3, and T4 locations, whereas in the bilingual group significant differences were noted during the 1500L task at the F4 location, as is shown in figure 2.18. These locations are responsible for short-term memory, working memory, attention, and executive control of behaviour, respectively.

Statistically independent tests were performed between the monolinguals and bilinguals during the 650L task. Graphical representations of the event-related changes in the bilingual Tamil 650L, English 650L, and English 1500L tasks are displayed in figures 2.19–2.21, respectively. Significant differences are noted in the Fp1 and Fp2 locations in the alpha band; the F3, Fp1, O1, and P4 locations in the beta band; F4 and O1 in the theta band; and F8, T3, and T4 in the gamma band. These locations are responsible for sentence and word generation, lexical searching, executive control behaviour, working memory, word encoding, syntactic processing, memory retrieval, declarative memory encoding, memory encoding, semantic processing, reasoning, semantic memory retrieval, short-term memory, spatial memory, episodic long-term memory, semantic categorisation, etc. The event-related changes in the alpha, beta, theta, and gamma bands during the 650L task are shown in figures 2.22–2.25, respectively.

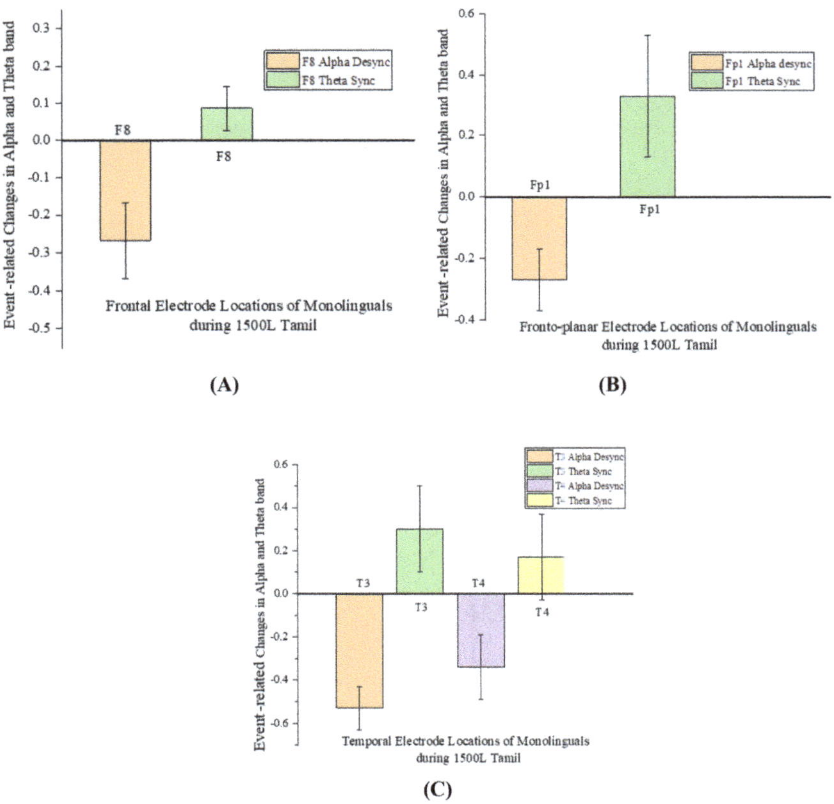

Figure 2.18. Event-related changes in the monolingual group during the 1500L task at (A) F8, (B) Fp1, and (C) T3 and T4.

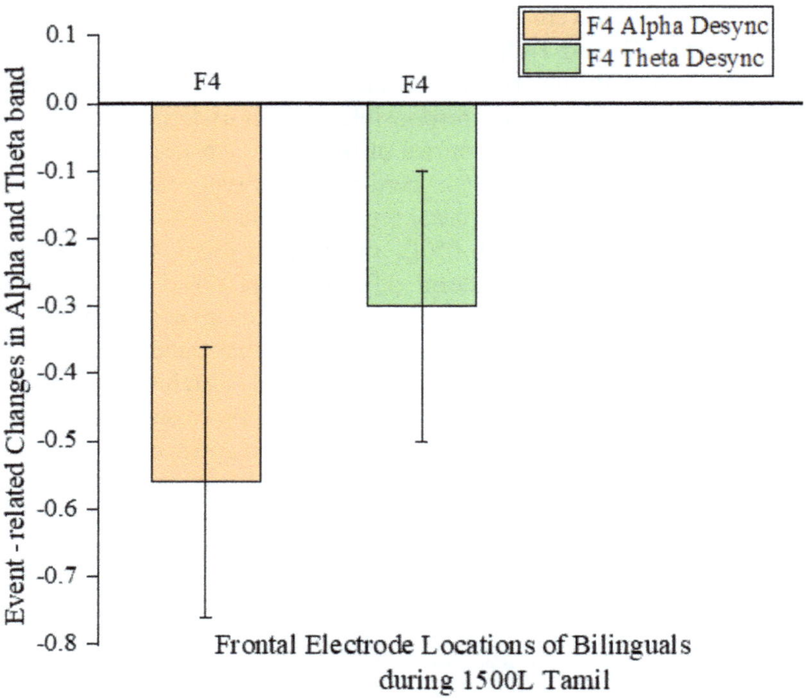

Figure 2.19. Event-related changes in the bilingual group during Tamil 1500L at F4.

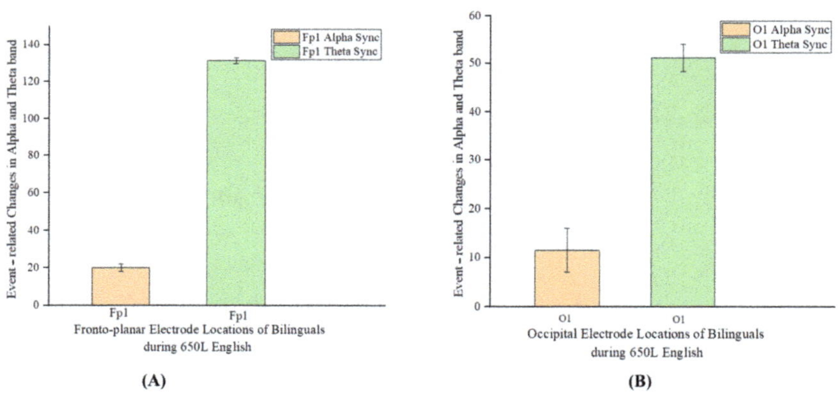

Figure 2.20. Event-related changes in the bilingual group during English 650L at (A) Fp1, and (B) O1.

Statistically independent tests were performed between the monolingual and bilingual groups during the 650L task. A significant difference was noted in the P3 and T3 locations in the alpha band, the T4 location in the beta band, the P3 location in the theta band, and the Fp1 and T5 locations in the gamma band. These locations are primarily responsible for episodic long-term memory, sentence and word generation, declarative memory encoding, working memory, semantic processing, syntactic processing, semantic categorisation, executive control behaviour, semantic

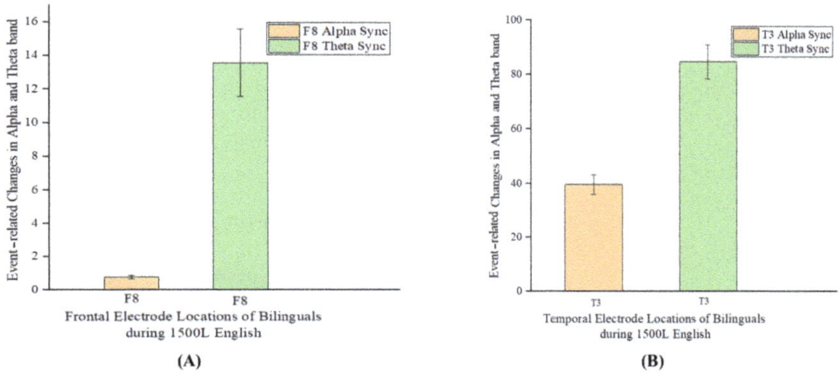

Figure 2.21. Event-related changes in the bilingual group during English 1500L at (A) F8, and (B) T3.

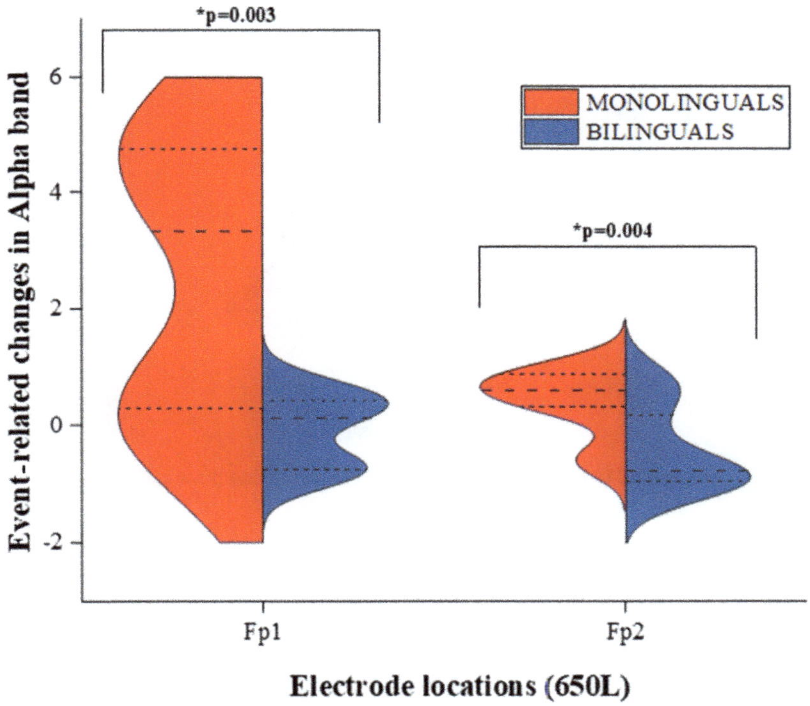

Figure 2.22. Event-related changes in the alpha band during 650L.

memory retrieval, short-term memory, spatial memory, memory encoding, reasoning, word encoding, and memory retrieval.

The event-related changes in the alpha, beta, theta, and gamma bands during the 1500L task are shown in figures 2.26–2.29, respectively. From figure 2.30, it can be seen that there was no inter-hemispheric connectivity between frontal electrode locations (F7, F3 with F8, F4) for the monolingual group in the 650L task for the alpha band, whereas for the bilingual group at the same lexical level an

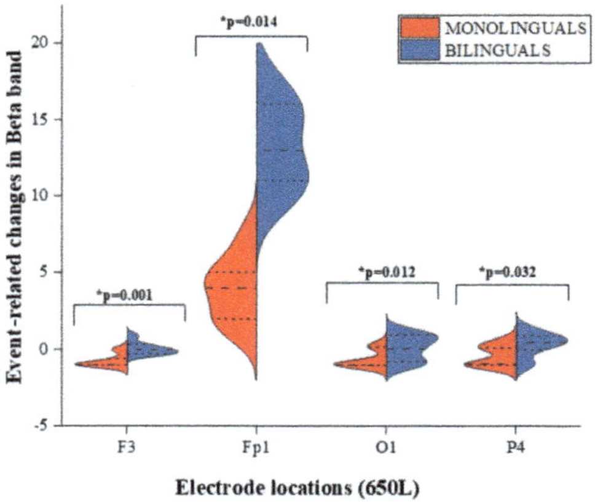

Figure 2.23. Event-related changes in the beta band during 650L.

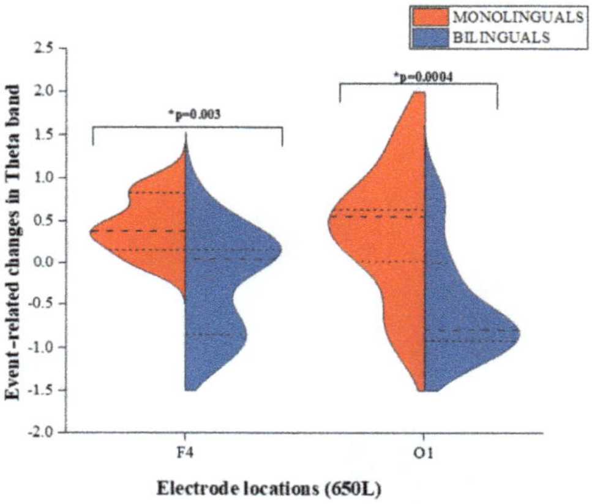

Figure 2.24. Event-related changes in the theta band during 650L.

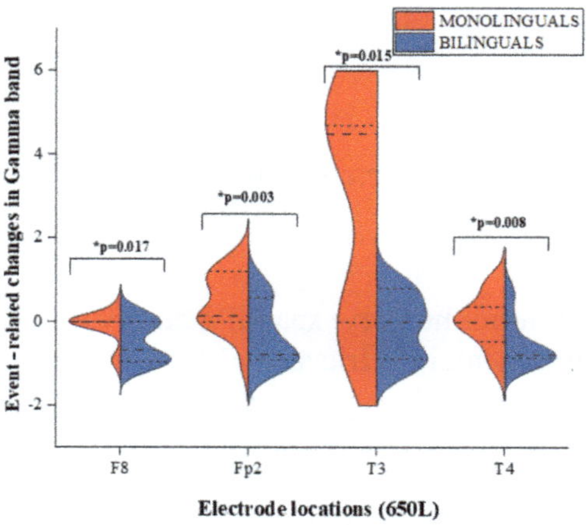

Figure 2.25. Event-related changes in the gamma band during 650L.

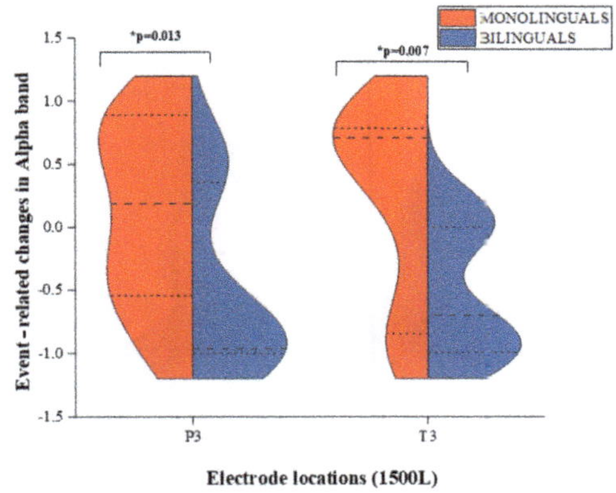

Figure 2.26. Event-related changes in the alpha band during 1500L.

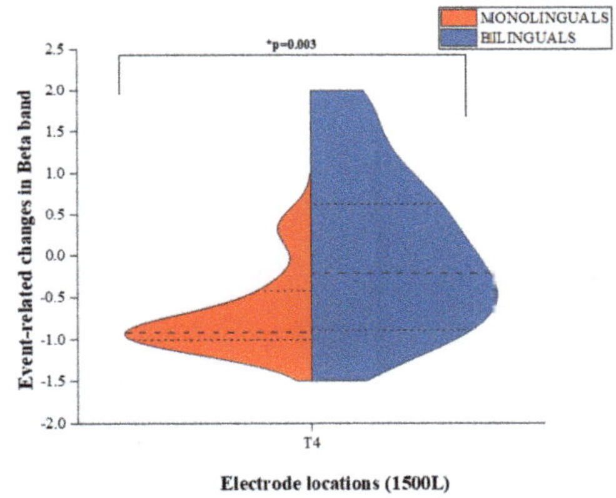

Figure 2.27. Event-related changes in the beta band during 1500L.

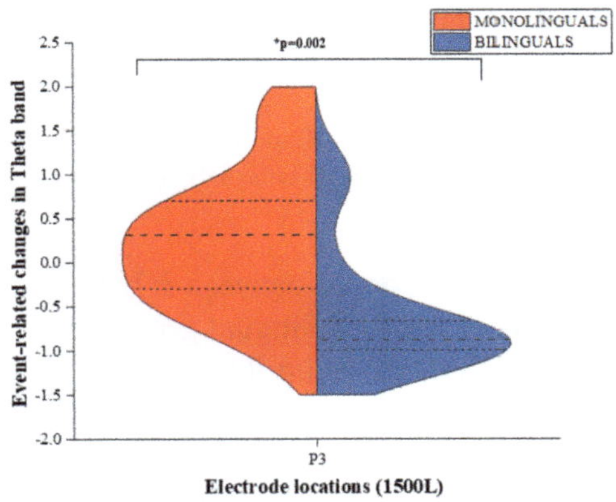

Figure 2.28. Event-related changes in the theta band during 1500L.

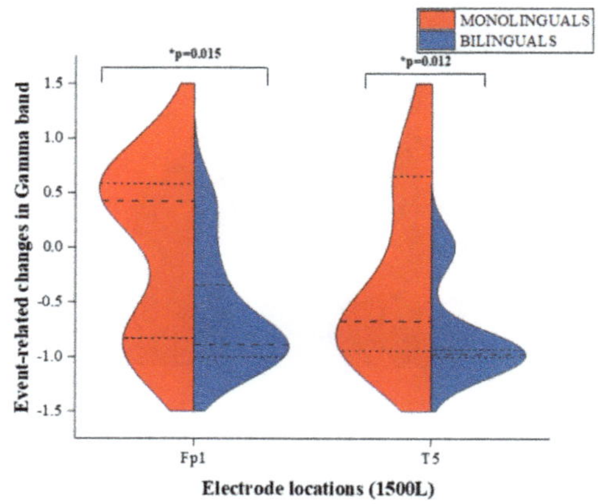

Figure 2.29. Event-related changes in the gamma band during 1500L.

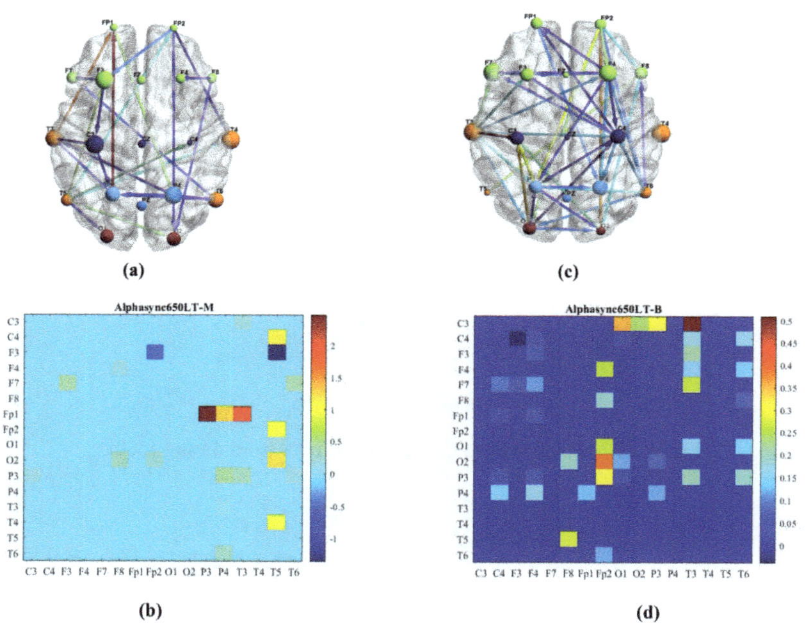

Figure 2.30. Alpha synchronisation during the 650L Tamil task: (a) brain connectivity of monolinguals, (b) correlogram of monolinguals, (c) brain connectivity of bilinguals, and (d) correlogram of bilinguals.

inter-hemispheric connectivity was noted between F7, Fz, F3 and F7. In addition, the mutual information transfer for the bilingual group was from T3 (BA 42) to F7 and F3, whereas for the monolingual group it was from T3 to Fp1. A very distinct information transfer was noted at parietal lobe electrode locations (P3 and P4), which correspond to BA 39 (angular gyrus), a part of Wernicke's area, an area that gets activated during reading-related tasks. In monolinguals the mutual information transfer was from P4 to P3, while for bilinguals it was from P3 to P4.

In monolinguals the P3, T5, and Fp1 regions acted as a hub, whereas in bilinguals P3, P4, C3, C4, O1, O2, Fp1, and Fp2 acted as hub. In monolinguals, there is no inter-hemispheric transfer of information between O1 and O2, but connectivity is found between T5 (BA 37) and O1 (BA 18), which is responsible for word generation and retrieval, single-letter processing, and semantic categorisation with respect to language processing. The transfer of information is noted in bilinguals from T3 (BA 42) and T6 (BA 36) to O1, and then to O2 (BA 18). It should be noted that BA 18 is responsible for response to the visual word form, whereas BA 37 is involved in lexico-semantic associations and is related with visual functions. As O1 (left) and O2 (right) belong to the same area (BA 18), there was a mutual information transfer that is noted in the bilingual group but is not found in the monolingual group. Fp1 (left) and Fp2 (right), belonging to area BA 10, are involved in complex language processing such as syntactic processing and comprehension of metaphor (i.e., related words).

The left hemisphere is critical for language processing, while the right hemisphere also contributes to language comprehension [29]. No connectivity was noted between Fp1 and Fp2 for both groups in the 650L task alpha band, whereas for the 1500L task information transfer was noted from Fp1 to Fp2 for both groups. T3, P3, and P4 transferred information to Fp1 for monolinguals in the 650L task, as was also noted for bilinguals 650L. In bilinguals, mutual information was relayed from Fp1 to P4 (visual spatial processing) but this was noted only for the 650L task alpha band. Apart from that, mutual information was carried from Fp2 to F8, T6, P4, O1, O2, and P3 (left hand). In monolinguals the information passed from Fp2 to F3 and P4, and from T5 to Fp2. In bilinguals, at the C4 electrode location, the node strength was highly actively engaged to all the electrodes, while for monolinguals the node strength was less and not evidently active in all the electrodes. Node strength represents the strength of a particular electrode. The node strength for T4 (BA 21) was similar in both mono- and bilinguals, where this region is involved in the semantic and selective processing of text. This area was active even though it is not engaged with respect to connectivity, while it was actively connected during the 1500L task for both groups. A correlogram represents the correlated mutual information from the various electrode locations: when comparing the correlograms of the 650L task for monolinguals, Fp1 was highly correlated with P3, P4, and T4; whereas, for bilinguals, Fp2-O2, O1-C3, and T3-C3 are highly correlated. The alpha synchronisation during the 1500L Tamil task is shown in figure 2.31.

In monolinguals, F4 acts as a hub for receiving information from P3, C3, C4, T3, and T6. In addition to this, Fp1 and Fp2 are actively engaged in information transfer from other electrode locations for Fp1, T3, P3, and Fp2 with F4, P3, and T4. This was not noted for the bilingual group. At a high lexical level, transfer was noted from Fp1 to Fp2 in bilinguals. Also, information is relayed to T3, C3, C4, O1, and P3 from F4 (BA 8), which is primarily responsible for language processing and language translation and also responsible for visuospatial attention. An active point of mutual information (MI) was noted at O1 (BA 18), which acts as a hub for receiving information. This was not noted for monolinguals. This degraded the accuracy of the task performance of monolinguals at a high lexical level. P4 was not actively connected to any other electrodes except for receiving information from T3

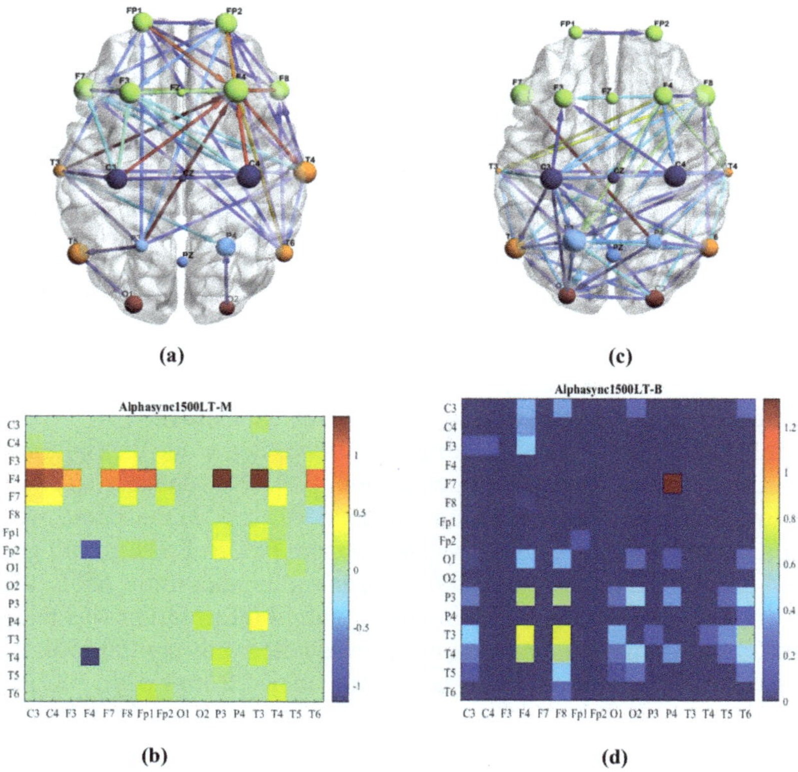

Figure 2.31. Alpha synchronisation during the 1500L Tamil task: (a) connectivity of monolinguals, (b) correlogram of monolinguals, (c) connectivity of bilinguals, and (d) correlogram of bilinguals.

and O2 for monolinguals, whereas for bilinguals at P3 information was received from F4, P4, C3, T5, O1, and O2; moreover, T6-P4-P3 were noted only for them. T4 (BA 21) was not actively engaged in the low-lexical-level task. This area is responsible for semantic processing, and was actively engaged during the high-lexical-level task (1500L) for both groups. Information was transferred from F8 to C3, O1, P3, T4, T5, and T6 for bilinguals alone. F8 (BA 45) is responsible for reasoning complex verbal functions such as in the processing of metaphors and reasoning processes. This improved the accuracy of related words for bilinguals. Based on the correlogram for MI (1500L), information at F4 is highly correlated with C3, C4, F3, F7, Fp1, Fp2, P3, T3, and T6 for monolinguals, where F4 (BA 8) is responsible for language processing and translation. In monolinguals, the information was the same at these electrodes, which degraded the task performance at high lexical level (1500L), while for bilinguals F7 and P4 were highly correlated.

The beta synchronisation for both monolinguals and bilinguals in the 650L and 1500L tasks is shown in figures 2.32 and 2.33, respectively. Here, there was no connectivity noted between Fp1 and Fp2. However, in monolinguals information was relayed to Fp2 from C3, F3, F8, T4, whereas for bilinguals at the same lexical level information was transferred from Fp2 to C3 and P3. For monolinguals, there

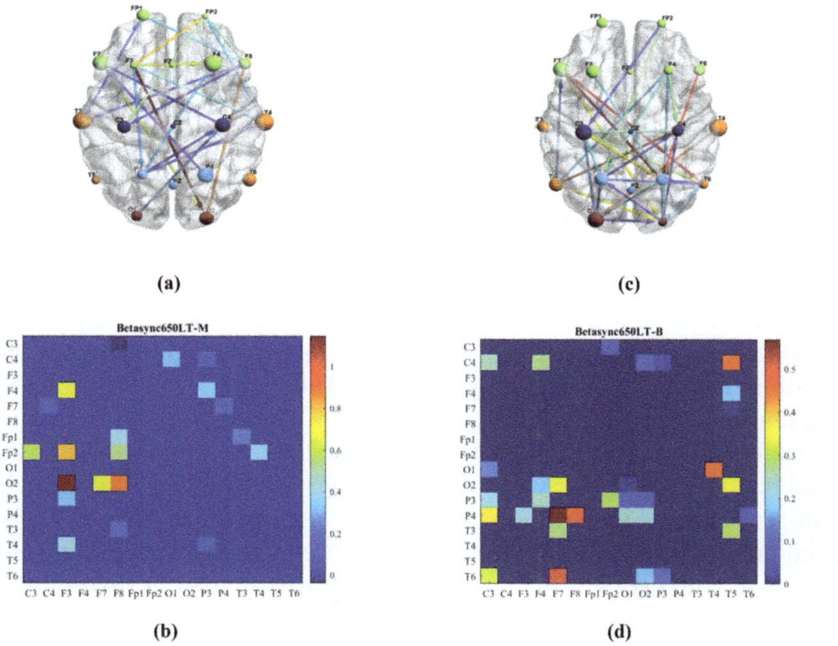

Figure 2.32. Beta synchronisation during the 650L Tamil task: (a) connectivity of monolinguals, (b) correlogram of monolinguals, (c) connectivity of bilinguals, and (d) correlogram of bilinguals.

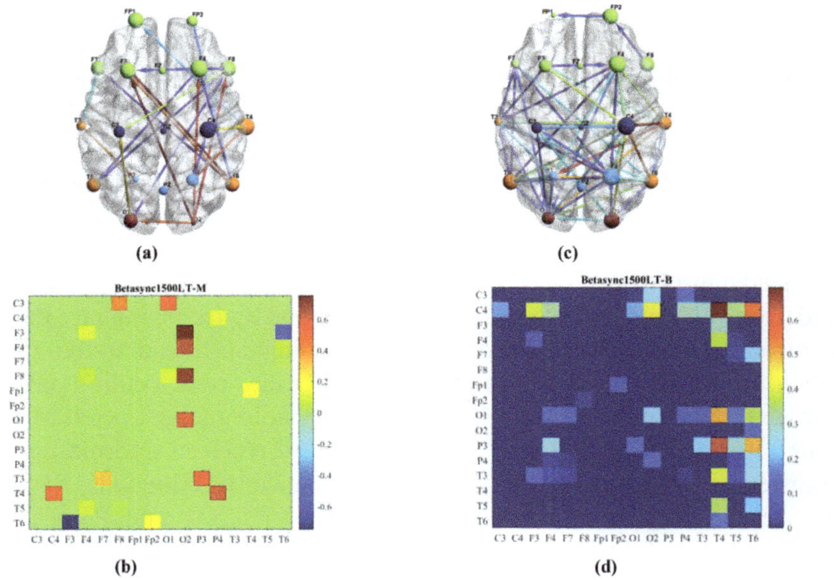

Figure 2.33. Beta synchronisation during the 1500L Tamil task: (a) connectivity of monolinguals, (b) correlogram of monolinguals, (c) connectivity of bilinguals, and (d) correlogram of bilinguals.

was transfer of information between F3, F4, and Fz, whereas in bilinguals there was no transfer of information between the frontal electrode locations (i.e., F3, F4, Fz, F7, F8). The transfer of information is noted from F8 to Fp2 in the monolingual group, whereas this is noted for the 1500L task in bilinguals. F7 received information from P4 and C4 for monolinguals, whereas information was transferred to P3, T6, and O2 from F7 in bilinguals. Beta synchronisation was noted at F7 and F4 for monolingualsm, whereas for bilinguals it was at the left frontal electrodes alone (i.e., F3 and F7). The right frontal electrodes had high node strength for both monolinguals and bilinguals. High beta synchronisation was noted at T3, T4 for monolinguals, and T3 received information from F8 and relayed to Fp1, whereas for bilinguals the node strength at T3 was not as high as for monolinguals; it received information from F7. For monolinguals, the T4 electrode location received from P3 and F3 and relayed to Fp2.

A greater complexity of brain connectivity has been previously noted in the occipital region of bilinguals when compared with monolinguals, which helps in the efficient processing of stimuli [30]; the same pattern was noted in the present work in the beta band, where the node strength at the occipital electrode locations (O1 and O2) was high, and O1, which acted like a hub for receiving information from other locations, namely the frontal (F4 and F7), parietal (P4), and temporal (T4 and T5) electrodes. Furthermore, this brain connectivity in the beta band improved task performance [30].

Connectivity between Fp1 and Fp2 is seen in bilinguals whereas it is not found in monolinguals. Transfer of information is noted from F4 to F3 in monolinguals, whereas in bilinguals the information flow was from F3 to F4. In monolinguals, F3 received information from O2 and relayed to T6. The node strength of O1 is less compared with monolinguals. In addition, it was well connected with T5, T3, F7, F4, P4, T4, and T6 and transferred information to C3 and P3. In monolinguals, T3 received information from F7 and P3, whereas in bilinguals, T3 received from F7, F3, F4, P4, and T5 and relaye information to O1, P3, and C4. The theta synchronisation for both monolinguals and bilinguals in the 650L and 1500L tasks is shown in figures 2.34 and 2.35, respectively.

In monolinguals, there is no connectivity noted between Fp1 and Fp2. Also, there is no inter-hemispheric connectivity as noted for Fp2, where information was received from C4 and transferred to T6. By contrast, for bilinguals information transfer from Fp1 to Fp2 was noted. Further, in bilinguals the node strength was less and the information was relayed to the parietal lobe electrode locations (P3 and P4). Even though the node strength is less at O1 in monolinguals, it acted as a hub for receiving information from F3, F8, T3, and T4. P4 received information from T4 and transferred to O2 alone among the monolinguals. In bilinguals, P4 acted as a hub for receiving information from C3, C4, F4, F7, O1 and P3. Fp2 relayed information to F3 and then to T3, whereas Fp2 relayed information to T6 and T6 received information from C4 and F4. It should be noted that, in monolinguals, C4 acted as a hub in monolinguals. But in bilinguals, even though it has a greater node strength there was no active connections noted. Theta synchronisation (node strength) was high at F4, Fp1, Fp2, O2, P4, and T6 for bilinguals during the

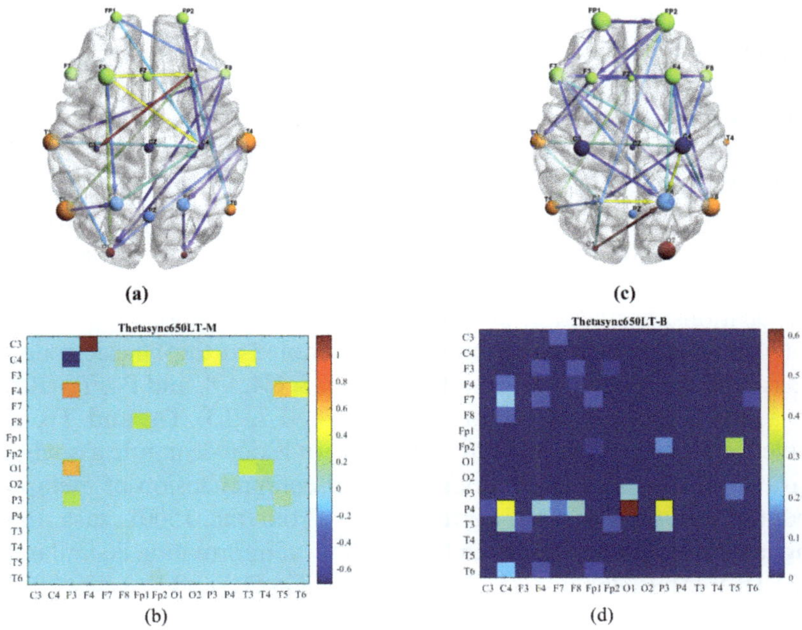

Figure 2.34. Theta synchronisation during the 650L Tamil task: (a) connectivity of monolinguals, (b) correlogram of monolinguals, (c) connectivity of bilinguals, and (d) correlogram of bilinguals.

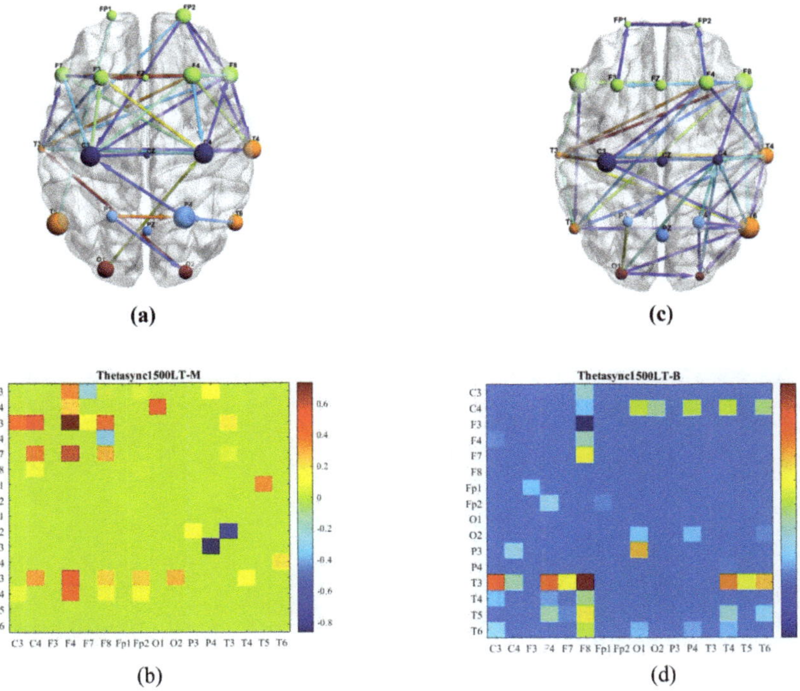

Figure 2.35. Theta synchronisation during the 1500L Tamil task: (a) connectivity of monolinguals, (b) correlogram of monolinguals, (c) connectivity of bilinguals, and (d) correlogram of bilinguals.

650L task in the theta band, but this was not noted for the monolingual group. T6 acted as a hub for receiving MI from C4, Fp1, and F4 for bilinguals.

The gamma synchronisation for both monolinguals and bilinguals in the 650L and 1500L tasks is shown in figures 2.36 and 2.37, respectively. Connectivity is noted between Fp1 to Fp2 for bilinguals in the 1500L task, but the node strength was less when compared to the 650L task. This connectivity was not seen in the 1500L task theta band for the monolingual group. Information transfer happened from T6 to P4 in the monolingual group's 1500L task theta synchronisation. Although the node strength of T5 in monolinguals is high, no transfer was noted with any other electrode locations. In addition to this, there are no connections found between T5 and T6. In bilinguals, theta synchronisation was noted at the T6 electrode location. It acted as a hub for receiving information from C3, C4, F8, and P4. T5 (BA 37) also acted as a link to receive information from F4, F7, T3, T4, and T6. BA 37 is responsible for word recognition and is involved in lexico-semantic associations and also in attention to semantic relations (T5) and comprehension of metaphor. This improved the accuracy of task performance. From the 1500L task theta band monolingual correlograms, it is noted that the flow of information is similar in F3-C3, C4, F4, F8 (BA 45); F7-C4, F4, F8; T3-F4; T4-F4; C4-O1; and Fp1-T5. F8 (BA 43) is a part of Broca's area, involved in complex verbal processing functions, which reflects verbal fluency, and is also involved in word generation, lexical searching (since the

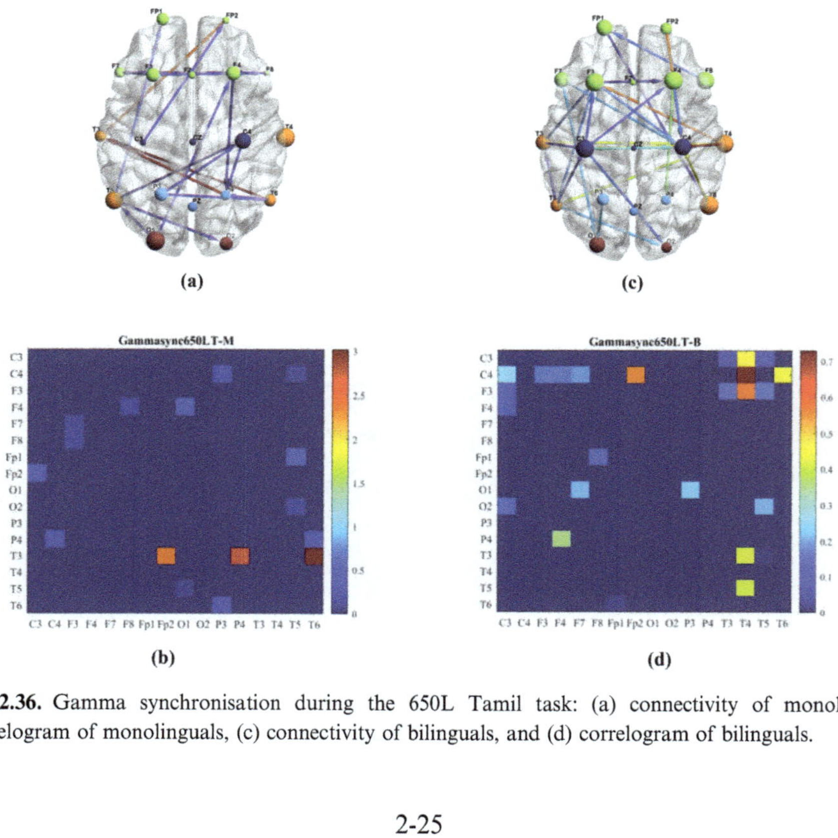

Figure 2.36. Gamma synchronisation during the 650L Tamil task: (a) connectivity of monolinguals, (b) correlogram of monolinguals, (c) connectivity of bilinguals, and (d) correlogram of bilinguals.

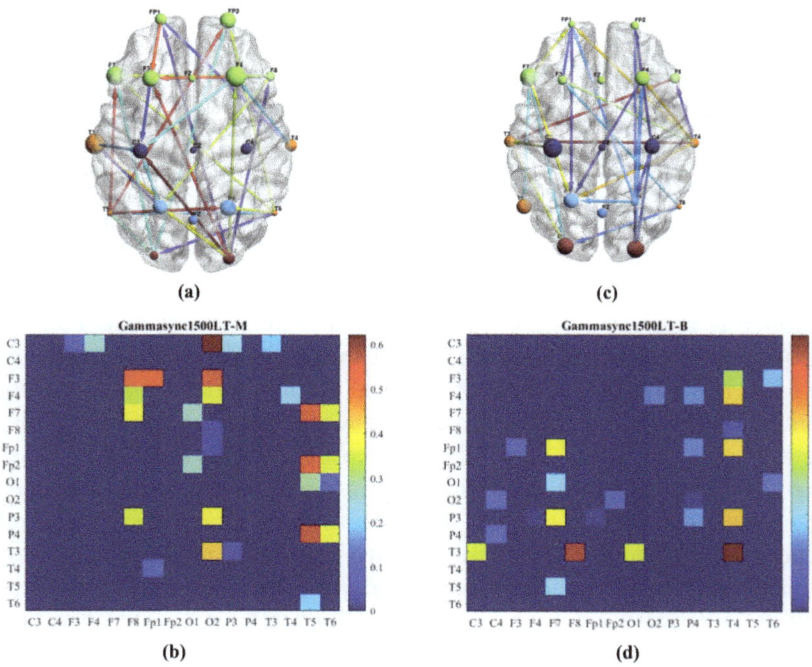

Figure 2.37. Gamma synchronisation during the 1500L Tamil task: (a) connectivity of monolinguals, (b) correlogram of monolinguals, (c) connectivity of bilinguals, and (d) correlogram of bilinguals.

information was the same, monolinguals here performed badly), and inflection. In the bilingual correlograms, a similar information flow is found at T3-C3, F4 (BA 8), F8 (BA 45), and T4.

Memory encoding in humans leads to a decrease in gamma synchronisation [31]. In the monolingual group for the 650L task, all frontal electrode locations were connected. In the bilingual group, F3 acted as a hub for the inflow of information from T4, C3, and T5. In the monolinguals, T5 acted as a hub to send information to O2, C4, and Fp1; T3 acted as a hub to receive information from inter-hemispheric electrode locations T6, P4, and Fp2. In the bilingual group for the 650L task, C4 acted as a link for the flow of information in F7, F4, F3, and Fp1. In the monolinguals, P3 and P4 were connected and received information from T6, whereas there was no active participation found in the bilingual group for task 650L: P3 relayed information to O1, and P4 received information from F4. The inter-hemispheric connection from F8 to Fp1 and then Fp1 to T6 is noted in the bilingual 650L, whereas in the monolingual 650L there is no such connection. C4 received information from T5 and P3, and relayed information to P4 in monolingual form. However, in the bilingual group C4 acted as a hub and received information from F4, F3, F7, T6, C3, and T4. The node strength of T4 was actively engaged with C4 and F3 in bilinguals. In the monolingual group there was no active engagement noted in the T4 location, even though the node strength was similar to the bilingual 650L task.

F4 received information from P4 and T4, and relayed information to C3. In the bilingual group 1500L task, F4 received information from T4 and P4, but relayed information to P3; this could be the reason for the improved task performance in bilinguals, as P3 is associated with language processing such as reading-related activities. In the monolingual group, Fp2 received information from T5, O1, and T6, whereas in bilinguals intra-connectivity is noted, i.e., Fp2 to O2 and from C4 to Fp2. P3 acted as hub of information from F7, Fp1, F4, T4, and P4 in bilinguals, whereas in monolinguals P3 received information from F8 and O2 and relayed to C3. In monolinguals Fp1 relayed to F3 and transferred to C3, whereas in bilinguals the information was received from F7, F3, P4, and T4 and relayed to P3. The node strength of O1 and O2 for the 1500L task in the bilingual group was much higher than the 650L task, whereas this is not noted in monolinguals. In the corresponding correlogram, F3, F4, P3, and P4 are very actively engaged in monolinguals, which leads to a rise in cognitive load. T3 acted as a hub in bilinguals, whereas in monolinguals, even though the node strength was high, it did not function as a hub.

The *cognitive load index (CLI)* is the ratio of the average power of the frontal theta band to the parietal alpha band. It has been demonstrated that there is an increase in frontal theta frequency activity, along with a decrease in parietal alpha frequency activity, with an increasing mental load related to memory tasks [32]. Graphical representations are depicted in figures 2.38–2.40.

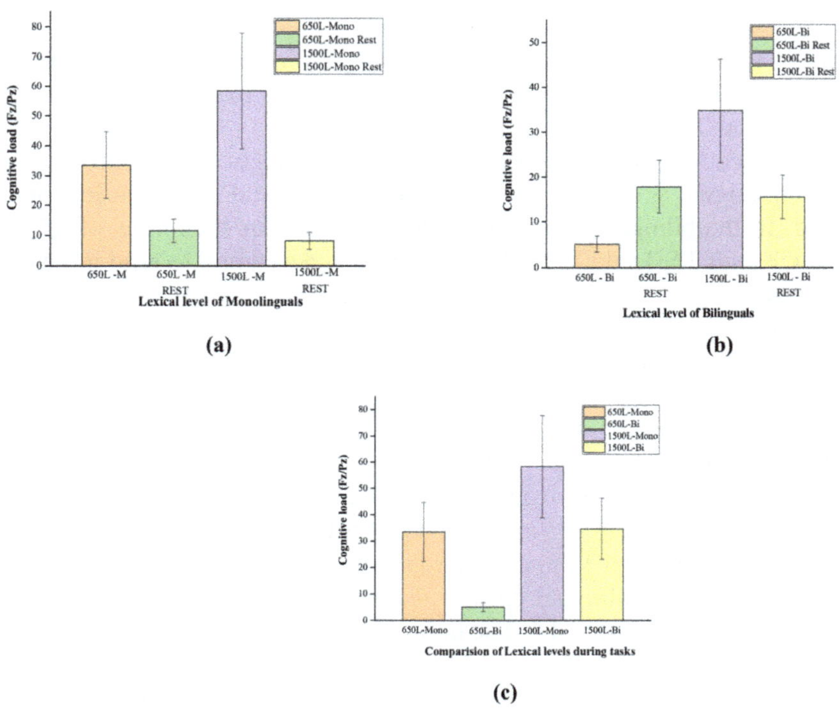

Figure 2.38. CLI (Fz/Pz) for the lexical level of (a) monolinguals, (b) bilinguals, and (c) during tasks.

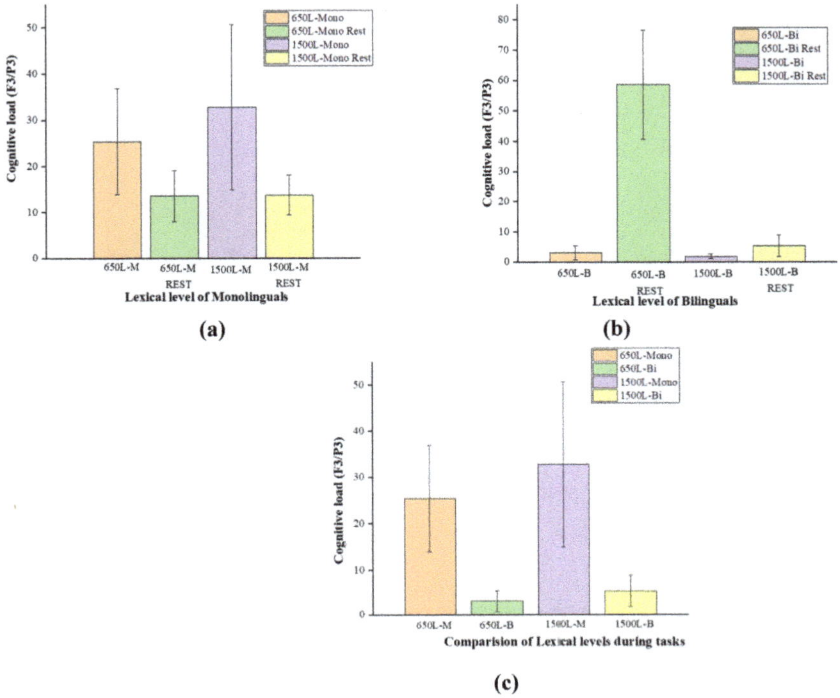

Figure 2.39. CLI (F3/P3) for the lexical level of (a) monolinguals, (b) bilinguals, and (c) during tasks.

2.4 Discussion

Two LDTs (650L and 1500L) were analysed for both monolingual and bilingual groups using EEG, as it provides better temporal resolution during information processing [33], and because the variation in EEG bands across each lobe is relevant for understanding cognitive processes and control [34, 35]. Alpha-band power reduction was noted in the language task performance in the language processing area [36]. The event-related changes resulted in an alpha reduction in alpha power for monolinguals at the O1 and P4 electrode locations in the 650L task, whereas for the 1500L task it was noted at the F8, FP1, T3, and T4 electrode locations. In the case of bilinguals, a significant reduction in alpha power was noted only at the F4 electrode location during the 1500L task [36]. Bilinguals show high alpha power when compared to monolinguals during rest, which indicates a high association of cognitive control [33]. During the 1500L task, alpha power increases were noted at the F8, T3, FP1, and O1 locations for bilinguals, which was not noted for the 650L task. This indicates that as task difficulty increases, the alpha power increases, giving better cognitive control and resulting in better task performance. In addition, the beta band increases during language knowledge tasks, indicating the dynamic upholding of associated cognitive networks [37]. When comparing the beta-band activity, the event-related beta power was significantly higher for bilinguals at the F3, FP1, O1, P4, and T4 locations for both LDTs when compared to monolinguals. Furthermore, an increase in theta power optimistically correlates to working

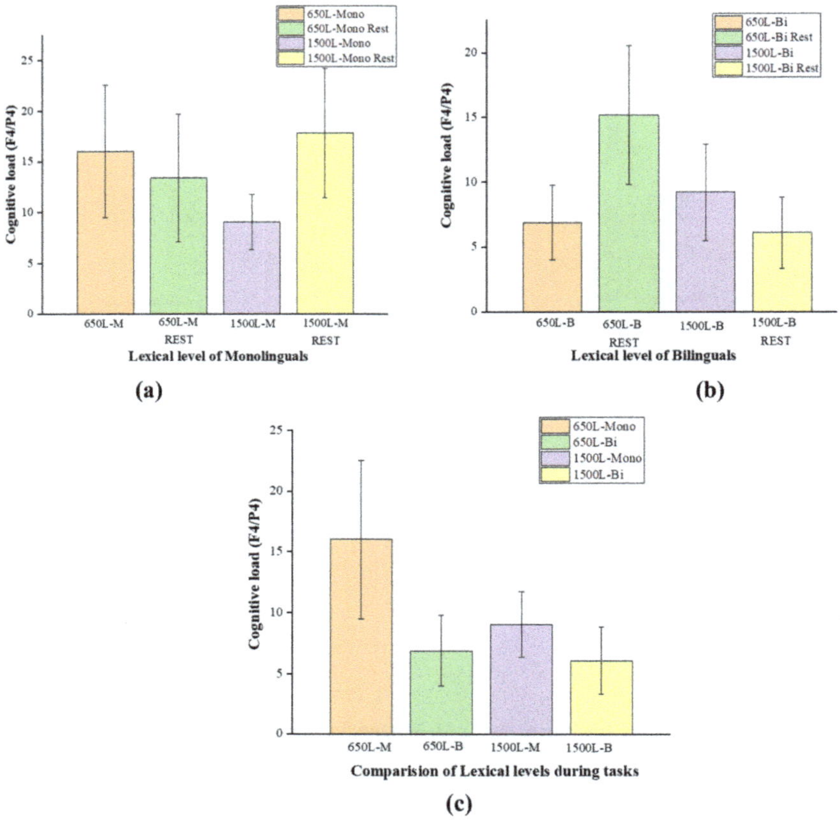

Figure 2.40. CLI (F4/P4) for the lexical level of (a) monolinguals, (b) bilinguals, and (c) during tasks.

memory demand [38–40]. During one LDT (1500L), the theta power was notably high at the F8, FP1, T3, and T4 electrode locations for monolinguals, whereas for bilinguals it was high at the F8 and T4 electrode locations, which relate to area BA 45, corresponding to working memory. This was noted for both mono- and bilinguals only during high-lexical-level processing (1500L) tasks and not for low-lexical-level processing (650L).

In a bilingual system, P3 acts as a repository for data available from F7, Fp1, F4, T4, and P4; while in a monolingual system, P3 gathers data from F8 and O2 and transfers that to C3. Even though data are acquired from F7, F3, P4, and T4 and relayed to P3 in bilinguals, they are divulged to F3 and transmitted to C3 in monolinguals. In monolinguals, there is a high degree of correlation between the points T6, Fp2, and F7; in bilinguals, there is relatively mild interconnectivity between the locations T4, F3, F4, F8, P4, and Fp1. Even though the node strength is prominent in monolinguals, T3 does not serve as a centre irrespective of the fact that it is functional in bilinguals. Elevated gamma activity is associated with an increase in linguistic and attention capability [41]: the 1500L bilingual node strength of the O1 and O2 locations was seen to be considerably greater than the 650L bilingual, although this has not been recognised in monolinguals. Beta and gamma power increases were noted for bilinguals, which led to improved accuracy in task performance.

2.5 Conclusion

In this chapter, changes in the cognitive load work for both monolinguals and bilinguals during high- and low-lexical levels were investigated. In terms of task performance, bilinguals are more accurate than their monolingual peers, even though the mean reaction times of bilinguals are higher. Further, significant differences were found for the accuracy of all non-word, related, and unrelated words, but in the mean reaction times non-words are identified as significantly different. While comparing the event-related changes between monolinguals and bilinguals, from the prime electrode locations F3, F4, F8, Fp1, Fp2, O1, P4, T3, and T4 significant changes are found during the low-level 650L task, whereas significant differences were found while performing the high-level 1500L task in electrode locations Fp1, P3, T3, T4, and T5, which are responsible for the language memory, attention, and semantic handling. This research can be extended further by investigating participants with various psychological assessment tasks, and, by evaluating the outcomes through various connectivity measures, phase synchronisation and desynchronization, asymmetry index, and relative spectral entropy can be compared.

References

[1] Bialystok E, Craik F I and Luk G 2012 Bilingualism: consequences for mind and brain *Trends Cogn. Sci.* **16** 240–50

[2] http://libguides.nsu.edu/c.php?g=413931

[3] https://psychologistworld.com/memory/cognitive-load-theory

[4] Wong B, Yin B and O'Brien B 2016 Neurolinguistics: structure, function, and connectivity in the bilingual brain *BioMed Res. Int.* **2016** 7069274

[5] Kumar P, Anandan K, Balasubramanian G and Veezhinathan M 2013 Analysis of cognitive load for bilingual subjects based on lexile measures *2013 IEEE 12th Int. Conf. on Cognitive Informatics and Cognitive Computing (Piscataway, NJ, July 2013)* (IEEE) pp 320–3

[6] Leppink J, Paas F, Van der Vleuten C P, Van Gog T and Van Merriënboer J J 2013 Development of an instrument for measuring different types of cognitive load *Behav. Res. Methods* **45** 1058–72

[7] Friedman N, Fekete T, Gal K and Shriki O 2019 EEG-based prediction of cognitive load in intelligence tests *Front. Hum. Neurosci.* **13** 191

[8] Higby E, Kim J and Obler L K 2013 Multilingualism and the brain *Annu. Rev. Appl. Linguist.* **33** 68–101

[9] Friesen D C, Chung-Fat-Yim A and Bialystok E 2016 Lexical selection differences between monolingual and bilingual listeners *Brain Lang.* **152** 1–13

[10] Quinteros Baumgart C and Billick S B 2018 Positive cognitive effects of bilingualism and multilingualism on cerebral function: a review *Psychiatr. Q.* **89** 273–83

[11] Bialystok E and Craik F I 2010 Cognitive and linguistic processing in the bilingual mind *Curr. Dir. Psychol. Sci.* **19** 19–23

[12] Bialystok E and Poarch G J 2014 Language experience changes language and cognitive ability *Z. Erziehungswiss.* **17** 433–46

[13] Costa A and Sebastián-Gallés N 2014 How does the bilingual experience sculpt the brain? *Nat. Rev. Neurosci.* **15** 336–45

[14] Pliatsikas C and Luk G 2016 Executive control in bilinguals: a concise review on fMRI studies *Biling.: Lang. Cogn.* **19** 699–705

[15] Kong A P H, Abutalebi J, Lam K S Y and Weekes B 2014 Executive and language control in the multilingual brain *Behav. Neurol.* **2014** 527951

[16] Kroll J F, Bobb S C and Hoshino N 2014 Two languages in mind: bilingualism as a tool to investigate language, cognition, and the brain *Curr. Dir. Psychol. Sci.* **23** 159–63

[17] James V A 2017 The bilingual brain *J. Counsel. Psychol.* **1** 1 (https://digitalcommons.gardner-webb.edu/jcp/vol1/iss2/1)

[18] Kukke S N, de Campos A C, Damiano D, Alter K E, Patronas N and Hallett M 2015 Cortical activation and inter-hemispheric sensorimotor coherence in individuals with arm dystonia due to childhood stroke *Clin. Neurophysiol.* **126** 1589–98

[19] Ashokumar M, Bala J R, Geethanjali B and Veezhinathan M 2017 Visualizing the functional connectivity of bilingual and monolingual brain during multitasking *2017 IEEE 16th Int. Conf. on Cognitive Informatics and Cognitive Computing (ICCI* CC) (July 2017)*

[20] Sukeerthi S, Veezhinathan M and Geethanjali B 2020 Analysing the cognitive load for monolinguals using EEG *2020 6th Int. Conf. on Advanced Computing and Communication Systems (ICACCS)* pp 253–60

[21] Balasubramanian G, Kanagasabai A, Mohan J and Seshadri N G 2018 Music induced emotion using wavelet packet decomposition—an EEG study *Biomed. Signal Process. Control* **42** 115–28

[22] Fraga González G, Smit D J, Van der Molen M J, Tijms J, Stam C J, De Geus E J and Van der Molen M W 2018 EEG resting state functional connectivity in adult dyslexics using phase lag index and graph analysis *Front. Hum. Neurosci.* **12** 341

[23] Krause C 2000 Auditorily elicited event-related desynchronization (ERD) and synchronization (ERS) as a method for studying cortical correlates of cognitive processes *Rev. Esp. Neuropsicol.* **2** 77–91

[24] Geethanjali B, Adalarasu K, Jagannath M and Seshadri N G 2018 Music-induced brain functional connectivity using EEG sensors: a study on Indian music *IEEE Sens. J.* **19** 1499–507

[25] Pavithran P G, Arunkumar K, Seshadri N G, Singh B K, Mahesh V and Geethanjali B 2019 Index of theta/alpha ratio to quantify visual-spatial attention in dyslexics using electroencephalogram *2019 5th Int. Conf. on Advanced Computing and Communication Systems (ICACCS) (March 2019)(Piscataway, NJ)* (IEEE) pp 417–22

[26] Grant A, Dennis N A and Li P 2014 Cognitive control, cognitive reserve, and memory in the aging bilingual brain *Fron. Psychol.* **5** 1401

[27] Aftanas L, Varlamov A, Pavlov S, Makhnev V and Reva N 2001 Event-related synchronization and desynchronization during affective processing: emergence of valence-related time-dependent hemispheric asymmetries in theta and upper alpha band *Int. J. Neurosci.* **110** 197–219

[28] Diaz M T and Eppes A 2018 Factors influencing right hemisphere engagement during metaphor comprehension *Front. Psychol.* **9** 414

[29] Solomon E A, Kragel J E, Sperling M R, Sharan A, Worrell G, Kucewicz M and Kahana M J 2017 Widespread theta synchrony and high-frequency desynchronization underlies enhanced cognition *Nat. Commun.* **8** 1–14

[30] Dan A and Reiner M 2017 Real time EEG based measurements of cognitive load indicates mental states during learning *J. Educ. Data Min.* **9** 31–44
[31] https://psytoolkit.org/experiment-library/ldt.html
[32] Bice K, Yamasaki B L and Prat C S 2020 Bilingual language experience shapes resting-state brain rhythms *Neurobiol. Lang.* **1** 288–318
[33] Sadaghiani S and Kleinschmidt A 2016 Brain networks and α-oscillations: structural and functional foundations of cognitive control *Trends Cogn. Sci.* **20** 805–17
[34] Miller E K, Lundqvist M and Bastos A M 2018 Working memory 2.0 *Neuron* **100** 463–75
[35] Wang P, He Y, Maess B, Yue J, Chen L, Brauer J and Knösche T R 2022 Alpha power during task performance predicts individual language comprehension *NeuroImage* **260** 119449
[36] Lewis A G, Schoffelen J M, Schriefers H and Bastiaansen M 2016 A predictive coding perspective on beta oscillations during sentence-level language comprehension *Front. Hum. Neurosci.* **10** 85
[37] Tang M, Zhao X, Chen B and Zhao L 2021 EEG theta responses induced by emoji semantic violations *Sci. Rep.* **11** 10092
[38] Luo Y, Zhang Y, Feng X and Zhou X 2010 Electroencephalogram oscillations differentiate semantic and prosodic processes during sentence reading *Neuroscience* **169** 654–64
[39] Dini H, Simonetti A and Bigne E *et al* 2022 EEG theta and N400 responses to congruent versus incongruent brand logos *Sci. Rep.* **12** 4490
[40] Soares S M P, Kubota M, Rossi E and Rothman J 2021 Determinants of bilingualism predict dynamic changes in resting state EEG oscillations *Brain Lang.* **223** 105030
[41] Tarullo A R, Obradović J, Keehn B, Rasheed M A, Siyal S, Nelson C A and Yousafzai A K 2017 Gamma power in rural pakistani children: links to executive function and verbal ability *Dev. Cogn. Neurosci.* **26** 1–8

IOP Publishing

Affective Computing in Healthcare
Applications based on biosignals and artificial intelligence
M Murugappan

Chapter 3

Detection of psychological stress using principal component analysis of phonocardiography signals

Amandeep Cheema and Mandeep Singh

Psychological stress and its associated mental health conditions affects a large proportion of the world population, impairing quality of life and resulting in high socioeconomic impacts on society. The onset of the recent COVID-19 pandemic worsened the global situation, and hence it has become imperative to find ways to detect psychological stress in a timely manner. The present chapter uses phonocardiography (PCG) signals, an easy-to-acquire biosignal suitable in homecare-based frameworks for psychological stress detection. The study uses signals acquired from 51 healthy male subjects, and the stressor used is not a laboratory-based stressor but a real-life institute examination. The S1–S1 interval of PCG signals is computed using an electrocardiogram-referencing method and used for time–frequency domain, non-linear, non-stationary signal decomposition using empirical mode decomposition (EMD) to unravel the complex characteristics of the PCG signals. Thereafter, the decomposed signal data matrix is used for principal component analysis (PCA) and formation of principal components. The features extracted from PCA of the decomposed signal are used for classification. The outcome of the study is evaluated, and the average accuracy, sensitivity, and specificity achieved for classification is 87.25%, 90.38%, and 84.23%, respectively. The novelty of this study is in exploring the potential of applying PCA to the outcomes of EMD for the relatively new field of PCG-signal-based psychological stress detection. The proposed framework may be useful in telemedicine in order to increase the outreach of expert healthcare diagnosis in rural areas and in underdeveloped economies.

3.1 Introduction

The World Health Organization (WHO) defines mental health as a state of well-being in which an individual is able to realise his or her potential, can cope with normal life

doi:10.1088/978-0-7503-5182-9ch3

stresses, can work productively, and contribute to their community [1]. The importance of mental health is evident from the definition of health as per the constitution of the WHO, which states that health is not merely the absence of disease but a state of complete physical, mental, and social well-being [2]. The physical, mental, and social health of an individual have a complex interdependence [3]. Approximately 450 million people around the world suffer from some form of mental disorder [4]. Most mental disorders can be effectively treated and the associated suffering can be minimised; however, between 76% and 85% of people receive no treatment for their disorder [5]. Globally, mental health conditions impose an enormous burden on society, and account for 1 in every 5 years lived with disability, causing more than US$1 trillion per year economic loss [6]. Due to this, it has become imperative to detect psychological stress in a timely manner in order to improve the quality of human life and reduce any associated socioeconomic burden. Moreover, experts warn of an unprecedented wave of the mental health crisis due to the recent COVID-19 pandemic as it has resulted in increased psychological stress and a spike in people seeking help regarding associated mental health issues [7–10].

Stress is the response of the brain and body to any demand. Any challenge, including performance at work, a significant change in life, or a traumatic event, can be perceived as stressful and are termed as stressors. When faced with a stressor, the body enters flight or fight mode, which increases heart rate, breathing rate, tenses muscles, and increases brain activity. Cortisol is released due to stress, exposure to which is linked to a broad range of problems, including metabolic syndromes, obesity, cancer, mental health disorders, cardiovascular disease, and increased susceptibility to infections [11]. Diseases and human pathologies, including diabetes mellitus, inflammatory bowel disease, and rheumatic diseases, can be regarded as by-products of endocrine reactions, which play an important role in the general adaptation syndrome and stress responses [12, 13].

This study presents a phonocardiography (PCG)-based framework for computer-aided psychological stress detection, and is a step in the direction of using machine learning, signal-processing techniques, and digital technologies to provide tele-medicine-based mental health services. Study of the existing literature shows that the PCG signals are primarily used for foetal heart-rate monitoring [14], fundamental heart sounds segmentation [15], and abnormal heart sound murmur detection [16]. However, the field of PCG-signal-based stress detection remains yet unexplored. Prior work on stress detection includes the applicability of electrocardiogram (ECG)-based heart-rate variability (HRV) signals [17], electroencephalogram (EEG) signals [18] and imaging [19–22], and photoplethysmography (PPG) and pulse rate variability [22, 23] for stress detection. The fusion of various modalities, including skin temperature variability, PPG, blood volume pulse (BVP), pupil diameter, electrodermal activity, EEG, and ECG, have been used in various studies for psychological stress detection [24–27].

Recent works in the field of psychological stress detection include a study [28] that utilises a multi-sensing approach using EEG and ECG signals acquired from 24 young individuals in age group from 18 to 23 years old. The study uses *K*-means clustering, and thereafter supervised machine-learning approaches are utilised to provide a patient-specific approach for stress detection. A study [29] used electromyographic signals to detect stress in automobile drivers. The findings of the study indicate the potential of using statistical features, including variance and standard deviation, with support vector machine (SVM) classifiers with a cubic kernel function for the purpose of detecting stress in drivers, which may be a significant cause in many accidents. Another study conducted on automobile drivers [30] used ECG HRV-based features for stress detection. This study utilises data acquired from an Apple watch, a wearable device with health sensors. The authors emphasised the importance of various HRV-based features for stress detection. Another study [31] also utilised wrist-based smartband sensors to acquire four signals—electrodermal activity, BVP, inter-beat interval (IBI), and skin temperature—to detect stress in older adults. The use of features from these four signals in combination showed a high accuracy in stress detection. Another interesting work [32] analysed various posts and comments shared by individuals on social media platforms using natural-language processing to extend concepts of sentiment analysis for detection of stress. This study used machine-learning models and a BERT language model for the purpose of stress detection. However, the approach of utilising PCG signals to detect stress is relatively new: to which end this study aims to explore use of principal component analysis (PCA) on PCG signals to detect psychological stress.

This chapter is composed of four sections, where the present section 3.1 has comprised an introduction. Section 3.2 of this study details the methodology, which contains dataset acquisition and pre-processing details, and outlines the signal decomposition technique used for feature extraction, the classifiers, and performance metrics used in the study. Section 3.3 gives the results and discussion, followed by the concluding remarks in section 3.4.

3.2 Methodology

The present study aims to detect psychological stress from PCG signals by computing the IBI signal using an ECG-gating method. This IBI signal is decomposed using an empirical mode decomposition (EMD) method, and intrinsic mode functions (IMFs) are then obtained. Following this, the principal components are extracted by using the PCA algorithm on the IMFs. These principal components are used for the classification of stressed and non-stressed states, as shown in figure 3.1.

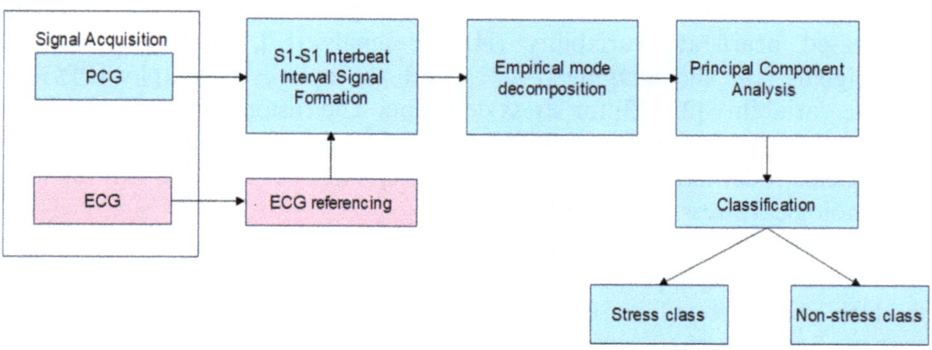

Figure 3.1. Block diagram showing methodology of psychological stress detection using PCG signals.

3.2.1 Signal acquisition

In previous studies, PCG signals have been used in applications for abnormal heart sounds/murmur detection and foetal heart-rate monitoring; however, the research area of focussing PCG signals to detect stress is relatively new. Therefore, to the best of our knowledge, there are no publicly accessible datasets for psychological stress detection using the IBI signal of PCG signals. The challenges of detecting psychological stress from PCG signals depicting mechanical activity of the heart are greater still because any dataset has to be recorded under the guidance of a physician, with related approvals from Institutional Ethics Committees. The acquisition is done in accordance with the guidelines from the Task Force of the European Society of Cardiology and North American Society of Pacing and Electrophysiology regarding the minimum duration of acquisition (5 min) for proper fiducial point information and minimum sampling frequency (250 Hz). Accordingly, in this study, a 5 min duration signal acquisition is undertaken at a sampling frequency of 256 Hz. Therefore, the process of data acquisition involves simultaneous ECG and PCG signal acquisition for 5 min duration.

The PCG and ECG signals are temporally related, with the S1 peak of the PCG signal appearing immediately after the R peak of the ECG signal [33]. Therefore, in the present study, PCG and ECG signals are simultaneously acquired; the ECG here is not used for stress detection but as a reference signal to detect the S1 peak in the PCG. Various studies [15, 34–36] have elaborated on methods to detect the S1 peak of PCG signals without using this ECG-reference method. However, in this study, the focus is on utilising PCG signals to detect stress and not on the fundamental heart sound (S1 and S2) segmentation, therefore to ease the process of finding the S1 peak accurately for construction of the IBI signal, we utilise a simultaneously acquired ECG signal.

The data were acquired from 54 healthy, male, adult students of the Thapar Institute of Engineering and Technology, India. However, data of subjects under medication or with a medical history were eliminated from the records, and so signals from 51 subjects were here used for this study. In order to record the PCG and ECG signals simultaneously, Physiopac, a dual-channel acquisition device by Medicaid with a sampling frequency 256 Hz, was used in the present study. This device has a PCG sensor attached on its channel 1 and ECG limb electrodes attached on channel 2, which ensures simultaneous PCG and ECG signal acquisition. The acquisition system used in the present study consists of one PCG sensor and four strap electrodes for ECG signal acquisition. The placement position of the PCG sensor was taken as the fifth intercostal space along the left mid-clavicular line, and ECG strap electrodes were attached to the limbs of subjects using bioelectrode gel for better conductivity.

The protocol adopted for this study is explained as follows.

Data acquisition was performed about 2 hr before a university exam, at around 11 am (for a university exam starting at 1 pm). In order to avoid diurnal variations, baseline readings were also recorded around 11 am on another day after the participants of the study had returned home after exams.

The inclusion criteria were as follows:

(1) Any adult male student of the Thapar Institute of Engineering and Technology having an institute examination the next day.
(2) Agrees to give two readings: R1, approximately 2 hr before an institute exam conducted the same day; R2, a baseline reading recorded once the participant had returned to the institute from home after exams.
(3) Eligible and willing to participate in the study.
(4) No medical history.
(5) Not currently on any type of medication.

The primary outcome of the study is detecting psychological stress using PCG signals, and the primary end point is recording R2 baseline readings.

A State-Trait Anxiety Inventory-Y1 (STAI-Y1) self-report questionnaire was filled by each participant before the data acquisition. The STAI form has 20 statements to evaluate how the participant feels right now (i.e., in the present moment). It is a four-point Likert scale, where 1 indicates 'not at all', 2 indicates 'somewhat', 3 stands for 'moderately so', and 4 stands for 'very much so' in response to the statements. It deals with a so-called States Anxiety Scale (S-Anxiety) and shows high alpha reliability coefficients under unavoidable conditions of psychological stress. The STAI S-Anxiety questionnaire used in this study is reported to show high reliability under psychologically stressful conditions and is suitable for real-life stressors, including job interviews, important examsm, and dental procedures [37]. The scores of the S-Anxiety scale increase under psychologically stressful conditions and reduce after relaxation [33]. As per the developers of this STAI scale, the affective states considered in the stress class include tension, nervousness, apprehension, and worry [37]. Examinations are a prominent real-life stressor for students of this age group. For this study, a non-stress baseline state is considered when students have returned from holidays after exams, as is used in previous studies [38, 39].

The steps included during the data-acquisition procedure are as follows:

- Informing the subject about the purpose of the study and taking written consent.
- The subject filling a declaration form regarding any recent use of medication or any extant medical conditions.
- The subject answering the STAI questionnaire in order to evaluate their present psychological state.
- Data acquisition from the subject in the supine position with normal breathing.
- Placing of the PCG sensor on the fifth intercostal space along the left mid-clavicular line.
- Attaching of the ECG strap electrodes to the limbs of the subject using a bioelectrode gel.
- Recording simultaneous PCG and ECG signals for 5 min.

The records of any subjects on medication were removed from the study. The study received ethical clearance from the Institutional Ethics Committee.

Real-life stress situations threaten homeostasis, and previous studies [38–42] have used exams, dental procedures, and job interviews as real-life stressors. The artificiality and absence of negative emotions are limitations of using laboratory stressors, and therefore limit their potential in eliciting actual stress responses [38]. Therefore, the present study utilises an institute examination as a real-life moderate-intensity stressor, as used in previous studies [38, 39].

3.2.2 Inter-beat interval signal formation

An ECG signal depicts the electrical activity of the heart, whereas a PCG signal shows the mechanical activity of heart, which is dependent on the electrical heart activity. In this study, as aforementioned, the purpose of acquiring the ECG signal is to use as a reference to help detect the S1 peak in the simultaneously acquired PCG signal. This method of using simultaneously recorded ECG and PCG signals for fundamental heart sound detection of PCG signals is used as a gold standard in the literature [33]. Therefore, in the present study, the S1 peaks are also detected using this method.

The Pan–Tompkins algorithm is used for ECG R-peak detection, and thereafter windowing is done in order to locate the S1 peak of the PCG appearing just after the R peak of the ECG signal. This ensures reliable S1 peak detection. The IBI signals are then computed by calculating the time-duration between successive S1 peaks of the PCG signal. These IBI signals are used for further processing to detect psychological stress.

Figure 3.2(a) depicts an ECG signal with baseline wander; such an ECG signal will ordinarily be corrected and then used to find the S1 peaks in a PCG signal. Therefore, figure 3.2(b) depicts simultaneously acquired ECG and PCG signals,

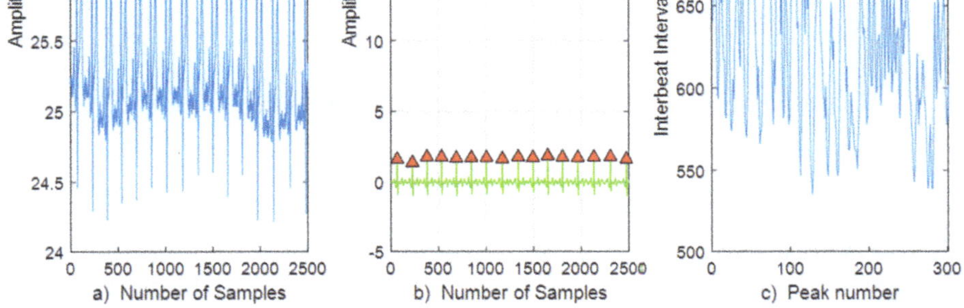

Figure 3.2. (a) Plot of ECG signal, (b) using ECG as a reference for detecting the S1 peak of the PCG signal (depicted in blue), and (c) extracted IBI signal.

with the peaks detected in red triangles. Here, the ECG signal has only one prominent peak—the R peak—whereas the PCG signal has two prominent peaks—S1 and S2—thereby making it difficult to detect the S1 peak and subsequently to compute the S1–S1 interval to form the desired IBI signal. Therefore, the temporal relation that exists between the ECG (i.e., the electrical activity of heart) and the PCG (i.e., the mechanical activity of heart) is utilised in this study to detect the S1 peak of the PCG using the ECG as a reference signal, as the S1 peak of the PCG appears immediately after the R peak of the ECG. The Pan–Tompkins algorithm is used for ECG R-peak detection and thereafter, windowing is done in order to locate S1 peak of PCG appearing just after the R peak of ECG signal. After detecting the S1 peaks of the PCG signal using the ECG as a reference, figure 3.2(c) of this study depicts a plot of the resulting IBI signal formed by computation of the time intervals between the successive S1 peaks of the PCG signal. All the signals used in the study have a minimum of 300 peaks, therefore, for uniformity in the signal analysis process, 300 peaks are considered for formation of IBI signals in the present study.

3.2.3 Empirical mode decomposition

Biological signals generally are non-linear and non-stationary, and require time–frequency domain analysis. Time–frequency domain signal decomposition is accomplished using the EMD technique, as this method is suitable for non-stationary and non-linear signals. The method is adaptive, data dependent, and takes no *a priori* assumptions, and hence has been extensively used in biomedical applications [43–45]. EMD decomposes the IBI signals, $Ib(t)$, into intrinsic mode functions (IMFs) using an iterative sifting technique [46], and includes the following steps:

1. Extraction of all extrema from $Ib(t)$.
2. Interpolation of maxima for forming an upper envelope, $Emax(t)$, and minima for forming a lower envelope, $Emin(t)$.
3. Obtaining the average of $Emax(t)$ and $Emin(t)$ using

$$M(t) = \frac{Emax(t) + Emin(t)}{2}. \tag{3.1}$$

4. Evaluating the difference between $Ib(t)$ and $M(t)$ as

$$Diff(t) = Ib(t) - M(t). \tag{3.2}$$

5. Checking if $Diff(t)$ satisfies two conditions of IMFs [42]; if yes, then proceed to step 6, and if no, then steps 1–4 are repeated until conditions are satisfied.
6. After finding the IMF, $D_1(t) = Diff(t)$, the residual, $R_1(t)$, is calculated as $R_1(t) = Ib(t) - D_1(t)$. The rest of the IMFs are computed from the residual

$R_1(t)$ by repetition of steps 1–6 until no further IMFs can be extracted from the final residual. After decomposition, the signal $Ib(t)$ can be denoted as

$$Ib(t) = \sum_{M}^{m=1} D_m(t) + R_m(t) \ , \tag{3.3}$$

where M is the number of IMFs extracted, $D_m(t)$ is the mth IMF, and $R_M(t)$ is the final residual.

The EMD technique suffers from the limitation of mode mixing; however, this problem is not significant for the present application as the EMD is not applied directly to the PCG signals, which comprise S1 and S2 peaks with overlapping spectra, but on the derived IBI signals from the PCG signals.

3.2.4 Principal component analysis

PCA is a mathematical tool used in the dimensionality reduction of datasets, while retaining most of the variation of the given dataset. The dimensionality reduction is achieved by identifying directions, named as principal components, where the data variation is maximum [47]. This algorithm includes computing of a covariance matrix, followed by eigenvalue and eigenvector decomposition; thereafter, eigenvectors are sorted according to decreasing order of eigenvalues and the original dataset is projected in the directions of the sorted eigenvectors. The majority of the data's variability will be depicted by the first few components [48].

This PCA technique has been utilised in many previous biomedical studies [48–50]. The advantages of applying the PCA algorithm to the outcome of EMD are described in detail in a previous study [51]. The present study utilises the principal components of the IMFs extracted using EMD as features for detection of psychological stress using PCG signals.

3.2.5 Classifiers

The aim of classifiers is to predict the accurate target class for each test sample based on a model trained using training samples. The classifiers used in this study are described as follows.

3.2.5.1 Support vector machine classifier

In this supervised learning classifier, the best separating hyperplane is constructed for classifying the data in order to maximise the margin between two classes. The data points that decide the hyperplane are termed as support vectors. The training set consists of X data points, $\{q_j, w_j\}_{j=1}^{Z}$, where $q_j \in \mathbb{R}^n$ is the jth input pattern and $w_j \in \mathbb{R}$ is the jth output pattern. The SVM classifier is given as [48]

$$q(w) = sign\left[\sum_{X}^{j=1} c_j q_j \varphi(w, w_j) + d\right]. \tag{3.4}$$

Here, c_j is a positive real constant, whereas d is a real constant, and $\varphi(w, w_j)$ is the kernel function used. The radial basis function (RBF) is a widely used kernel function for biomedical applications.

3.2.5.2 Random forest classifier

This supervised learning classifier combines multiple tree predictors, in which each tree is dependent on a randomly chosen vector value, ∂_p, distributed among all trees of a forest in the same manner. Every tree is grown using training data, and ∂_p leads to tree-structured classifiers, represented as [52]

$$\left\{t\left(x, \partial_p\right),\ p = 1,2\ldots.\right\}, \tag{3.5}$$

where x is the input vector. Thereafter, in this algorithm, the large number of trees generated casts a vote for the most popular class [52]. Random forest classifiers have been found to be suitable for biomedical applications [53, 54]. This study utilises a random-forest-based classifier in psychological stress detection using PCG signals.

3.2.5.3 Naïve Bayes classifier

A naïve Bayes classifier uses probability to determine the class $h \in \mathbb{N}_H = \{1,\ldots., H\}$ of every test sample, and every feature $\vec{t} = \{t,\ldots, t_N\}$ has a say in deciding the class. The prior probability, $\Pr(H)$, of every class is computed by calculating the frequency of every class in the training data or by assuming equiprobable classes. The likelihood estimate of each class is presented as follows [55]:

$$h = \mathrm{argmax}_{h \in \mathbb{N}_H} p(h|\vec{t}) = \mathrm{argmax}_{h \in \mathbb{N}_H} \Pr(h) p(\vec{t}|h). \tag{3.6}$$

This classifier is used in a wide range of applications, from text classification to colon cancer detection. In this study, a Naïve Bayes classifier is used for PCG-based psychological stress detection.

3.2.6 Performance metrics

To evaluate the efficacy of the developed method in a target population, the performance metrics selected in this study are accuracy, sensitivity, and specificity. The terms used for defining the performance metrics are explained below [56]:

- True positive (TP): If a condition is actually present in the subject and the developed method also produces a positive test result.
- True negative (TN): If a condition is actually not present in the subject and the developed method also produces a negative test result.
- False positive (FP): If a condition is actually not present in the subject but the developed method produces a positive test result.
- False negative (FN): If a condition is actually present in the subject but the developed method produces a negative test result.

The performance metrics used in this study are as follows:

- Accuracy: The ratio of the number of correct assessments to the total number of assessments, denoted as

$$\frac{\mathrm{TP} + \mathrm{TN}}{\mathrm{TP} + \mathrm{TN} + \mathrm{FP} + \mathrm{FN}}. \tag{3.7}$$

- Sensitivity: The ratio of number of the correct positive assessments to the total number of subjects having the condition, denoted as

$$\frac{\mathrm{TP}}{\mathrm{TP} + \mathrm{FN}}. \tag{3.8}$$

- Specificity: The ratio of the number of correct negative assessments to the total number of subjects not having the condition, denoted as

$$\frac{\mathrm{TN}}{\mathrm{TN} + \mathrm{FP}}. \tag{3.9}$$

3.3 Results and discussions

As has been detailed in the previous section, in the present study the PCG and ECG signals were simultaneously acquired from healthy male subjects of the institute, before an exam in a psychologically stressed state and after a subsequent holiday in a baseline state. The ECG-gating method is applied on the PCG signals to track the S1 peaks for construction of the S1–S1 IBI signal. The adaptive, data-driven EMD signal decomposition method, being suitable for non-linear and non-stationary signals, is applied on the IBI signal to cater to the non-linear dynamics of heart sounds. Thereafter, PCA is applied on the outcome of the EMD. The mean of the coefficients of the PCA is used in this study for further classification. A SVM classifier with a RBF kernel function is used. The records of any subjects taking medication or with a prior medical history were not included in the analysis.

The IBI signals, as shown in figure 3.2(c), are generated and then used for further analysis by applying EMD to generate IMFs. Additionally, the signals used in the study decompose to different numbers of IMFs; however, for uniformity in the signal analysis, seven-band decomposition is used and seven lowest-frequency IMFs are considered for the study. In order to consider these lower-frequency IMFs, the numbering of the IMFs is reversed, with IMFr1 termed as the lowest frequency IMF, in contrast to the convention as shown in figure 3.3. The resulting IMFs as an outcome of the EMD process are used as input for the PCA algorithm. A previous study [51] highlights the advantages of such an application of the PCA algorithm to the outcome of EMD. The PCA algorithm further reduces the seven-band decomposition system used in this study to six principal component coefficients, arranged in descending order of variance. The mean of this PCA coefficient (MPCoeff) is

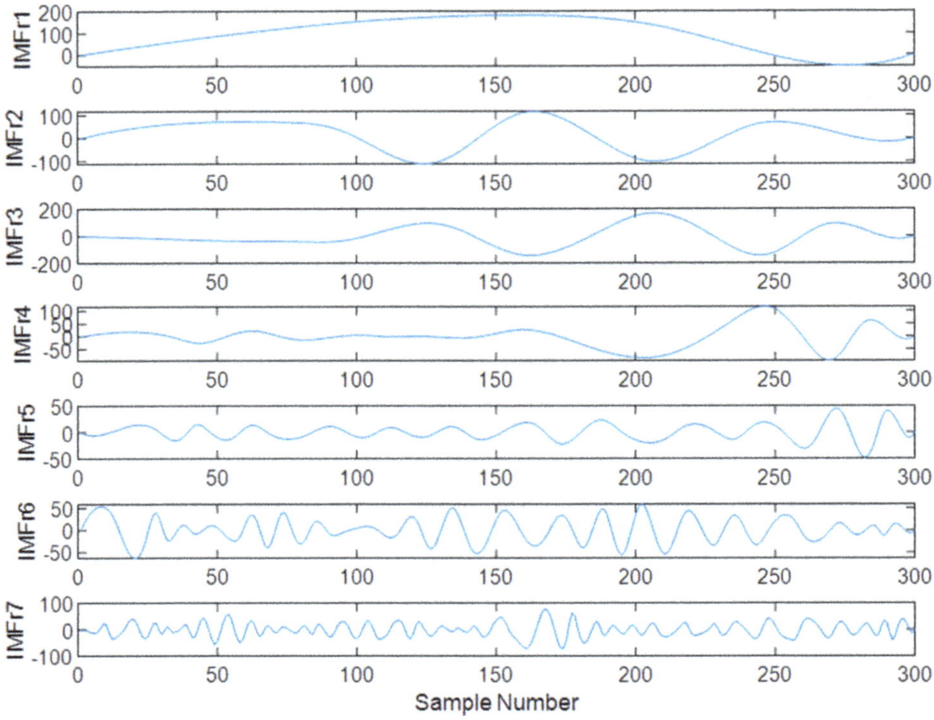

Figure 3.3. EMD method for extraction of IMFs.

Table 3.1. The mean ± standard deviation values of the extracted features.

Feature	Psychologically non-stressed baseline state (mean ± standard deviation)	Psychologically stressed state (mean ± standard deviation)
MPCoeff1	0.013681 ± 0.01499	0.00581 ± 0.01171
MPCoeff2	0.003578 ± 0.004663	0.003055 ± 0.009322
MPCoeff3	0.000822 ± 0.00763	0.000248 ± 0.004844
MPCoeff4	0.000046 91 ± 0.006339	0.001545 ± 0.004195
MPCoeff5	−0.000139 ± 0.008528	0.001524 ± 0.007749
MPCoeff6	0.0021259 ± 0.006337	0.001604 ± 0.006659

computed and used in this study for further evaluation. These coefficient values obtained for psychologically stressed and non-stressed states are depicted in table 3.1. The resulting values are used as the discriminating features to classify stressed and baseline signals.

From this, the average accuracy, sensitivity, and specificity obtained by applying this combination EMD and PCA for PCG-based stress detection is depicted in table 3.2.

Table 3.2. The performance parameters obtained for PCG-based stress detection using different classifiers.

Classifier used	Kernel function and kernel scale used	Average accuracy (%)	Average sensitivity (%)	Average specificity (%)
Naïve Bayes	—	73.53	80.38	66.77
Random forest	—	80.39	84.46	76.46
SVM	Linear	64.71	54.69	74.54
	Polynomial Order 2	77.54	72.85	82.23
	RBF Kernel scale: auto	87.25	90.38	84.23
ECG-based LF/HF method	—	76.47 (an increase signifies sympathetic dominance)	—	—

For this study, the SVM classifier with a RBF kernel function performed with an average accuracy of 87.25%, an average sensitivity of 90.38%, and an average specificity of 84.23%. The Naive Bayes classifier acts as the baseline classifier of the study and achieved 73.53% accuracy, whereas the Random Forest classifier achieved classification accuracy of 80.39% for classifying stress and non-stress signals. The results of this study depict the potential of using PCA on the outcome of EMD in order to detect stress from PCG signals. Moreover, an ECG-based low-frequency/high-frequency power ratio sympathovagal indicator method was accurate in 76.47% of the subjects; a comparison with the proposed methodology indicates the better discriminating potential of the PCG-based EMD-PCA method for classifying stress and non-stress category signals.

3.4 Conclusions

A novel methodology of using PCA on the outcome of EMD to detect states of psychological stress from PCG signals was introduced in this chapter. The stressor used in the study was a real-life institute examination scenario. Heart sound PCG signals were utilised for formation of inter-beat signals after detection of the S1 peaks and the duration between consecutive peaks. After application of EMD on the IBI signals, the IMFs were formed and the PCA applied on these modes. The findings of this study suggest the potential of this EMD-PCA methodology for detecting stress using PCG signals. This research opens new avenues in the field of psychological stress detection using combinations of techniques. In future, work may be done in the fields of state and trait anxiety differentiation. The framework of using PCG for stress detection needs to be evaluated on large datasets in order to make it suitable for use in a homecare setting or for screening in the case of the non-availability of expert diagnosis.

Acknowledgements

This work was supported by the Department of Science and Technology (DST), India, under the project titled 'Design and development of phonocardiography based psychological stress classifier' (project number—SR/WOS-B/202/2016).

References

[1] World Health Organization 2004 Promoting Mental Health: Concepts, Emerging Evidence, Practice (Summary Report) https://apps.who.int/iris/bitstream/handle/10665/42940/9241591595.pdf

[2] World Health Organization 1946 Constitution of the World Health Organization https://apps.who.int/gb/bd/pdf_files/BD_49th-en.pdf#page=6

[3] World Health Organization 2001 The World Health Report 2001: Mental Health: New Understanding, New Hope https://apps.who.int/iris/handle/10665/42390

[4] Msw Á C, Navarro-Pérez J and Mestre M-V 2020 Challenges and barriers in mental healthcare systems and their impact on the family: a systematic integrative review *Health Soc. Care Community* **28** 1366–79

[5] Wang P S, Aguilar-gaxiola S, Alonso J, Angermeyer M C, Borges G, Bromet E J and Bruff R 2007 Use of mental health services for anxiety, mood, and substance disorders in 17 countries in the WHO world mental health surveys *Lancet* **370** 841–50

[6] Mnookin S *et al* 2016 World Bank Group/World Health Organization high-level meeting on making mental health a global development priority, *WBG/IMF Spring Meetings* (Washington, D.C.: World Bank Group and GWU)

[7] Baldwin D S, Gordon R and Marlowe K 2021 The roles of a psychiatrist in the COVID-19 pandemic *Clinics in Integr. Care* **4** 100036

[8] Wan W 2020 Washington Post: 'The coronavirus pandemic is pushing America into a mental health crisis' https://www.washingtonpost.com/health/2020/05/04/mental-health-coronavirus/#

[9] Pfefferbaum B and North C S 2020 Mental health and the COVID-19 pandemic *N. Engl. J. Med.* **383** 510–2

[10] Duan L and Zhu G 2020 Psychological interventions for people affected by the COVID-19 epidemic *Lancet Psychiatry* **7** 300–2

[11] Russell G and Lightman S 2019 The human stress response *Nat. Rev. Endocrinol.* **15** 525–34

[12] Selye H 1946 The general adaptation syndrome and the diseases of adaptation *J. Clin. Endocrinol.* **6** 117–230

[13] Mohd R 2008 Salleh, life event, stress and illness *Malays. J. Med. Sci.* **15** 9–18 (PMID: 22589633)

[14] Kovacs F, Horváth C, Balogh Á and Hosszú G 2011 Extended noninvasive fetal monitoring by detailed analysis of data measured with phonocardiography *IEEE Trans. Biomed. Eng.* **58** 64–70

[15] Chen T, Yang S, Ho L, Tsai K, Chen Y, Chang Y, Lai Y, Wang S, Tsao Y and Wu C 2017 S1 and S2 heart sound recognition using deep neural networks *IEEE Trans. Biomed. Eng.* **64** 372–80

[16] Latif S, Usman M, Rana R and Qadir J 2018 Phonocardiographic sensing using deep learning for abnormal heartbeat detection *IEEE Sens. J.* **18** 9393–400

[17] Castaldo R, Montesinos L, Melillo P, James C and Pecchia L 2019 Ultra-short term HRV features as surrogates of short term HRV: a case study on mental stress detection in real life *BMC Med. Inform. Decis. Mak.* **19** 12

[18] Asif A, Majid M and Anwar S M 2019 Human stress classification using EEG signals in response to music tracks *Comput. Biol. Med.* **107** 182–96

[19] Sharma N, Dhall A, Gedeon T and Goecke R 2013 Modeling stress using thermal facial patterns: a spatio-temporal approach *Humaine Association Conf. on Affective Computing and Intelligent Interaction* pp 387–92

[20] Chen T, Yuen P, Richardson M, Liu G and She Z 2014 Detection of psychological stress using a hyperspectral imaging technique *IEEE Trans. Affect. Comput.* **5** 391–405

[21] Baltaci S and Gokcay D 2016 Stress detection in human–computer interaction: fusion of pupil Dilation and facial temperature features *Int. J. Hum. Comput. Interact.* **32** 956–66

[22] Giannakakis G, Pediaditis M, Manousos D, Kazantzaki E, Chiarugi F, Simos P G, Marias K and Tsiknakis M 2017 Stress and anxiety detection using facial cues from videos *Biomed. Signal Process. Control* **31** 89–101

[23] Zubair M and Yoon C 2020 Multilevel mental stress detection using ultra-short pulse rate variability series *Biomed. Signal Process. Control* **57** 101736

[24] Palanisamy K, Murugappan M and Yaacob S 2013 Multiple physiological signal-based human stress identification using non-linear classifiers *Elektron. Elektrotech.* **19** 80–5

[25] Karthikeyan P, Murugappan M and Yaacob S 2011 ECG signals based mental stress assessment using wavelet transform *2011 IEEE Int. Conf. on Control System, Computing and Engineering (Penang, Malaysia)* pp 258–62

[26] Karthikeyan P, Murugappan M and Yaacob S 2012 EMG signal based human stress level classification using wavelet packet transform, trends in intelligent robotics, automation, and manufacturing. IRAM 2012 *Communications in Computer and Information Science* vol 330 (Berlin: Springer)

[27] Karthikeyan P, Murugappan M and Yaacob S 2012 A study on mental arithmetic task based human stress level classification using discrete wavelet transform *2012 IEEE Conf. on Sustainable Utilization and Development in Engineering and Technology (STUDENT) (Kuala Lumpur, Malaysia)* pp 77–81

[28] Gonzalez-Carabarin L, Castellanos-Alvarado E A, Castro-Garcia P and Garcia-Ramirez M A 2021 Machine learning for personalised stress detection: inter-individual variability of EEG–ECG markers for acute-stress response *Comput. Methods Programs Biomed.* **209** 106314

[29] Vargas-Lopez O, Perez-Ramirez C A, Valtierra-Rodriguez M, Yanez-Borjas J J and Amezquita-Sanchez J P 2021 An explainable machine learning approach based on statistical indexes and SVM for stress detection in automobile drivers using electromyographic signals *Sensors* **21** 3155

[30] Dalmeida K M and Masala G L 2021 HRV features as viable physiological markers for stress detection using wearable devices *Sensors* **21** 2873

[31] Nath R K and Thapliyal H 2021 Smart wristband-based stress detection framework for older adults with cortisol as stress biomarker *IEEE Trans. Consum. Electron.* **67** 30–9

[32] Nijhawan T, Attigeri G and Ananthakrishna T 2022 Stress detection using natural language processing and machine learning over social interactions *J. Big Data* **9** 33

[33] Wang X, Liu C, Li Y, Cheng X, Li J and Clifford G D 2021 Temporal-framing adaptive network for heart sound segmentation without prior knowledge of state duration *IEEE Trans. Biomed. Eng.* **68** 650–63

[34] Springer D B, Tarassenko L and Clifford G D 2016 Logistic regression-HSMM-based heart sound segmentation *IEEE Trans. Biomed. Eng.* **63** 822–32

[35] Papadaniil C D and Hadjileontiadis L J 2014 Efficient heart sound segmentation and extraction using ensemble empirical mode decomposition and kurtosis features *IEEE J. Biomed. Health Inform.* **18** 1138–52

[36] Zhang W, Han J and Deng S 2017 Heart sound classification based on scaled spectrogram and partial least squares regression *Biomed. Signal Process. Control* **32** 20–8

[37] Spielberger C D, Gorsuch R L, Lushene R, Vagg P R and Jacobs G A 1983 *Manual for the State-Trait Anxiety Inventory* (Palo Alto, CA: Consulting Psychologists Press)

[38] Lucini D, Norbiato G, Clerici M and Pagani M 2002 Hemodynamic and autonomic adjustments to real life stress conditions in humans *Hypertension* **39** 184–8

[39] Melillo P, Bracale M and Pecchia L 2011 Nonlinear heart rate variability features for real-life stress detection. Case study: students under stress due to university examination *Biomed. Eng. Online* **10** 96

[40] Dimitriev D A, Dimitriev A D, Karpenko Y D and Saperova E V 2008 Influence of examination stress and psychoemotional characteristics on the blood pressure and heart rate regulation in female students *Hum. Physiol.* **34** 617–24

[41] Corah N L, Gale E N and Illig S J 1979 Psychological stress reduction during dental procedures *J. Dent. Res.* **58** 1347–51

[42] Mccarthy J and Goffin R 2004 Measuring job interview anxiety: beyond weak knees and sweaty palms *Pers. Psychol.* **57** 607–37

[43] Pachori R B, Avinash P, Shashank K, Sharma R and Acharya U R 2015 Application of empirical mode decomposition for analysis of normal and diabetic RR-interval signals *Expert Syst. Appl.* **42** 4567–81

[44] Pachori R B, Kumar M, Avinash P, Shashank K and Acharya U R 2016 An improved online paradigm for screening of diabetic patients using RR-interval signals *J. Mech. Med. Biol.* **16** 1–23

[45] Ari S and Saha G 2008 Classification of heart sounds using empirical mode decomposition based features *Int. J. Med. Eng. Inform.* **1** 91–108

[46] Huang N E, Shen Z, Long S R, Wu M C, Shih H H, Zheng Q, Tung C C and Liu H H 1998 The empirical mode decomposition and the Hilbert spectrum for nonlinear and non-stationary time series analysis analysis *R. Soc.* A **454** 903–95

[47] Ringnér M 2008 What is principal component analysis? *Nat. Biotechnol.* **26** 303–304

[48] Martis R J, Acharya U R, Mandana K M, Ray A K and Chakraborty C 2012 Application of principal component analysis to ECG signals for automated diagnosis of cardiac health *Expert Syst. Appl.* **39** 11792–800

[49] Polat K and Güneş S 2007 Detection of ECG arrhythmia using a differential expert system approach based on principal component analysis and least square support vector machine *Appl. Math. Comput.* **186** 898–906

[50] Langley P, Bowers E J and Murray A 2010 Principal component analysis as a tool for analyzing beat-to-beat changes in ECG features: application to ECG-derived respiration *IEEE Trans. Biomed. Eng.* **57** 821–9

[51] Pinheiro E, Postolache O and Girão P 2012 Empirical mode decomposition and principal component analysis implementation in processing non-invasive cardiovascular signals *Measurement (Lond)* **45** 175–81

[52] Breiman L 2001 Random forests *Mach. Learn.* **45** 5–32

[53] Mohapatra S K and Mohanty M N 2020 Big data analysis and classification of biomedical signal using random forest algorithm *New Paradigm in Decision Science and Management. Advances in Intelligent Systems and Computing Advances in Intelligent Systems and Computing* vol 1005 (Singapore: Springer)

[54] Masetic Z and Subasi A 2016 Congestive heart failure detection using random forest classifier *Comput. Methods Programs Biomed.* **130** 54–64

[55] Xu S 2018 Bayesian naïve Bayes classifiers to text classification *J. Inf. Sci.* **44** 48–59

[56] Schwenke C and Schering A G 2014 True positives, true negatives, false positives, false negatives *Wiley StatsRef: Statistics Reference Online*

[57] Suykens J A K and Vandewalle J 1999 Least squares support vector machine classifiers *Neural Process. Lett.* **9** 293–300

Chapter 4

Affective computational advertising based on perceptual metrics

Soujanya Narayana, Shweta Jain, Harish Katti, Roland Goecke and Ramanathan Subramanian

We present ACAD, an Affective Computational ADvertising framework expressly derived from perceptual metrics. Differing from advertising methods that either ignore the emotional nature of (most) programmes and advertisements (ads), or are based on axiomatic rules, our framework incorporates findings from a user study examining the effect of within-programme ad placements on ad perception. A linear programme formulation seeking to achieve (a) genuine ad assessments, and (b) maximal ad recall is then proposed. The effectiveness of the framework is confirmed via a validation user study, where ACAD-induced ad placements are found to be optimal with respect to objectives (a) and (b) against competing approaches.

4.1 Introduction

Video advertising has grown by leaps and bounds thanks to multimedia publishers like Vimeo and YouTube and popular movie streaming services such as Netflix and Hulu. As humans are emotional beings, video advertisements (ads) are thus designed to evoke specific emotions in viewers, employing a variety of narrative tools to effectively convey a message. Ad designers intend that these emotions become associated with the advertised product (message), and that they influence subsequent consumer behaviour[1].

Ads are not only used for promoting brands to increase their commercial viability, but also to influence consumers' health beliefs and behaviours. Ads (commercials) are typically interspersed within longer, often-emotional programmes to occasionally distract viewers as well as generate revenue for content publishers. Advertising in broadcast television involves presentation of relevant ads at fixed temporal locations

[1] 'Emotional ads work best': https://www.neurosciencemarketing.com/blog/articles/emotional-ads-work-best.htm.

doi:10.1088/978-0-7503-5182-9ch4

in the programme, but a manual mix-and-match strategy would not scale to online content where millions of programme videos (PVs) and ads exist. Algorithmic video-in-video advertising (VIVA) formulations [1, 2] attempt to jointly select appropriate ads from an inventory, plus to determine their insertion locations within a programme. VIVA as a computational problem needs to balance the conflicting goals of (a) minimal viewing experience (VX) disruption, and (b) maximal ad impact, so that viewers readily recall ads and associated messages over the long term.

CAVVA, or computational affective advertising [1], works by matching programme scenes and ads with respect to valence (val; positive or negative emotional feeling) and arousal (asl; extent of physiological activation) [3], so that VX and ad recall are maximised. CAVVA rules model two axioms, namely, (i) the emotional inertia hypothesis [4], which argues that programme emotion lingers and influences evaluation of subsequent ads, and (ii) the general tendency of humans to maintain a positive mood. These assumptions preclude CAVVA from inserting ads that strongly contrast with the programme val; for example, a horror movie trailer will rarely be inserted within a sitcom programme via the CAVVA framework (see section 4.5). Differing from the CAVVA framework outlined in [1], which is based on advertising theories, we here expressly examine affective ad evaluation from a user study involving strongly positive and negative programmes and ads. The effects of inserting similar/opposite-val ads within emotional programmes are studied to formulate ad-insertion rules, which are realised via linear integer programming to derive our novel Affective Computational ADvertising (ACAD) strategy. ACAD's effectiveness is validated via a second user study. Figure 4.1 summarises our work, which makes the following research contributions:

- In contrast to postulate-based advertising strategies [1, 2], the ACAD formulation is derived from a user study examining the influence of affective ad placements within a positive/negative programme. This user study reveals that (a) negative ads are better recalled and receive genuine ratings when embedded at the tail of the PV, and (b) ads incongruent to the programme's mood are better recalled overall.

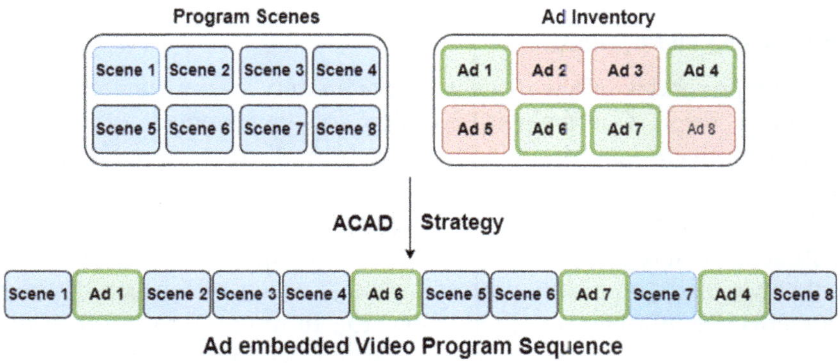

Figure 4.1. ACAD overview. Given an emotional programme video comprising multiple scenes (blue ovals), and an ad inventory (green ovals), ACAD employs linear integer programming to select and embed the requisite number of ads (in red) at optimal temporal locations to synthesise a VPS. Ad selections (in red) and placements are determined as a function of (a) ad valence ratings, and (b) the degree of emotional dissimilarity-plus-content similarity between ads and programme scenes.

- Integer linear programming is employed to select the optimal inventory ads and their insertion locations based on the user-study findings. This formulation embeds ads within programmes considering (i) val ratings of the programme scenes and ads, and (ii) semantic scene–ad similarities. Therefore, low-level (semantic) and high-level (emotional) scene–ad relevance are modelled in the embedding process.
- A validational user study is performed to evaluate ACAD against competing methods. This study reveals (i) ACAD's efficacy at eliciting genuine ad evaluations and better ad recall, and (ii) a trade-off between ad recall and VX, which should serve as a design guide for future affective advertising works.

4.2 Related work

To position the novelty of our work with respect to the literature, we review related work on (a) affective ad analysis, (b) the influence of programme mood on affective ad evaluation, and (c) computational advertising.

4.2.1 Advertisements as affective stimuli

Ads are inherently emotional, and emotions play a critical role in effectively conveying a message to viewers regarding lifestyle choices. Emotions can mediate consumer attitudes towards advertised brands [5–7], and an advertising strategy that achieves favourable brand (message) evaluation can benefit content publishers and advertisers alike [1]. Adopting a circumplex model [3] where emotions are characterised via the val and asl attributes, an affective ad dataset is proposed in [8] and ad affect predicted by examining the content and users. An eye-tracking study [9] concludes that ad emotions are primarily conveyed via a few central scene characters and the visual scene design. The positive impact of emotional cues towards ad and movie scene recall is confirmed in [10] and [11].

4.2.2 Advertising and healthcare

Advertising represents a unique strategy for community awareness, mainly due to its wide customer reach. Comprehensive design and development of advertisement content can motivate behavioural change in several areas of public health. Ads conveying negative health consequences are perceived to be effective in increasing knowledge and awareness, for instance in changing the attitudes and beliefs of college students with regards to smoking [12]. Ads designed with a strongly negative emotional style, and graphically portraying the ill effects of tobacco on the human body, are effective in tobacco use reduction [13]. In response to health-related ads, an increase in the resolve to wear seat belts [14] and alcohol abuse prevention [15] are also observed. Anti-smoking messages that evoke strong emotional arousal, particularly the ill-health effects of smoking, are found to be more memorable [16]. Overall, advertising plays a key role in shaping a health-conscious and responsible society.

4.2.3 Programme influence on ad perception

As ads are interspersed within programmes, the impact of programme mood on ad evaluation has been studied extensively. Programme context, characterised by audio-visual and emotional programme–ad (dis)similarity, impacts ad evaluation. Kamins *et al* [17] focus on how commercial liking, and consequently user purchase intent, is affected by programme mood; they observed an effect of emotional inertia, i.e., happy ads are perceived favourably within a happy programme while sad ads are better liked in a sad context. Broach *et al* [4] note that both programme asl and val impact ad perception. Specifically, positive ads are evaluated favourably within a highly arousing positive programme or a mildly arousing negative programme. These findings strengthen the emotional inertia theory [18], as lingering emotions under high asl adversely impacts focus on opposite-val ads; the greater cognitive resources available under low asl result in ads being viewed as more positive/negative within a sad/happy programme. Nevertheless, only positive ads are studied in [4].

Varied findings exist regarding user evaluation of ads (in)congruent to the programme mood. A study involving only two programmes and two ads [19] concludes that it may be optimal to show promotional ads within positive programmes, and messaging campaigns within negative programmes. Other studies nevertheless point to increased recall of incongruent ads; for example, Feltham and Arnold [20] note that when one watches an arousing programme, emotionally inconsistent ads tend to stimulate internal processing and are therefore better recalled. Similarly, Furnham and Goh [21] note that health-and-safety-related messages are better recalled within a sitcom programme. The positive influence of programme asl on ad recall, where users are free to watch or skip ads, is noted in [22]. Shapiro *et al* [23] argue that programme asl and val independently influence ad recall. Asl impacts information processing capacity (deeper processing under low asl, shallow processing under high asl), while val influences the nature of processing (logic-based but superficial under high val, and attentive to detail under low val). As information processing is key to brand evaluation and attitude, this study has design implications for computational VIVA strategies. A very recent study examines the influence of music video mood on emotionally (in)congruent ads and concludes that positive ads are more favoured by users while watching less-arousing videos, while negative ads are deemed more persuasive under high asl.

4.2.4 Strategic video-in-video advertising

To exploit the surge in Internet video and benefit both content publishers and advertisers, computational advertising strategies have been proposed. An appraisal of the computational advertising field [24] emphasises the need to account for consumer behaviours during advertising design, execution, and evaluation. However, VIVA approaches typically examine user behaviours only at the evaluation stage. VideoSense [2] inserts ads at temporal points of low involvement (e.g., shot discontinuities), and presents ads which are audio-visually similar to the preceding video scene. The twin objectives of optimal ad selection and placement are modelled via non-linear integer programming (NLIP). While subjective evaluations are presented to validate the approach, emotional programme–ad relevance is ignored in VideoSense.

The CAVVA framework [1] improves over VideoSense by modelling emotional relevance for programme–ad matching. Matching rules are derived from [4], and by postulating that the embedded ads should (a) minimally perturb user emotional state and help attain/maintain a positive mood, and (b) maximally engage viewers. Consistently, low-val ads are inserted after negative-val scenes, while high-val ads are embedded between positive-val scenes. Ad selections and placements are achieved via NLIP, and CAVVA achieves superior VX and ad recall to VideoSense. Rules modelling emotional inertia preclude CAVVA from embedding ads incongruent to programme mood.

4.2.5 Inference summary and research questions

We note from the literature that ads are effective in mediating consumer attitudes towards brands, and in influencing their behaviour towards adopting healthy lifestyle choices. Programme mood is known to influence ad perception, and automated VIVA methods have been developed by modelling programme–ad relevance. In this regard, (a) while a few works have measured ad-induced user behaviours, user assessments have hardly been incorporated for VIVA design; (b) even as marketing studies have examined the effects of programme mood on affective ad evaluation, very few VIVA works embed ads based on programme–ad emotional relevance; and (c) VIVA methods either focus on content-based or mood-sustaining advertising. Embedding ads strongly incongruent to the programme mood is therefore not possible.

To address these issues, we expressly perform an exploratory user study involving both positive and negative programmes and ads to understand (a) the impact of programme mood on ad evaluation and recall, and (b) whether certain temporal placements are desirable for positive- and negative-val ads. The findings convey that optimal commercial evaluation and recall are achieved when (i) low-val ads are placed towards the programme tail, and (ii) inserted ads are emotion-wise dissimilar but content-wise similar to the (preceding) scenes. The study employed to derive ACAD rules is described below.

4.3 Materials and methods

To examine the influence of programme mood on ad evaluations, we performed a user study with two programmes (one happy and another sad) embedded with both positive and negative emotional ads, as described below.

4.3.1 Materials

Programmes: For this work, we utilised the affective ad dataset and two PVs presented in [8]. The first PV is a sequence from the movie *In Pursuit of Happiness* (hereafter *IPOH*) in the drama genre, while the other PV is Episode 1 from the *Friends* Season 2 sitcom. Both PVs comprise eight scenes and are of roughly similar lengths (mean scene length of 110 ± 44 s for *IPOH* versus 119 ± 69 s for *Friends*). These two PVs were considered as they depicted self-contained episodes and were representative of online videos[2]. One can infer from [8] that both PVs are sufficiently arousing. While the *Friends* PV is happy-mood inducing, the *IPOH* PV detailing the travails of a father and son is sad-mood eliciting.

Ads: To examine how emotional ads are perceived within an emotional programme, we used 14 ads: seven high asl-high val (HAHV) and seven high asl-low val (HALV) ads from [8]. The HAHV ads are promotional in nature, while the HALV ads are public messages conveying the ill effects of unhealthy and hazardous lifestyle choices such as overspeeding, smoking, and drug and physical abuse.

Video programme sequences: As both programmes and the selected ads are deemed to be sufficiently arousing, we exclusively examined the effect of programme and ad val on commercial evaluation. For the user study, four (two HAHV + two HALV) of the 14 ads were randomly chosen and inserted within each PV. Consistent with the VideoSense [2] and CAVVA [1] methods, we embedded ads uniformly across each PV. As both PVs had seven scene-change points where ads could be inserted, chosen ads were placed at change points 1, 3, 5, and 7. Cumulatively, we examined four different ad-placement configurations, depicted in figure 4.2, where HV (LV) ads were placed at the *head* (*tail*), *tail* (*head*), *ends* (*middle*), and *middle* (*ends*) of the PV. These four configurations summarise *meaningful* placements of the two HV + two LV ads given four insertion locations (in total $^4P_4$ possibilities). The ads were 0.5–1 min long ($\mu = 45$ s, $\sigma = 14.5$ s). The ad-embedded programmes or video programme sequences (VPSs) were $\approx$ 18 min long ($\mu = 18.3$, $\sigma = 0.6$ min).

4.3.2 Participants

Twenty-four university students (15 male) aged between 18 and 39 years ($\mu = 23.4$, $\sigma = 4.9$) conversant with English-language programmes participated in the study. This demographic accounts for 21% of the global audience accessing online video websites[3], who advertising approaches should most effectively target. All users were provided with a definition of stimulus-related terms such as PV and VPS, and the val and asl emotional attributes. Participants provided written informed consent as per ethics committee approval and were paid a token fee for their time and effort.

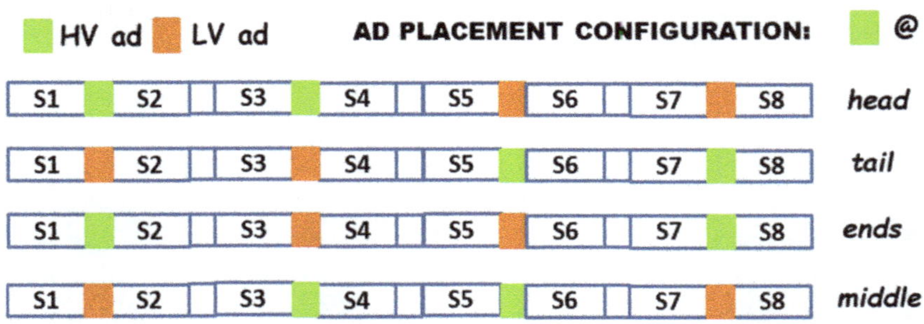

Figure 4.2. Ad-placement strategies examined for our user study. S1–S8 denote the eight PV scenes.

[2] Mean YouTube video length = 11.7 min (as of December 2018). Source: Statista.com.

[3] As per hootsuite.com.

4.3.3 Procedure

The *IPOH* and *Friends* VPSs were presented on a computer screen. Upon viewing, users rated each ad on a 1–5 scale for val (very unpleasant–very pleasant) and asl (boring–exciting) via a radio button. On VPS completion, users rated the PV for asl and val, and the ad-embedded VPS for VX on a 1–5 scale (very bad–very good). To test visual ad recall, viewers were shown thumbnails of the 14 inventory ads, and asked to identify the four viewed ads in any order. This protocol resulted in $24 \times 2 \times 4 = 192$ user asl and val ratings being available for ads, and $24 \times 2 = 48$ scores being available for programme asl and val, ad recall, ad asl, and ad val per placement condition and the VPS VX. Including preparation time and a break between the two VPSs, $\approx$50 min were required for the experiment. We will share the user-study data and the ACAD implementation for research purposes upon request.

4.3.4 User data analyses

In this section, we examine (i) asl and val ratings for PVs, (ii) within-programme ad evaluations in terms of asl, val, and recall scores, focusing on both general and placement-specific trends, and (iii) ad-placement effects on VPS VX.

4.3.4.1 Arousal and valence ratings for programme videos

Figure 4.3 presents the mean val (left) and asl (right) user ratings for the two PVs. The *IPOH* and *Friends* PVs, respectively, elicited mean val scores of 3 and 4.4, which were significantly different as per an unequal variance *t*-test ($t(46) = 4.827$; $p < 0.000001$). Both PVs evoked similar asl ratings: 3.6 for *IPOH* versus 3.8 for *Friends* ($t(46) = 0.714$; n.s.). These observations are similar to [8], and the *Friends* and *IPOH* programmes are termed as happy and sad PVs, respectively.

4.3.4.2 Impact of programme video mood on advertisement arousal and valence ratings

To understand how programme-induced mood impacts ad evaluations, we examined user asl and val ratings for HV and LV ads inserted within the happy and sad PVs.

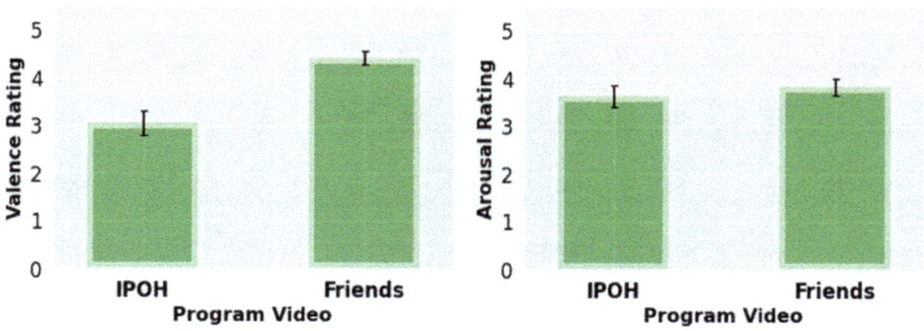

Figure 4.3. Mean val (left) and mean asl (right) ratings obtained for the two PVs. Error bars denote unit standard error of mean.

Figure 4.4 presents the mean asl and val scores received by the HV and LV ads within the positive and negative programmes. With respect to val (figure 4.4, left), HV ads expectedly elicited higher val ratings than LV ads within both programmes. HV ads elicited mean val scores of 4 ± 0.2 and 3.9 ± 0.3 when shown within the sad and happy PVs, indicating that HV ads were perceived as more pleasant in a sad PV. Conversely, LV ads evoked a mean val score of 1.6 ± 0.3 and 1.7 ± 0.1 within the *IPOH* and *Friends* PVs, implying that LV ads were seen as less unpleasant in a happy programme. However, perceived differences in ad val for the happy and sad programmes were insignificant, as per a one-way analysis of variance (ANOVA) test ($F(1, 188) = 0.06$; n.s).

In terms of asl impressions (figure 4.4, right), LV ads evoked higher asl *vis-à-vis* HV ads in general. HV ads shown in the *IPOH* and *Friends* PVs received asl ratings of 3.2 ± 0.3 and 2.7 ± 0.2, respectively, while corresponding LV ads achieved higher asl scores of 3.7 ± 0.3 and 3.8 ± 0.2. A two-way ANOVA confirmed the main effect of ad val ($F(1, 188) = 18.77$; $p < 0.00001$), but the negligible impact of programme val ($F(1, 188) = 1.34$; n.s) on asl scores. *Post-hoc t*-tests, however, revealed slightly different asl scores for HV ads within the happy and sad PVs ($t(94) = -1.75$; $p = 0.083$).

4.3.4.3 Advertisement recall analysis

Visual ad recall critically influences brand attitude [1, 10]. Figure 4.5(left) presents ad recall for the happy and sad PVs irrespective of ad val. The heat map depicts the

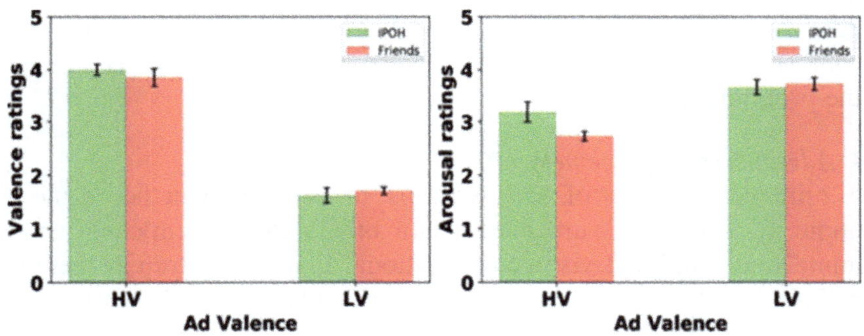

Figure 4.4. Mean ad val and asl ratings when shown within the two PVs. Error bars denote unit standard error of mean.

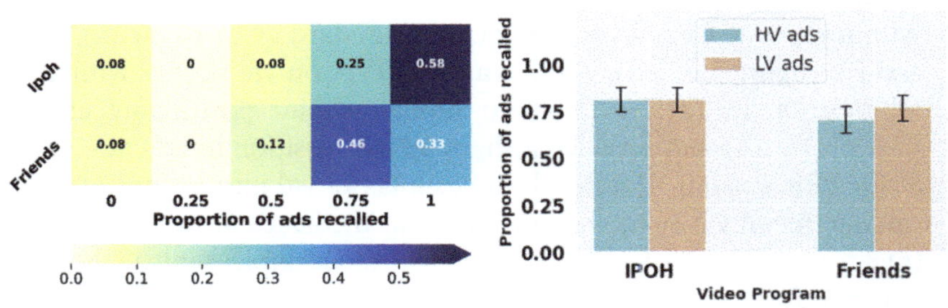

Figure 4.5. Ad recall. Left: Heat map showing fraction of users for varying ad recall rates. Right: Programme-wise recall rates for high- and low-val ads. Error bars denote standard error of mean.

proportion of users achieving a given ad recall rate for the happy and sad programmes. Evidently, ad recall rates were higher for the sad programme. Fifty-eight percent of users recalled all ads within the sad programme, while only 33% of users remembered all ads in the happy programme. Figure 4.5(right) presents programme-wise recall of the HV and LV ads. As in figure 4.5(left), superior recall of both HV and LV ads is achieved for the sad PV (mean recall rate, or MRR, of 0.81 for both HV and LV ads), as compared to the happy PV (MRR of 0.77 for LV versus 0.71 for HV ads). ANOVA tests to examine the effects of PV and ad val on ad recall did not reveal any effects.

4.3.4.3.1 Discussion

Observations from the user study are largely consistent with prior findings. With respect to ad asl and val ratings, LV ads are more arousing in general. Negative ads elicited higher asl scores, as per [8], and this holds even within a programme's context, as seen in figure 4.4(right). In terms of val, HV ads elicited higher scores when shown within a sad programme, while LV ads evoked higher val scores within a happy programme. That ads are better remembered in the negative programme context is also known; prior studies [25, 26] note that negative mood induces better recall and greater attention to detail [23]. Greater memorability for negative stimuli [25, 26] explains why LV ads are better recalled irrespective of programme mood. That HV ads are better recalled in the sad PV context can be attributed to the contrastive effect noted in prior studies [20, 21]. While these trends suggest that a promotional ad may have more impact when shown in an arousing sad programme, we set out to examine if certain placements are more optimal for HV and LV ads given the programme mood.

4.3.4.4 Advertisement placement effects

As the primary objective of this work is to examine whether some within-programme ad placements are better than others for ads (in)congruent to the programme mood, and to devise a computational advertising strategy therefrom, we examined if ad evaluations differed for the varied placements shown in figure 4.2.

4.3.4.4.1 Arousal and valence impressions

Ad positioning induced marginally different user emotional ratings, as detailed below.

(i) **Valence:** Figure 4.6 presents val scores elicited for varied ad placements within the two PVs (error bars denote standard error of mean). Within the sad PV (figure 4.6, left), a two-way ANOVA on val ratings with ad val and ad position as factors failed to reveal any ad positioning effect (F (3, 88) = 1.37; n.s), but revealed a slight ad val–position interaction effect (F (3, 88) = 2.39; $p = 0.074$). HV ads induced better val impressions at the tail and middle (mean val = 4.2 for both) than at the head (mean val = 3.9) or ends (mean val = 3.7). LV ads were deemed most unpleasant at the tail (mean val = 1.3), and least unpleasant at the head (mean val = 2.2), and this difference was marginally significant ($t(46) = -1.933$; $p = 0.06$); no differences were noted between the ends or middle placements (mean val = 1.5).

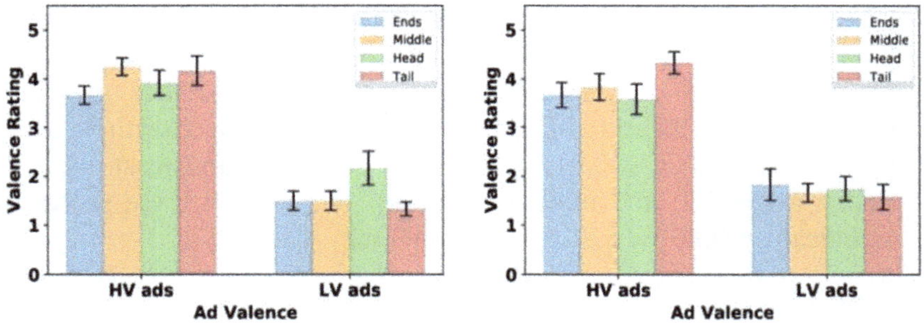

Figure 4.6. Ad val scores by position in sad (left) and happy (right) PVs.

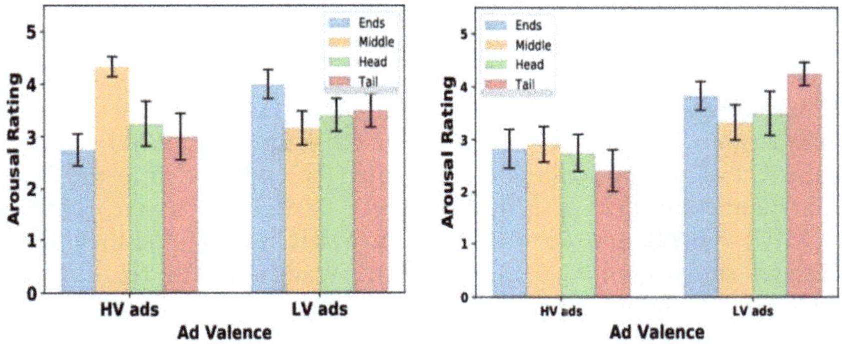

Figure 4.7. Ad asl scores by position in sad (left) and happy (right) PVs.

Within the happy PV (figure 4.6, right), a two-way ANOVA again failed to reveal any effect of ad positioning but revealed a significant ad val–position interaction effect (F (3, 184) = 3.3107; $p < 0.05$). HV ads were deemed more positive at the tail (mean val = 4.3) than at the middle (mean val = 3.8), ends (mean val = 3.7), or head (mean val = 3.6). Slightly different val distributions were noted for the tail and head positions ($t(46) = 1.947$; $p = 0.066$), and also for the tail and ends ($t(46) = 1.956$; $p = 0.063$). LV ads were perceived as most negative when placed at the tail (mean val = 1.6), and least negative at the ends (mean val = 1.8), with the head (mean val = 1.75) and middle (mean val = 1.7) positions achieving moderately negative evaluations. The val score differences among these positions were however insignificant.

(ii) **Arousal:** Figure 4.7 presents asl ratings elicited for varied ad placements within the negative and positive PVs, with error bars denoting standard error of mean. Within the sad PV (figure 4.7, left), a two-way ANOVA revealed a significant ad val–position interaction effect (F (3, 184) = 4.614; $p < 0.005$). HV ads evoked most asl in the middle (mean asl = 4.3), and least asl at the ends (mean asl = 2.8). Middle ad ratings differed significantly with respect to the ends ($t(46) = 4.423$; $p < 0.0005$), head ($t(46) = 2.315$; $p < 0.05$), and tail ($t(46) = 2.766$; $p < 0.05$). LV ads evoked most asl at the ends (mean asl = 4.0), and least asl in the middle of the PV (mean asl = 3.2). Within the happy PV (figure 4.7, right), ANOVA revealed an ad val–position interaction effect (F (3, 184) = 4.44; $p < 0.005$). HV ads in the middle (mean asl = 2.9) and tail (mean asl = 2.4) elicited distinct asl ratings ($t(46) = -2.943$; $p < 0.01$). LV ads evoked most and least asl at the tail (mean asl = 4.3) and middle (mean asl = 3.3), and these scores differed significantly ($t(46) = 8.983$; $p < 0.000001$).

4.3.4.4.2 Ad recall

For both the sad (figure 4.8, left) and happy (figure 4.8, right) programmes, we noted a marginal impact of ad positioning on recall. For the sad PV, ANOVA revealed a significant ad val–position interaction effect on visual recall (F (3, 40) = 3.18; $p < 0.05$). Highest recall of HV ads was noted in the VPS middle (MRR = 1), and lowest at the ends (MRR = 0.67). For LV ads, recall was higher at the tail (MRR = 1) than the middle (MRR = 0.58) and head (MRR = 0.75) positions. LV ad recall rates differed marginally for the tail versus middle ($t(46) = 2.076$; $p = 0.093$), and for tail versus head ($t(46) = 2.236$; $p = 0.076$). For the happy PV, ANOVA revealed a marginal effect of ad positioning on recall rate (F (3, 40) = 2.35; $p = 0.087$), but a significant interaction effect (F (3, 40) = 3.06; $p < 0.05$). HV ads were recalled best at the tail (MRR = 0.92), and worst at the ends (MRR = 0.33), and these recall rates differed significantly ($t(46) = -3.13$; $p < 0.05$). LV ads were also recalled best at the tail (MRR = 0.92) and worst in the middle (MRR = 0.58), but the differences were marginal.

4.3.4.4.3 Viewing experience

As the CAVVA [1] framework is designed to perform ad insertions that sustain user mood to ensure a pleasant VX, we examined if VX scores differed with varying ad placements. Figure 4.9 summarises the impact of HV ad placements within the sad and happy programmes (see figure 4.2 for inferring corresponding LV ad placements). For the sad PV, superior VX (mean VX = 2.8) was reported when HV (LV) ads were placed at the VPS head (tail), with the other three configurations eliciting identical mean VX scores of 2.5. Within the happy PV, very similar VX scores were reported for different configurations; overall, the VX score differences were insignificant.

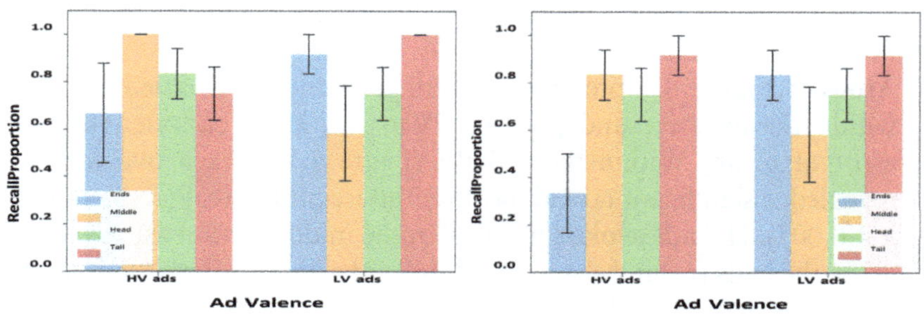

Figure 4.8. Ad recall by position in sad (left) and happy (right) PVs. Error bars denote standard error of mean.

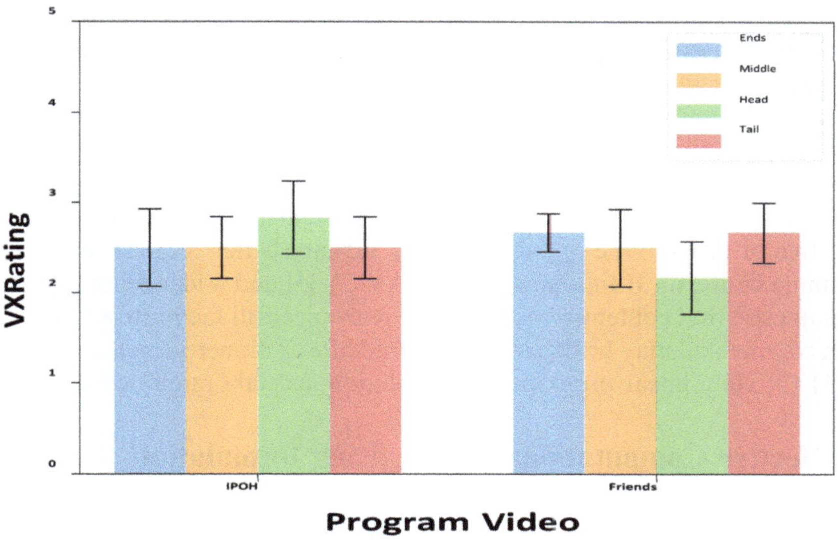

Figure 4.9. VX for HV ad placements within the two PVs. Error bars denote standard error of mean.

4.3.5 Inferences and Affective Computational ADvertising design rules

Our analysis reveals that within-programme ad placements have some effect on affective impressions and recall rates, with ANOVA tests largely revealing a marginal effect of ad positioning, or an interaction effect between ad val and positioning. Interestingly, trends common to both HV and LV ads are apparent irrespective of programme mood, such as (a) HV ads being perceived as most pleasant when placed at the VPS tail or middle, and LV ads perceived as most unpleasant when placed at the VPS tail; (b) HV ads being recalled best at the VPS middle and tail, and LV ads achieving best recall at the VPS tail; and (c) HV ads evoking maximal asl when placed in the middle of the VPS.

Overall, our study confirms that both programme mood and ad-placement impact ad evaluation and recall. Ad-placement effects convey that it may be beneficial to present (especially LV) ads later in the VPS, as the middle and tail embeddings generally achieve genuine val ratings than at the ends or the head. As our study involves presentation of ads strongly (dis)similar to the programme mood, our findings suggest that users are able to evaluate ads more genuinely upon sufficient programme exposure. Programmes are likely to maximally attract viewers at the beginning, as they begin to engage with the content; ads presented under such high-asl conditions are not adequately processed by users as per findings in [4]. With sufficient programme exposure, users tend to transit to a moderately aroused state, where both positive and negative messages are well received, as conveyed by minimal VX variations across placements.

Given that the success of an advertising/awareness campaign hinges on a positive message being viewed most favourably, and conversely a negative message being viewed most unfavourably by consumers, we hypothesise that a computational VIVA framework should generate ad embeddings that achieve the most genuine val evaluations. Secondly, the ads should also have maximum recall rates, so that they influence purchase intent [1]. Consistently, the ACAD strategy should result in (a) genuine ad val evaluations, and (b) maximal ad recall. This imposes several rules. (1) That LV ads should be embedded at the VPS tail where they achieve the most genuine assessments and maximum recall; HV ads are also well received in the VPS middle where they evoke high asl and achieve good recall. (2) Ads incongruent to the programme mood are well recalled (figure 4.5, right); LV ads achieve high recall irrespective of programme mood, while HV ads are better recalled in the negative programme context. (3) In line with the CAVVA [1] and VideoSense [2] strategies, we hypothesise that content-based ad-scene relevance will facilitate ad recall (e.g., a kitchen commercial may be better remembered after a dinner scene). ACAD realises rules (1)–(3) via a linear programme formulation, as elaborated below.

4.4 Affective Computational ADvertising formulation

Let $\{S_1, S_2, \ldots, S_N\}$ denote the N programme scenes onto which ads can be inserted at M slots ($M = N - 1$ if scene transition points are candidate insertion slots). Let $\{A_1, A_2, \ldots, A_P\}$ denote the P inventory commercials from which K ads are to be chosen, so as to embed an equal number of HV and LV ads in the programme. We introduce selection-cum-insertion binary variables $y_{ij} \in \mathrm{R}^{N \times P}$, where $y_{ij} = 1$ if ad A_j follows programme scene S_i and $y_{ij} = 0$ otherwise. Let Y be a $N \times P$ matrix containing these binary variables. As our study involves arousing programmes and ads, we only consider val scores in the programme scene–ad matching process. Let val^{Si} and val^{Aj} denote the val evoked by scene S_i and ad A_j, where $val^{Si}, val^{Aj} \in [0, 1]$. Further, let $val^S \in \mathrm{R}^N$ and $val^a \in \mathrm{R}^P$, respectively, denote the vectors denoting scene and ad val scores. Our objective is then to come up with the matrix Y so as to maximise the reward function $RF(val^S, val^A, \alpha, \beta)$ with trade-off parameters α, β, where

$$RF(val^S, val^A, \alpha, \beta) = \alpha \sum_{i=1}^{M} i \sum_{j=1}^{P} y_{ij}\left(1 - val^{A_j}\right) + \beta \sum_{i=1}^{M} \sum_{j=1}^{P} y_{ij}\left(\mid val^{S_i} - val^{A_j} \mid\right) rel\left(S_i, A_j\right) \tag{4.1}$$

$$\text{s. t. } \sum_{j=1}^{p} y_{ij} = 1 \ \forall\, i; \ \sum_{i=1}^{M} \sum_{j=1}^{p} y_{ij} K; \ \sum_{i=1}^{[M/K]} y_{ij} = 1 \ \forall\, j \text{ and } \alpha + \beta = 1.$$

Here, $rel(S_i, A_j)$ models the content-wise similarity between scene S_i and ad A_j. Decoding equation (4.1), the α term enforces LV ads, for which $(1 - val^{Aj})$ is high, to be embedded later in the VPS. The β term encourages emotionally dissimilar (so that $val^{Si} - val^{Aj}$ is large) but content-wise similar scene–ad combinations. The constraints, in order, specify that (a) only one ad can be filled per ad-slot, (b) the total number of embedded ads is K, and (c) the inserted ads be uniformly distributed over the VPS, as in [1, 2], requiring one ad to be placed over every $[M/K]$ slots, where

$\lceil . \rceil$ denotes the *ceil* function operator. Equation (4.1) represents a binary integer linear programme, which is solved via algorithm 4.1.

4.4.1 Brute-force Affective Computational ADvertising algorithm

Algorithm 4.1 presents a brute-force implementation of the ACAD formulation. The inputs to the algorithm are the scene and ad val vectors, number of ads to be inserted, number of available ad slots, and the scene–ad similarity matrix. The algorithm outputs an optimal ad-embedded VPS, denoting which ad is to be inserted at which ad slot. The optimal sequence *opt allo* of length M is initialised to zero (Step 1). Step 2 considers all K ad combinations that can be chosen from P candidates. To avoid bias, only those combinations involving an equal number of HV and LV ads are deemed valid. On choosing K ads, their optimal VPS placements need to be computed (Step 3). Here, we consider all permutations of K ads via matrix L and retain only those placements which satisfy constraint (c). Each row of L gives a matrix Y satisfying all constraints of equation (4.1). The reward function (RF) is then computed, and the maximum RF value updated (Step 5). Steps 4 and 5 are repeated for all valid ad combinations and permutations (Step 6).

Input: Programme scenes val $\{val^S_1, val^S_2, \ldots, val^S_N\}$, inventory ads val $\{val^A_1, val^A_2, \ldots, val^A_P\}$. Number of ads to insert: K and number of ad slots: M, Relevance matrix $rel(S_i, A_j)$ denoting the relevance score between scene i and ad j, Parameters α and β.

Output: Optimal ad-embedded VPS schedule.

1. Initialise a one-dimensional array *opt allo*, which denotes the optimal ad sequence, with M zeros.
2. Create a matrix C with ${}^PC_K$ rows and K columns, whose rows consist of all possible subsets of $\{1,\ldots,P\}$ with K elements. Retain only those rows in C, which have a balanced sampling of HV and LV ads from the inventory.
3. For each row r in C which denotes a valid ad sampling, create a matrix L with $M!$ rows and M columns, where each row is a permutation of the ad choices in r. We fill these M slots with K ads, such that constraint (b) is satisfied.
4. For each row j in L, compute the reward function $RF(val^S, val^A, \alpha, \beta)$ as per equation (4.1).
5. Compute $max(RF)$ and update *opt allo* as the ad sequence corresponding to row j.
6. Repeat (4) and (5) for each row in C to obtain optimal *opt allo*.

Algorithm 4.1: Brute-force ACAD implementation. Algorithm 4.1's complexity is exponential in terms of the number of inventory ads and ad slots. This is not serious in practice, as in a typical VPS (e.g., Youtube-streamed videos), the number of ads and ad slots are limited in number. Efficient ways to solve binary integer programmes such as *branch-and-bound* exist and are easily solved by solvers like Gurobi [27]. Another efficient way to solve equation (4.1) is to relax the linear programme, allowing y_{ij} to assume real values in [0, 1]. The solution obtained thereof may not be optimal, and we will attempt to efficiently solve equation (4.1) in future.

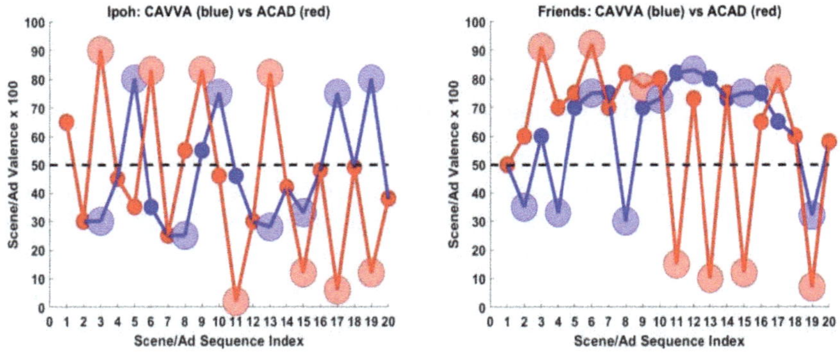

Figure 4.10. CAVVA (blue) and ACAD (red) VPS val profiles for the *IPOH* (left) and *Friends* (right) programmes. Eight ads are inserted within a 12-scene PV. Small, solid balls denote scenes, while large, hollow balls denote the inserted ads.

To compute the scene–ad similarity matrix, we employed the Places365 Resnet152 model [28]. Forty uniformly sampled key frames from each video scene and ad, denoted as $\{K_s\}$ and $\{K_{ad}\}$, are input to the Resnet and 512-D fc7 features extracted. The similarity between key-frame pairs is then computed via cosine distance, and $rel(S_i, A_j)$ denotes the mean similarity among 40 pairs. Figure 1.10 presents exemplar video scene–ad key-frame pairs and their similarity scores. The Resnet model effectively captures similarities in scene structure (cafe-kitchen scenes for left-top pair) and face/body orientation, and enables selection of semantically similar but emotionally dissimilar ads to follow scenes in ACAD.

4.4.2 Computational affective advertising versus Affective Computational ADvertising scheduling

The key difference between the CAVVA [1] and ACAD formulations is that while CAVVA leverages emotional inertia to embed ads that minimally perturb the user's emotional state and VX, ACAD seeks to insert ads strongly incongruent to the programme mood to elicit genuine ad assessments and maximal recall. To examine the differences in VPSs generated by these two VIVA methods, we added four scenes to both the *Friends* and *IPOH* PVs used in section 4.3.1 so that the new *Friends* and *IPOH* programmes were, respectively, about 24 and 18 min long. Eight ads—four each of HV and LV—were then embedded onto these PVs (with 11 ad slots) via the CAVVA and ACAD methods. These ads were selected from distinct inventories for the two programmes (see section 4.3.1).

Figure 4.10 presents val profiles (on a scale of 100) of the generated CAVVA and ACAD VPSs for the sad and happy programmes. Scene/ad val scores input to the ACAD and CAVVA algorithms were computed as the average of the ratings provided by three experts. Smaller, solid balls denote programme scenes, while the larger, hollow balls represent the eight embedded ads. Scenes/ads having a val score of >50 are deemed HV, and others LV. From the generated VPSs, we make the following observations:

- Clearly, CAVVA attempts to generate smooth VPS val profiles to maintain emotional inertia. This is especially evident for the *Friends* VPS (figure 4.10, right), where HV ads are added between scenes of similar val so as to sustain a positive mood. For the *IPOH* programme (figure 4.10, left), which contains a number of LV scenes, LV ads are added next to LV scenes so as to enable viewers to transition to a happy emotional state through the prior scene–ad–next scene sequence.
- Similar to ACAD, CAVVA was constrained to include both HV and LV ads in the generated VPS, different from its natural behaviour. Under such conditions, CAVVA attempts to embed HV (LV) ads in the sad (happy) programmes, so that the resulting VPS val profile is as 'less spiky' as possible. Further, the emphasis on VX results in LV ads being embedded earlier rather than later in the VPS. This behaviour adversely impacts ad val assessment and recall, as discussed in section 4.5.2.
- Contrastingly, ACAD favours the generation of VPSs with spiky val profiles, consistent with our hypothesis that ads emotionally different to preceding scenes are evaluated and recalled better. The ACAD *Friends* and *IPOH* VPSs exhibit 'bumpy' val profiles. The ACAD formulation also forces LV ads to be embedded at the VPS tail.

Recall that the RF specified by equation (4.1) comprises trade-off parameters α and β. While higher α enforces the embedding of LV ads towards the VPS tail, β emphasises an embedding scheme wherein programme scenes are followed by emotionally dissimilar but semantically similar ads. To examine the impact of this trade-off, we generated ACAD VPSs with $\alpha = \beta = 0.5$ and $\alpha = 0, \beta = 1$. Val profiles for the corresponding VPSs are, respectively, shown in red and blue in figure 4.11. When ACAD solely focuses on semantic-plus-emotional ad-scene matching (blue curve), LV ads are also added towards the VPS head (figure 4.11, right). Little difference is noted between the red and blue ACAD VPSs generated for the *IPOH*

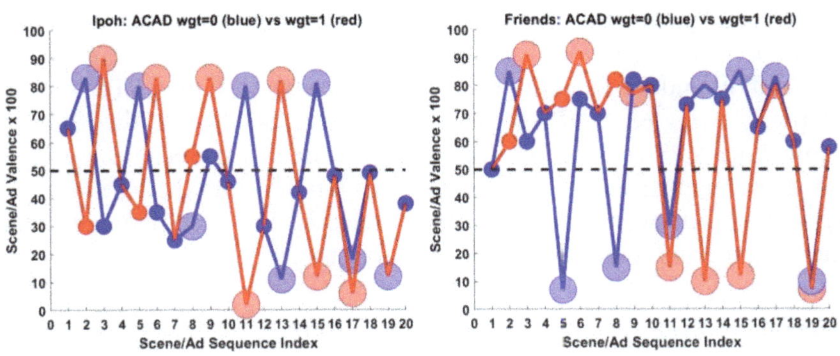

Figure 4.11. Val profiles for the *IPOH* and *Friends* ACAD VPSs with $\alpha/\beta = 1$ (red) and 0 (blue). Eight ads (hollow balls) were inserted within a PV comprising 12 scenes (solid balls).

programme (figure 4.11, left). Nevertheless, the red curves, denoting a positioning–relevance trade-off, achieve optimal ad assessments and recall, as evidenced by the following validational user study.

4.5 Validational study and hypotheses

To confirm if the ACAD rules indeed enable optimal ad assessments and recall, we performed a validational user study comparing the CAVVA and ACAD methods against a simplistic ('Trivial') VIVA approach. Differing from the CAVVA and ACAD approaches, which enforce a uniform distribution of ads across the VPS (constraint (*c*) in equation (4.1)), the Trivial method works by placing multiple ads at the VPS head and middle. The CAVVA and ACAD VPSs shown in figure 4.11 were used in this study. The Trivial method randomly selects four HV plus four LV ads, following which four ads each are randomly arranged before programme scenes 1 and 7, respectively. In line with the design of CAVVA and ACAD, we expected the following:

- ACAD to achieve superior ad evaluations and recall.
- CAVVA to induce the optimal VX.
- Both these methods to perform better than Trivial embedding in the above respects.

4.5.1 Materials and methods

Programmes and ads: The *Friends* and *IPOH* PVs with 12 scenes each (section 4.3.1) were used in this validational study. Forty-eight ads (24 HAHV and 24 HALV) from [8] were used. To avoid memory effects, we created distinct ad inventories for the two programmes; both inventories comprised 24 ads (12 HV plus 12 LV). VPSs with eight ad embeddings were then generated for the two PVs via the ACAD, CAVVA, and Trivial approaches, and presented to users.

Users: Twenty-four university students (14 male and 10 female), naive to the purpose of the study and different from the participants in section 4.3.2, viewed and assessed the above VPSs (two programmes × three VIVA schemes = six VPSs). It took about 1 hr to cumulatively view the *Friends* and *IPOH* VPSs, and users were paid a token fee for their time and effort.

Protocol: Each user viewed the *Friends* VPS generated by one VIVA method and the *IPOH* VPS generated via another approach. The VPS viewing order was counterbalanced across users to ensure that (i) all VPSs had the same number of viewings, and (ii) and an equal number of users viewed the happy VPS first and vice-versa. Upon viewing each VPS scene and ad, users had to rate them for val (1–5 scale); following VPS completion, they were required to (i) recall the eight viewed ads from thumbnails from the 24 inventory ads, and (ii) rate the VPS VX. Six users cumulatively viewed two instances of each of the six VPSs, resulting in 16 ad-specific and two VPS-specific scores for recall and VX per user.

4.5.2 Results

Figure 4.12 presents the user-study results, with error bars denoting standard error. With respect to ad val evaluations (first two bar plots from the left), the ACAD and

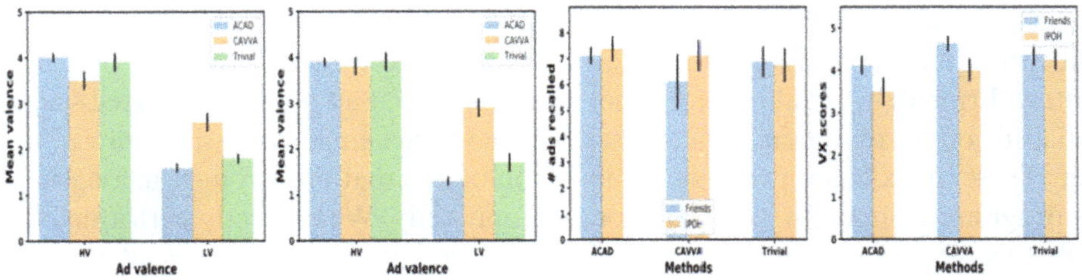

Figure 4.12. Validational study: (left to right) Ad val ratings for positive and negative VPSs, ad recall, and VX scores for the different VIVA methods.

Trivial methods achieved more genuine assessments than CAVVA (higher val scores for HV ads and lower scores for LV ads). For the *Friends* VPS, ACAD, CAVVA, and Trivial HV ad embeddings received mean val ratings of 4, 3.5, and 3.9; the val scores for ACAD and CAVVA differed marginally as per a two-sample t-test (t (14) = 1.857; $p = 0.093$). LV ads inserted via ACAD evoked the lowest mean val score of 1.6; the mean CAVVA and Trivial ad scores were 2.6 and 1.8, respectively. Distinct val scores were evoked for ACAD versus CAVVA LV ads (($t(14) = -4.058$; $p < 0.005$)), and for CAVVA versus Trivial LV ads ($t(14) = 3.237$; $p < 0.01$).

For the sad *IPOH* VPS, HV ads embedded via all three VIVA methods evoked similar val scores (mean val scores of 3.9, 3.8, and 3.9 for ACAD, CAVVA, and Trivial, respectively), but distinct ratings were noted for LV ads (mean val scores of 1.3, 2.9, and 1.7 for ACAD, CAVVA, and Trivial). Distinct val ratings were noted for ACAD versus CAVVA ads ($t(14) = -7.439$; $p < 0.0001$), and slightly distinct ratings for ACAD versus Trivial ($t(14) = -1.857$; $p < 0.096$). Overall, while the HV ad val ratings were unaffected by the VIVA approach, ACAD-embedded LV ads elicited more genuine val scores than other methods.

With respect to ad recall, more ads were generally recalled for the *IPOH* VPS (MRRs of 7.4, 7.1, and 6.8 ads for ACAD, CAVVA, and Trivial, respectively), but greater recall variations were noted for the *Friends* VPS (MRRs of 7.1, 6.1, and 6.9 ads for ACAD, CAVVA, and Trivial). A slight difference in *IPOH* ad recall was noted for ACAD versus Trivial ($t(14) = 2.017$; $p = 0.065$), while distinct recall rates were noted for ACAD versus CAVVA ($t(14) = 2.397$; $p < 0.05$) methods in the *Friends* programme. In terms of VX, the CAVVA-generated *Friends* VPS received the highest scores (mean VX = 4.6) followed by Trivial (mean VX = 4.4) and ACAD (mean VX = 4.1), while the Trivial *IPOH* VPS (mean VX = 4.3) received higher scores than CAVVA (mean VX = 4) and ACAD (mean VX = 3.5). Overall, (i) ACAD achieves higher ad recall at the cost of VX (due to scene–ad emotional dissimilarity), and (ii) when constrained to include ads strongly opposite to programme mood, CAVVA may not necessarily achieve the optimal VX.

4.6 Summary and conclusions

Advertisements are known to mediate brand evaluations in consumers, and also to influence their health beliefs and lifestyle choices, making them a critical component of healthcare messaging. However, the programme context within which an ad is presented to the viewer influences the ad evaluation by users; prior studies have noted that health-and-safety-related messages are better received in a positive programme context. Prior VIVA studies have either exclusively focused on content-based scene–ad similarity or on marketing principles that favour sustaining a positive mood in the user. These approaches preclude the insertion of ads that are strongly incongruent to the programme mood, which is the focus of our study. We expressly performed a user study to assess the impact of emotionally (in)congruent programmes on ad evaluation.

Based on exploratory and validational user studies, each involving 24 users, we showed that (i) the ACAD VIVA strategy devised from user impressions rather than axiomatic rules is flexible and can effectively accommodate ads strongly incongruent to programme mood, and (ii) ACAD induces genuine ad evaluations and superior recall in users as compared to CAVVA. While the ACAD rules were derived from a user study involving two short programmes and a small number of ads, these rules are nevertheless generalisable, as confirmed by the validational study involving longer programmes, a larger number of ads, and an independent set of users. The validational study also revealed a trade-off between ad recall and VX, which should guide future designs. A limitation of our work is that we ignore the asl dimension for ad evaluation, and this will be investigated in future. Other improvements as part of future work include (i) designing a more efficient ad-embedding strategy than a brute-force approach, and (ii) evaluating ACAD in real-life situations where scene and ad ratings are computed via automated methods.

References

[1] Yadati K, Katti H and Kankanhalli M 2014 CAVVA: computational affective video-in-video advertising *IEEE Trans. Multimedia* **16** 15–23

[2] Mei T, Hua X and Li S 2009 VideoSense: a contextual in-video advertising system *IEEE Trans. Circuits Syst. Video Technol.* **19** 1866–79

[3] Russell J 1980 A circumplex model of affect *J. Pers. Soc. Psychol.* **39** 1161–78

[4] Broach V, Page T J and Wilson R 1995 Television programming and its influence on viewers' perceptions of commercials: the role of program arousal and pleasantness *J. Advert.* **24** 45–54

[5] Holbrook M B and Shaughnessy J O 1984 The role of emotlon in advertising *Psychol. Mark.* **1** 45–64

[6] Holbrook M B and Batra R 1987 Assessing the role of emotions as mediators of consumer responses to advertising *J. Consum. Res.* **14** 404–20

[7] Pham M T, Geuens M and Pelsmacker P D 2013 The influence of ad-evoked feelings on brand evaluations: empirical generalizations from consumer responses to more than 1000 TV commercials *Int. J. Res. Mark.* **30** 383–94

[8] Shukla A, Gullapuram S S, Katti H, Kankanhalli M, Winkler S and Subramanian R 2020 Recognition of advertisement emotions with application to computational advertising *IEEE Trans. Affect. Comput* **13** 781–92

[9] Shukla A, Katti H, Kankanhalli M and Subramanian R 2018 Looking beyond a clever narrative: visual context and attention are primary drivers of affect in video advertisements *ACM Int. Conf. on Multimodal Interaction* pp 210–9

[10] Friestad M and Thorson E 1993 Remembering ads: the effects of encoding strategies, retrieval cues, and emotional response *J. Consum. Psychol.* **2** 1–23

[11] Subramanian R, Shankar D, Sebe N and Melcher D 2014 Emotion modulates eye movement patterns and subsequent memory for the gist and details of movie scenes *J. Vis.* **14** 31
[12] Murphy-Hoefer R, Hyland A and Rivard C 2010 The influence of tobacco counter marketing ads on college students' knowledge, attitudes, and beliefs *J. Am. Coll. Health* **58** 373–81
[13] Donovan R J, Boulter J, Borland R, Jalleh G and Carter O 2003 Continuous tracking of the australian national tobacco campaign: advertising effects on recall, recognition, cognitions, and behaviour *Tob. Control* **12** ii30–9
[14] Sutton S R and Eiser J 1984 The effect of fear-arousing communications on cigarette smoking: an expectancy-value approach *J. Behav. Med.* **7** 13–33
[15] Stainback R D and Rogers R W 1983 Identifying effective components of alcohol abuse prevention programs: effects of fear appeals, message style, and source expertise *Int. J. Addict.* **18** 393405
[16] Terry-Mcelrath Y, Wakefield M, Ruel E, Balch G I, Emery S and Szczypka G *et al* 2005 The effect of antismoking advertisement executional characteristics on youth comprehension, appraisal, recall, and engagement *J. Health Commun.* **10** 127–43
[17] Kamins M, Marks L and Skinner D 2013 Television commercial evaluation in the context of program induced mood: congruency versus consistency effects *J. Advert.* **20** 1–14
[18] Meyers-Levy J and Sternthal B 1993 A two-factor explanation of assimilation and contrast effects *J. Mark. Res.* **30** 359–68
[19] Aylesworth A B and MacKenzie S B 1998 Context is key: the effect of program-induced mood on thoughts about the ad *J. Advert.* **27** 17–31
[20] Feltham T and Arnold S 1994 Program involvement and ad/program consistency as moderators of program context effects *J. Consum. Psychol.* **12** 51–77
[21] Furnham A and Goh M 2013 Effects of program-advertisement congruity and advertisement emotional appeal on memory for health and safety advertisements *J. Appl. Soc. Psychol.* **12** 44
[22] Moorman M, Neijens P and Smit E 2007 The effects of program involvement on commercial exposure and recall in a naturalistic setting *J. Advert.* **04** 125–41
[23] Shapiro S, Macinnis J D and Park W C 2013 Understanding program induced mood effects: decoupling arousal from valence *J. Advert.* **31** 15–26
[24] Yun J T, Segijn C M, Pearson S, Malthouse E C, Konstan J A and Shankar V 2020 Challenges and future directions of computational advertising measurement systems *J. Advert.* **49** 446–58
[25] Kensinger E A 2009 Remembering the details: effects of emotion *Emot. Rev.* **1** 99–113
[26] Rimmele U 2011 Emotion enhances the subjective feeling of remembering, despite lower accuracy for contextual details *J. Vis.* **11** 553–62
[27] Gurobi Optimization L. Gurobi Optimizer Reference Manual; 2021. Available from: http://gurobi.com
[28] Zhou B, Lapedriza A, Khosla A, Oliva A and Torralba A 2017 Places: a 10 million image database for scene recognition *IEEE Trans. Pattern Anal. Mach. Intell* **17** 296

IOP Publishing

Affective Computing in Healthcare
Applications based on biosignals and artificial intelligence
M Murugappan

Chapter 5

Machine-learning-based emotion recognition in arousal–valence space using photoplethysmogram signals

Md Nazmul Islam Shuzan, Moajjem Hossain Chowdhury, Md Shafayet Hossain, Md Sakib Abrar Hossain and Muhammad E H Chowdhury

Modelling human emotions is one of the biggest challenges in the field of affective computing research. Proper monitoring and modelling of human emotions will unlock new ways of tracking the mental health of users. A good model will allow the users to properly manage their stress levels. However, human emotions are inherently complex, and hence they are often represented in multiple dimensions. To relate changes in emotional state with physiological changes in the body, much research has been conducted that uses various physiological signals to denote emotional states. Among those, photoplethysmogram (PPG) signals present a very interesting option. Since PPG signals can be acquired non-invasively using cost-effective devices, the utilisation of PPG signals for emotion recognition has many practical applications. In this work, PPG signals are used to classify the state of arousal and valence of subjects. Arousal relates to the general level of excitement that is experienced by a person (such as anger and calm). Valence, on the other hand, denotes the level of happiness experienced by a person (such as contentment and sadness). These two dimensions of emotion will allow us to capture a wide range of emotional states. The Dataset for Emotion Analysis using Physiological dataset has been used in this work for the classification of arousal and valence. Time-domain, frequency-domain, and statistical features were extracted from PPG signals and their derivatives. Multi-collinearity was reduced by removing highly correlated features. These features were used to train machine-learning (ML) models, which were evaluated using fivefold cross-validation. In particular, the XGBoost model outperformed every other model and achieved an accuracy of 81.03% and 82.98% for the classification of arousal and valence, respectively. The models outperform current state-of-the-art techniques in emotion classification. These models can thus be used for emotion recognition using wearable devices, and hence improve mental healthcare.

doi:10.1088/978-0-7503-5182-9ch5

5.1 Introduction and background

Emotions are mental states that are triggered by neurophysiological alterations and are related to thoughts, feelings, behavioural reactions, and a level of satisfaction or dissatisfaction [1–3]. Mood, temperament, personality, disposition, and ingenuity are all inter-related with human emotion, which is usually disclosed through facial expressions, voice, text, and gestures, and have a direct impact on biological signals [4–8]. Despite significant advancements in human–computer interaction, detecting the true state of human emotions has remained a very vexing question, which has consequently hindered diagnostic tools from attaining a good understanding of people [9–11]. Taking this into account, an accurate grasp of human sentiments can have enormous benefits in terms of comprehending today's complex world. As emotions change rapidly and easily, recognising short periods of feeling is becoming an increasingly crucial field of research.

Human emotions are difficult to model because they are complicated outcomes associated with many key components. Previously, two approaches have been regularly used. The first is by recognising emotions by separate names, such as joy, sadness, rage, happiness, fear, and so on. Although this approach is conceptually straightforward, it has issues portraying mixed emotions that are impossible to class as a single case. Further, such an approach fails to quantify the intensity and degree of the given emotional state, such as measuring how happy one is. The second method involves labelling emotions on various levels, wherein each level signifies an emotional intensity, resulting in a series of continuous scales rather than a single scale. According to Russell's circumplex hypothesis [12], the most prevalent emotional aspects are valence and arousal. Valence (usually the horizontal axis) depicts the degree of pleasantness (such as contentment and sadness), whereas arousal (typically the vertical axis) shows the amount of excitement (such as anger and calm). Therefore, human emotions can be represented in a two-dimensional (2D) space based on their valence and arousal, as illustrated in figure 5.1. For example, a depressed person exhibits a low valence and low arousal value, but a happy person has a high valence and high arousal value. Therefore, identifying human emotion necessitates the use of two binary classifiers: valence and arousal.

Utilising facial images, voice tone, pulse rate, etc., different types of emotions have been studied using a variety of methods as technology has progressed [4, 5, 13]. Physiological signals, such as electromyogram (EMG), electroencephalogram (EEG), respiration pattern, electrocardiogram (ECG), and photoplethysmogram (PPG), are important in emotion detection [14–19], since they are spontaneous reactions that individuals cannot normally regulate/fake at their will [20, 21]. It is difficult to determine someone's true state of emotion from their exterior appearance if they do not reveal their sentiments through facial expressions, such as intentionally keeping a 'poker face', or restraining themselves from all sorts of verbal communications. On the other hand, physiological signals (EEG, EMG, ECG, PPG, etc.) are more reliable in detecting emotions since these are involuntary manifestations, which also tend to be impossible to fake.

Most of the proposed machine-learning and deep-learning-based solutions have performed well for automated emotion recognition in controlled testing. There is,

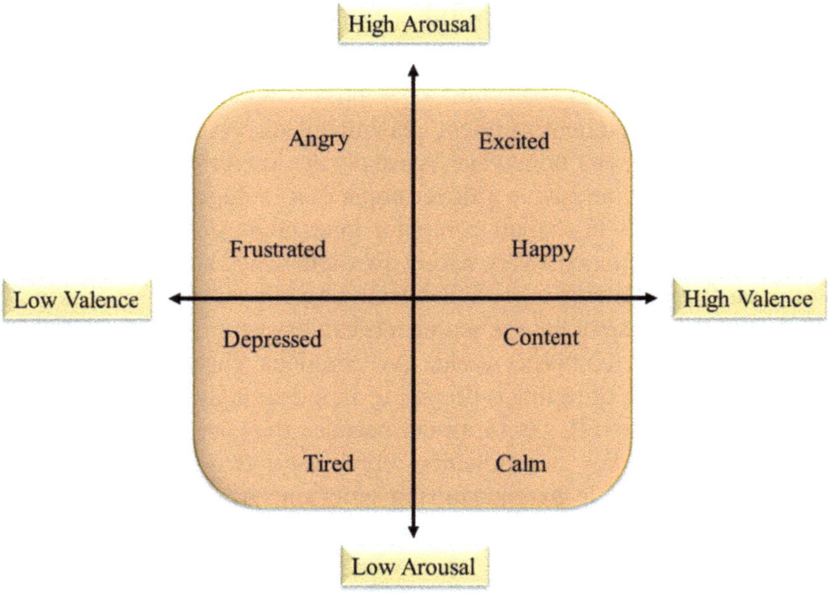

Figure 5.1. Emotion model based on arousal and valence. Adapted from [12].

nevertheless, a requirement to achieve excellent performance for emotion recognition even in an uncontrolled setting [22]. Emotion detection utilising physiological signals has become a hot topic at the current time, with various proposed methodologies [23–25]. Two basic approaches, i.e., categorising emotions based on hand-crafted features and extracting features using deep-learning frameworks, are now gaining popularity. Initially, emotion-recognition biosignal characteristics were derived directly using statistical computations and frequency properties. For greater performance, additional biosignals were used to extract more characteristics. To categorise emotions into different classes, the authors of [26] retrieved various hand-crafted features (110 in total) acquired from four-channel biosensors, which were used to record ECG, respiration, skin conductivity, and EMG signals. Legendre and Krawtchouk moments were proposed by Giakoumis *et al* [27] to extract contextual features, whereas in [28] EEG features were explored and investigated for the categorisation of emotions. Jenke *et al* [29] analysed EEG signal feature-extraction methods and identified characteristics that were suitable for emotion identification. Mert *et al* [30] suggested an emotion-identification system based on EEG data utilising multivariate extension empirical mode decomposition. Yoo *et al* [14] used a hand-crafted feature from four signals as input to an artificial neural network to categorise six emotions. Hassan *et al* [31] extracted statistical features from the power spectral density of amplitude versus occurrence distribution using electro-dermal activity (EDA), PPG, and EMG data. Variations in experimental settings and cognitive health factors present difficulties for EEG-based emotion recognition in practical applications. Ineffective emotional recognition and expression are prominent symptoms of Parkinson's disease (PD), the second most prevalent kind of neurodegenerative condition [32]. A so-called extreme learning machine was paired with a one-dimensional convolutional recurrent neural network (1D-CRNN) to create a model that was both reliable for detecting PD patients' emotions and amenable to cross-dataset learning with a wide range of emotions and experimental conditions [32].

A new one-dimensional CNN model was proposed in [33] to identify short-term emotions using a single PPG pulse. Their findings showed that the suggested pre-processing strategy may improve the accuracy of emotion identification by around 32%, and the model performed well on valence and arousal classification tasks, with a mean accuracy of 90.80% and 91.03%, respectively. Lee *et al* [34] combined statistical features and deep-learning features of PPG signals to classify arousal (binary class) and valence (binary class). Their work demonstrated state-of-the-art performance for emotion classification using PPG, with an accuracy of 80.9% and 82.1% for arousal and valence, respectively.

All of the above works utilised signals that require either expensive hardware or complex configurations for signal acquisition. There have been very few works that have used PPG for emotion classification (a major motivation of this study), despite the fact that PPG signals are easy to acquire, have cheaper hardware for signal acquisition, and are also available in wearable devices form. Hence, focusing on utilising PPG for emotion detection can enable more potential practical applications, and thus PPG signals are used in this work for the classification of arousal and valence. PPGs use an optical sensor to monitor changes in blood volume, with the fingertip being the most accurate measuring site. As the shape and values of PPG signals fluctuate from person to person in different emotional/physiological conditions, we chose PPG signals to detect human emotions [35], and, as such, we need to extract a lot of information from a small amount of data in order to detect short-term emotions. When we see a gruesome scene or are in a humiliating circumstance, for example, our hearts beat quicker than usual, and we may use PPG to evaluate blood pressure and stress levels [36]. In [37], two different autonomic nerve signals, known as SKT and PPG, were evaluated in order to obtain a 2D emotional feature vector (PPI and SKT amplitude), which was then used to classify happy and sad feelings.

In [38], the authors proposed to evaluate changes in the morphological aspects of finger PPG signals and feature time series that exist between happy and sad emotional states. In [39], it was proposed that entropy-based complex wavelet sub-band measures be used for the classification of a PPG into 14 different emotion categories. In [40], the authors made an effort to suggest an automatic emotion-recognition method that is capable of characterising PPG signals while a subject was being exposed to an emotional music video. Using Poincaré section measurements, their primary goal was to identify and categorise the dynamical characteristics of the PPG trajectories associated with the three distinct emotional categories of love, hate, and fun. In [41], the authors proposed a system for recognising emotions that would be based on deep learning. The researchers decided to break down the feelings to be identified into two distinct groups (good and negative) and four distinct groups (neutral, angry, happy, and sad). In their research, the authors fed the spectrogram of the PPG data into a BiLSTM model and a novel ResNet +BiLSTM model that they had devised for the purpose of emotion identification. In [42], the authors were able to record signals for emotion detection by using PPG as well as

EMG, deciding to use a bimodal structure to extract shared PPG and EMG representations in order to improve the performance of the recognition system. In comparison to the standard high/low binary classification, the arousal–valence mapping that was produced by this method was significantly more in depth.

As mentioned earlier, we here elect to use a two-parameter arousal and valence emotion model to capture emotions. Several time-domain, frequency-domain, and statistical features are extracted from PPG signals and their derivatives. Multi-collinearity is reduced by removing highly correlated features, and model complexity is further reduced by using feature-selection algorithms, which reduce the chance of overfitting the model as well. The features are then used to train and evaluate several machine-learning (ML) models. The best-performing classification models are selected for the binary classification of arousal and valence separately. To verify the efficacy of the model, we utilise a database for emotion analysis using the physiological signals (the Dataset for Emotion Analysis using Physiological, DEAP emotion dataset) [43], which comprises physiological data from a good number of test subjects. Our proposed models can be easily deployed in wearable devices for real-time emotion recognition utilising PPG signals.

The structure of this chapter is as follows. Section 5.1 analyses the limitations of earlier emotion-identification algorithms based on hand-crafted characteristics, and presents a way to characterise emotions using two parameters. The proposed approach based on PPG signals is described in section 5.2. The DEAP dataset, experimental setup, and experiment results are presented in section 5.3. The chapter is summarised and concluded in section 5.4.

5.2 Materials and methods

In this section, the overall methodology is explained. Figure 5.2 summarises the whole workflow of this investigation. The dataset was collected by using video to evoke a specific emotion in users. PPG signals were acquired during each session. The emotions of the users were then scored in the arousal–valence space, and the acquired data then pre-processed by removing high-frequency noise and motion artefacts (MAs). The processed signals were then fed to a feature-extraction pipeline, where time-domain (42), derivative-based (48), and frequency and statistical features (14) were extracted. Then, dimensionality reduction was used to reduce the complexity of the models. The feature matrix created is then trained and evaluated using a fivefold cross-validation technique to classify arousal and valence for a binary classification problem.

5.2.1 Dataset description

As aforementioned, the DEAP dataset was used in this work, which is a commonly used dataset in emotion-recognition studies. After obtaining authorisation, The dataset was first proposed by Koelstra et al [43]. There are two sections to the DEAP dataset: online ratings and participant ratings. Fourteen to sixteen volunteers rated 120 1 min music videos based on arousal, valence, dominance, and enjoyment in an online self-assessment. Second, the remaining 32 participants watched a subset of 40 films while monitoring various physiological signals and rated the videos on a scale of 1 to 9 for arousal, valence, dominance, and liking. We only used the PPG signals

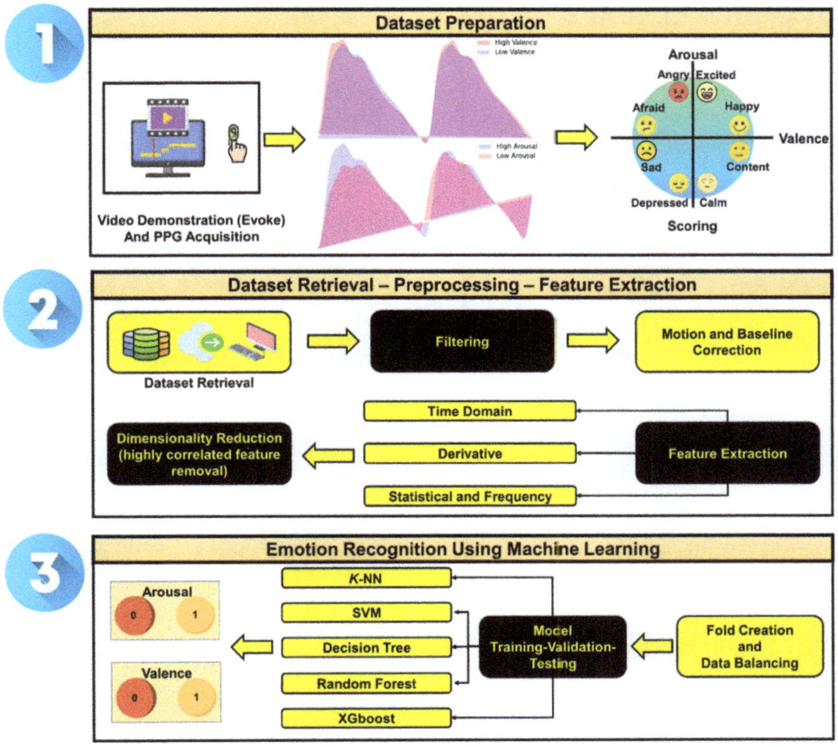

Figure 5.2. Overall methodology of the system.

from the DEAP dataset, which in total comprises PPG, EMG, EEG, and EDA, among other physiological signals. The dataset included 32 healthy individuals (50% female), from ages 19–37 (mean age 26.9). EEG and peripheral physiological signals (such as PPG) were captured on a dedicated recording PC with a Biosemi Active Two system (Pentium 4 CPU, 3.2 GHz). Stimuli were delivered to a recording PC through a specialised stimulus PC (Pentium 4, 3.2 GHz) that applied synchronisation markers directly to it. The Presentation software, from Neurobehavioral Systems, was used to display the stimuli and record the participants' assessments. The signals were initially sampled at 512 Hz. The dataset providers then down-sampled the PPG signals to 128 Hz.

We divided the arousal and valence groups based on a median value of 5 (low/high), since arousal and valence were measured on a scale of 1 to 9 and our goal was a binary identification. Table 5.1 summarises the dataset per category.

5.2.2 Data pre-processing

The DEAP dataset signals are first resampled to a fixed sample rate so that the model can be trained and evaluated on this dataset. In normal conditions, it is very common to have MAs and high-frequency noise in the acquired PPG signal. The MAs can range from spikes in data to distortion of the signal's fiducial points, which are shown in figure 5.3. These corruptions will obstruct the extraction of features from the signals. To

Table 5.1. DEAP dataset description per category.

Category/class	Samples
High arousal	4535
Low arousal	2529
High valence	4066
Low valence	2998
Total	7064

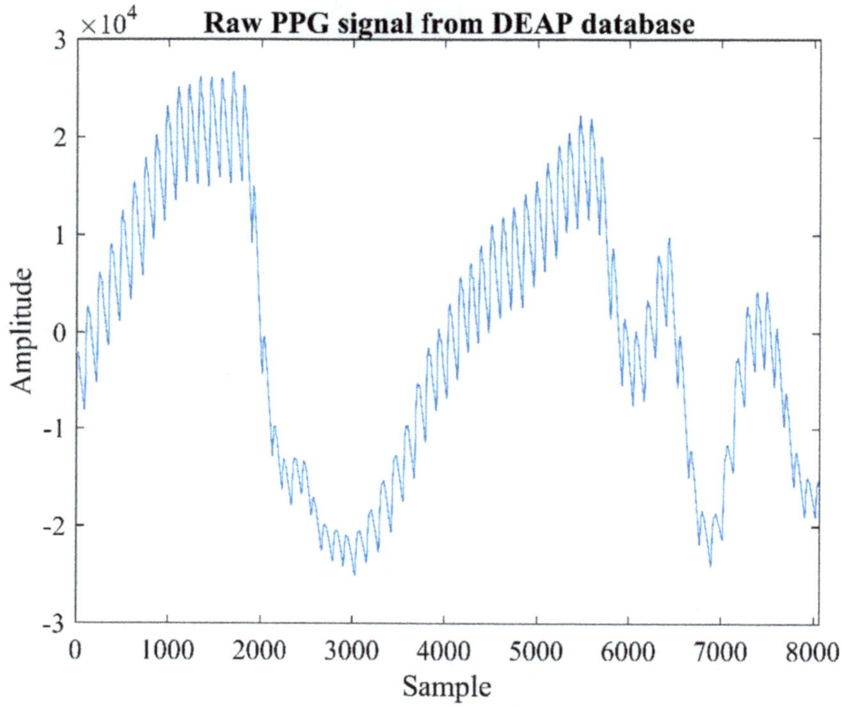

Figure 5.3. Raw PPG waveform for emotion analysis from the DEAP database.

rectify this, a low-pass filter is used to remove the noise. A low-pass Butterworth infinite impulse response zero-phase filter [44] was implemented in MATLAB; the filter was of sixth order and had a cut-off frequency of 25 Hz. To remove MAs from the PPG signal, variational mode decomposition [45] was found to be robust and quite effective in our previous work [46–48]. The same configuration was used in this work, as well, which is shown in figure 5.4. PPG signals with baseline wandering had their baseline corrected using a polynomial fit. A 10th-degree polynomial was used to find the baseline trend, which was then removed from the signal.

To achieve quick on-site emotion recognition, we attempted to examine PPG segments ranging in duration from 5 to 60 s. Small segments result in poor performance, while others may include more information but be too lengthy to be

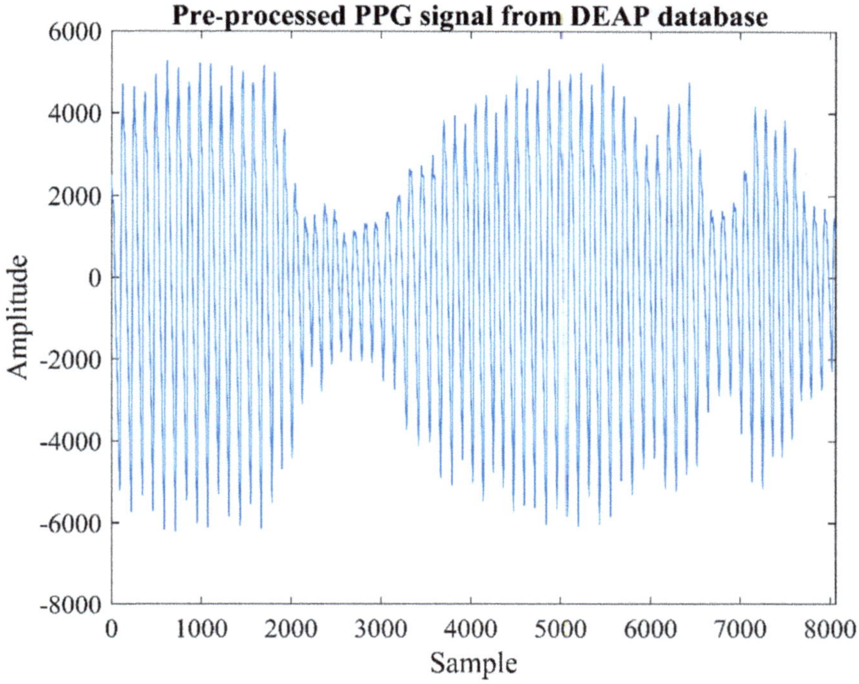

Figure 5.4. Pre-processed PPG signal for emotion analysis from the DEAP database.

detected on site. Accordingly, we considered both efficacy and efficiency before deciding to choose 10 s segments. We divided the signal into 10 s segments, starting at the beginning of each record. In a 60 s experiment, we were able to gather six non-overlapping segments. We thus acquired 7680 (=6 × 40 × 32) data samples from 32 participants, each having 40 trials and six segments in each trial.

5.2.3 Feature extraction

In this work, three different types of features were extracted from the PPG signals: time-domain, frequency-domain, and statistical features [46, 49, 50]. PPG signals are very rich in information. Their distinctive morphology allows for the extraction of various features in both the time domain and in various derivatives of the signal. Some typical features that can be extracted are the amplitude of the peak from the foot of the signal, the width of the pulse, the pulse interval, the peak-to-peak interval, and so on. Many other meaningful features were extracted using feature-extraction techniques in our previous work [50]. The time-domain features were extracted from both the PPG signal as well as its first and second derivatives, as depicted in figures 5.5(a) and (b). Statistical features were, however, only extracted from the PPG signal and not from its derivatives. The statistical features were obtained from [49, 51]. As a result, a total of 107 features were extracted and used in this work.

Table 5.2 list the 107 features that were extracted from the PPG signals. Here, 'sys' refers to the amplitude of the systolic peak and 'amp foot' denotes the amplitude of the

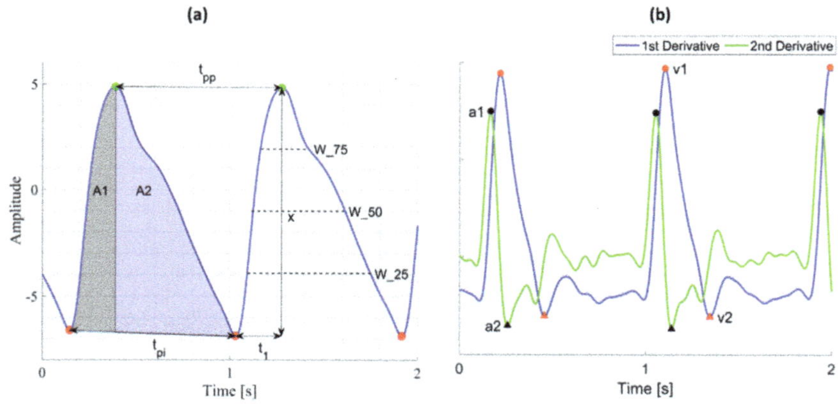

Figure 5.5. Extracting features from (a) the time domain, (b) and their first and second derivates from the PPG waveform. Adapted from [46]. CC BY 4.0.

Table 5.2. List of features extracted from PPG signals. Adapted from [46]. CC BY 4.0.

Feature Type	Feature Name		
Time-domain features (42 features)	mean(sys)	std(sys)	var(sys)
	mean(amp foot)	std(amp foot)	var(amp foot)
	mean(x)	std(x)	var(x)
	mean(t1)	std(t1)	var(t1)
	mean(tpi)	std(tpi)	var(tpi)
	mean(tpp)	std(tpp)	var(tpp)
	mean(t1/x)	std(t1/x)	var(t1/x)
	mean(t1/tpi)	std(t1/tpi)	var(t1/tpi)
	mean(x/(tpi-t1))	std(x/(tpi-t1))	var(x/(tpi-t1))
	mean(A1)	std(A1)	var(A1)
	mean(A2)	std(A2)	var(A2)
	mean(width_25)	std(width_25)	var(width_25)
	mean(width_50)	std(width_50)	var(width_50)
	mean(width_75)	std(width_75)	var(width_75)
PPG derivative features (48 features)	mean(v1)	std(v1)	var(v1)
	mean(tv1)	std(tv1)	var(tv1)
	mean(v2)	std(v2)	var(v2)
	mean(tv2)	std(tv2)	var(tv2)
	mean(a1)	std(a1)	var(a1)
	mean(ta1)	std(ta1)	var(ta1)
	mean(a2)	std(a2)	var(a2)
	mean(ta2)	std(ta2)	var(ta2)
	mean(v2/v1)	std(v2/v1)	var(v2/v1)
	mean(a2/a1)	std(a2/a1)	var(a2/a1)
	mean(tv1/tv2)	std(tv1/tv2)	var(tv1/tv2)
	mean(ta1/ta2)	std(ta1/ta2)	var(ta1/ta2)

(*Continued*)

Table 5.2. (*Continued*)

Feature Type	Feature Name		
	mean(tv1/ta1)	std(tv1/ta1)	var(tv1/ta1)
	mean(tv1/ta2)	std(tv1/ta2)	var(tv1/ta2)
	mean(tv2/ta1)	std(tv2/ta1)	var(tv2/ta1)
	mean(tv1/ta1)	std(tv1/ta1)	var(tv1/ta1)
Frequency and statistical features (14)	MaxFreq	MaxVal	MaxRatio
	Mean(sig)	Median(sig)	Std(sig)
	Mad(sig)	25th percentile of sig	75th percentile of sig
	Inter-quartile range of sig	Skewness(sig)	Kurtosis(sig)
	Signal_entropy(sig)	Spectral_entropy(sig)	

foot. The amplitude from the foot of a PPG signal to the systolic peak is referred to as 'x'. Other notations in the time domain and derivative features are depicted in figure 5.5, where the various features are annotated on the PPG signals. The mean, variance, and standard deviation of these features are calculated. In frequency and statistical features, 'MaxFreq' refers to the frequency at which the signal has maximum power and 'MaxVal' refers to that maximum power. 'MaxRatio' is the ratio between MaxVal and the power of the whole spectrum. 'Signal_entropy' refers to the Shannon's entropy of the signal. 'Spectral_entropy' refers to the normalised Shannon's entropy that is applied to the power spectrum density of the signal.

5.2.4 Feature reduction

To avoid influencing the feature-ranking algorithm, removal of strongly correlated features is conducted before feature ranking. Pairwise linear correlation is used to compute the correlation matrix between features. A feature with a correlation coefficient threshold of 0.95 is deemed heavily correlated, and one of them is removed from the feature vector [52]. Figure 5.6(a) shows the all-PPG signal-based

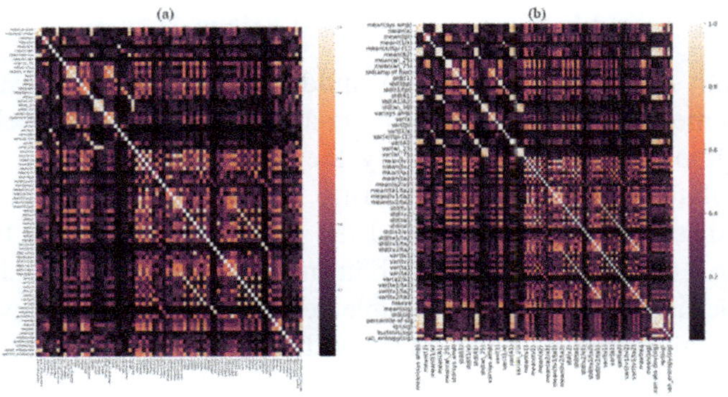

Figure 5.6. Heat map of correlation between (a) all 107 features, and (b) 78 features after removing highly correlated features.

features heat map, and figure 5.6(b) shows the features after eliminating highly correlated features. Seventy-eight features were left after removing these highly correlated features.

5.2.5 Data balancing

Training using an unbalanced dataset might result in a biased model since the dataset will not include an equal number of signals for the different classes. As a result, data augmentation for the training set can aid in attaining a similar number of signals in the various classes, resulting in reliable model development. To balance the datase, the synthetic minority oversampling technique (SMOTE) was used [53, 54].

In this experiment, the number of high-arousal and high-valence samples was 4535 and 4066, while the number of low-arousal and low-valence samples was 2539 and 2998, which is an imbalanced distribution. As a result, we employed the SMOTE technique to up-sample the data for the low-arousal and low-valence classes, thus balancing all classes of the training dataset.

5.2.6 Machine-learning models

The emotion-recognition task in this work is approached as two binary classification tasks. This is done by leveraging the arousal–valence theory of emotion. Hence, this task consists of binary classification of arousal and valence. As such, the experimental schemes can be stated as (i) low arousal versus high arousal, and (ii) low valence versus high valence. The feature matrix that is acquired from the PPG signal is then used to train five different ML models: a *K*-nearest neighbour model (*K*-NN), a support vector machine classifier (SVM), a decision tree, a random forest, and an XGBoost model. These models were trained and evaluated using fivefold stratified cross-validation. Stratification ensures that the distribution of the classes in all of the folds is the same. Ensuring this distribution means that the model should perform almost equally in all of the folds. Accordingly, the feature matrix was extracted from the DEAP database into five different folds and the models were trained five times; each time four folds were used for training, while the remaining one fold of data was used for testing. Then, the overall evaluation metrics were reported for each model. The five models trained in this work are listed below:

(I) ***K*-NN:** *K*-NN is a type of ML model that uses non-generalised learning. This means that it does not create a general internal model, rather it uses neighbouring points to classify the data. For new data, the distance is calculated for each neighbouring point. The one with the minimum distance is then examined and the new data is assigned the label which is most common in that neighbouring point. The biggest advantage of this model is that it is easy to implement and deploy. However, the biggest downfall is that with a higher number of features, the model will overfit.

(II) **SVM:** A SVM is a supervised learning algorithm where the model is trained using a symmetrical loss function. The SVM works by creating hyperplanes in a higher-dimensional space. This hyperplane allows for more accurate separation of the data. Its utilisation of various kernels allows for various adaptive decision boundaries. Furthermore, a SVM is very effective with large-dimensional data, i.e., feature matrices with a high number of features.

(III) **Decision tree:** A decision tree is a model that tries to predict the label by learning simple rules about its features. They can be seen as piece-wise function approximators. To this end, to create a decision tree that can model the relationship between features and labels, a greater depth for the trees are needed. Increasing the depth means more complex rules will be learned. This, however, sometimes causes the model to overfit as it tries to learn too much from the training data. However, the biggest pros of decision trees are that they are very easy to interpret. Furthermore, they do not require any feature normalisation or categorical encoding.

(IV) **Random forest:** A random forest is an ensemble of multiple decision trees. Here, multiple trees are created wherein each tree is trained on a slightly different training set, which is called a bootstrap sample. Along with that, each tree also only trains on a subset of features. These multiple trees will overfit their part of the training data. This ensures that each tree will emphasise different data and features. The subsampling of features and bootstrapping of data allows for a random forest to be trained in which the variance is low. This low variance yields a robust model.

(V) **XGBoost:** XGBoost is an ensemble model wherein multiple decision trees are used to predict the label. In XGBoost, multiple weak learners work together to create an overall robust model. Unlike the random forest ensemble, XGBoost tries to minimise both the bias and variance aspects of the model. The building of XGBoost is a sequential process where trees are added after each iteration. Furthermore, the model uses gradient descent (a technique that makes neural networks highly competent) to optimise the loss. These features together allow for the creation of a very robust model.

5.2.7 Evaluation criteria

In this work, five metrics are used to evaluate the model performance of the classifiers. Here 'TP', 'TN', 'FN', and 'FP' denote the number of true positives, true negatives, false negatives, and false positives, respectively. The five metrics are explained below:

(1) **Accuracy:** Accuracy is one of the basic metrics that is used to assess the performance of a classification model. Accuracy can be defined simply as the total number of correct guesses out of all the total samples. The metric is calculated using equation (5.1):

$$\text{Accuracy} = \frac{\text{TP} + \text{TN}}{\text{TP} + \text{TN} + \text{FP} + \text{FN}}. \tag{5.1}$$

(2) **Precision:** Precision is a metric that calculates how many positive classes were correctly classified out of all the predicted positive cases. This metric is

used to reduce the cases of false positives. This metric can be calculated using equation (5.2):

$$\text{Precision} = \frac{\text{TP}}{\text{TP} + \text{FP}}. \tag{5.2}$$

(3) **Recall:** Recall is a metric that calculates how many positive classes were correctly classified out of all the positive cases. This is very important in healthcare as in most cases it is imperative to not miss any positive cases. This metric can be calculated using equation (5.3):

$$\text{Recall} = \frac{\text{TP}}{\text{TP} + \text{FN}}. \tag{5.3}$$

(4) **F1 score:** The F1 score is a metric that takes into account both false positives and false negatives. It can be stated as a weighted average of precision and recall. This metric is especially important in assessing models with imbalanced datasets. This metric is calculated as shown in equation (5.4):

$$\text{F1 score} = 2 \times \frac{\text{Precision} \times \text{Recall}}{\text{Precision} + \text{Recall}} = \frac{2 \times \text{TP}}{2 \times \text{TP} + \text{FN} + \text{FP}}. \tag{5.4}$$

(5) **Receiver operating characteristic area under curve (ROC-AUC):** A ROC curve is a graph where the true-positive rate is plotted against the false-positive rate. The area under the curve is calculated to assess the performance of the model. The value of the ROC-AUC score ranges from 0.0 to 1.0, with 0.0 being the worst and 1.0 representing the best performance.

These five metrics were chosen based on evaluation criteria in the literature [33, 34]. The different models that were trained had their performance evaluated using these metrics. Following the literature on the classification of arousal and valence, the accuracy score is regarded as the top metric for the evaluation of the models.

5.3 Results and discussion

In this section, the results of the five different ML algorithms are given and their implications discussed. Table 5.3 shows the results of the binary classifiers for arousal and valence. In both cases, XGBoost outperforms all the other models by a large margin. *K*-NN, SVM, and the decision tree performed poorly in detecting high and low cases for arousal and valence. This is because these models are comparatively simpler when it comes to capturing the relationship between the predictors and labels. On the other hand, the random forest and XGBoost performed very well. The random forest uses many decision trees and forms an ensemble of their output to give predictions, and XGBoost uses a gradient descent to optimise the number of decision trees in the ensemble. Both are a type of ensemble model and hence can understand more complicated interactions between the features and labels. The

Table 5.3. Classification results for predicting arousal and valence.

Classifier	Accuracy	Precision	Recall	F1 Score	ROC-AUC
Arousal					
K-NN	62.77	66.13	62.77	63.53	68.15
SVM	60.83	64.90	60.83	61.64	66.47
Decision tree	66.90	67.90	66.90	67.27	65.36
Random forest	78.16	77.87	78.16	77.95	82.94
XGBoost	**81.03**	**80.87**	**81.03**	**80.47**	**85.76**
Valence					
K-NN	65.06	65.88	65.06	65.25	70.03
SVM	60.69	63.13	60.69	60.77	67.31
Decision tree	67.36	67.62	67.36	67.45	66.94
Random forest	78.75	78.66	78.75	78.64	85.82
XGBoost	**82.98**	**83.15**	**82.98**	**82.77**	**89.85**

The bold rows represent the best result.

XGBoost model performed the best in both cases. The hyperparameters for XGBoost have been obtained using Optuna. The best-performing XGBoost model had the following parameters: a 'learning_rate' of 0.027, 'reg_lambda' of 0.484, 'reg_alpha' of 0.0008, a subsample of 0.773, a 'colsample_bytree' of 0.948, 'max_depth' of 8, 'early_stopping_rounds' of 340 and 'n_estimators' of 7000. The other models had the following parameters:

- *K*-NN: *n_neighbors* = 5.
- SVM: *kernel* = 'rbf', *degree* = 3.
- Decision tree: *max_depth* = 8, *criterion* = Gini impurity.
- Random forest: *n_estimators* = 1000, *max_depth* = 10.

For binary classification of arousal, XGBoost achieved an accuracy of 81.03%, a precision of 80.87%, a recall of 81.03%, an F1 score of 80.47%, and a ROC-AUC score of 85.76%. Most of the metrics are above 80% and the ROC-AUC score was above 85%. For the classification of valence, XGBoost achieved an accuracy, precision, recall, F1 score, and ROC-AUC score of 82.98%, 83.15%, 82.98%, 82.77%, and 89.85%, respectively. In this case, the model achieved an excellent ROC-AUC of 90%.

Figure 5.7 depicts the ROC curves of the five models for the binary classification of arousal (figure 5.7(a)) and valence (figure 5.7(b)). The plots also include the calculated AUC. In the ROC curves, the true-positive rates are plotted against the false-positive rate.

As has been mentioned, ROC curves are important in diagnosing model performance of binary classifiers; the plots also include the calculated AUC. In ROC curves, the true-positive rates are plotted against the false-positive rate at different thresholds. Some manner, it could be seen as removing the signal from the noise. Further, the AUC of a ROC curve can be seen as an overall summarisation of the ROC curve. The AUC score represents the model's capability to separate the

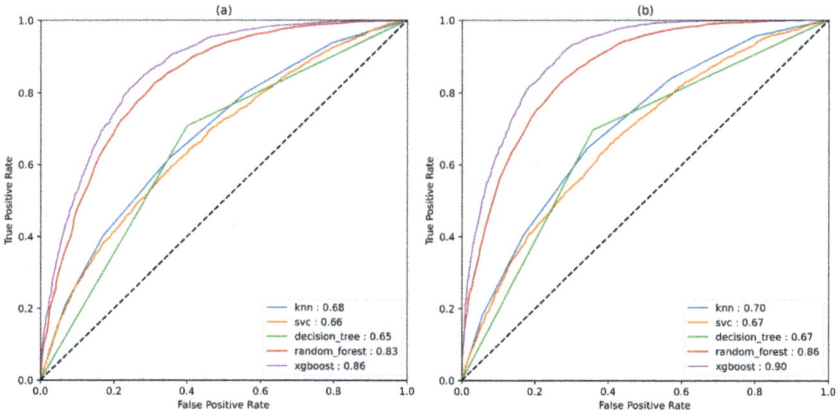

Figure 5.7. ROC curve for binary classification of (a) arousal, and (b) valence with AUC.

positive and negative classes. In our case, the positive class is high arousal/valence and the negative class is low arousal/valence. The ideal point of the ROC curve plot will be on the top-left corner of the graph. In that case, the model will have a 100% true-positive rate and a 0% false-positive rate: that is to say, all the positive instances will be predicted as positive and all the negative instances will be predicted as negative, and this model will have an AUC of 1. On the other hand, an AUC of 0 will mean that the model predicts all the positive instances as negative, and vice versa. When the AUC of a ROC curve is between 1 and 0.5, the model will have a good capability of differentiating between positive and negative samples. Most models' ROC curves fall in this zone as they predict more classes correctly than incorrectly. With an AUC of 0.5, the model is not able to separate the classes in any manner; the model is either predicting randomly or predicting one class repetitively. A '$y = x$' model is drawn to represent the performance of such a model. To summarise, it can be said that a higher ROC-AUC score gives a better performance and the model should lean towards the top-left of the graph as much as possible. Furthermore, ROC curves can be used to compare multiple models visually as the ROC-AUC score is a good indicator of a model's performance.

As depicted in figure 5.7(a), the curves of the XGBoost and random forest models tend more towards the top-left corner than the other three models. This is verified by the ROC-AUC scores of 0.83 and 0.86 attained by the random forest and XGBoost, respectively. The same pattern is seen in figure 5.7(b): XGBoost and random forest have the best performance, with curves that are close to the ideal curve, and ROC-AUC scores of 0.90 (XGBoost) and 0.86 (random forest).

Figure 5.8 depicts confusion matrices for the binary classification of arousal and valence for the best model (XGBoost). A confusion matrix is used to summarise the performance of a classifier, and is here used to visualise accuracy, precision, and recall. Furthermore, it can be used to directly compare the number of true positives, true negatives, false positives, and false negatives. In figure 5.8(a), a confusion matrix for arousal is shown. In this case, there are only 416 false negatives and 924 false positives. On the other hand, there are 4119 and 1605 true positives and true

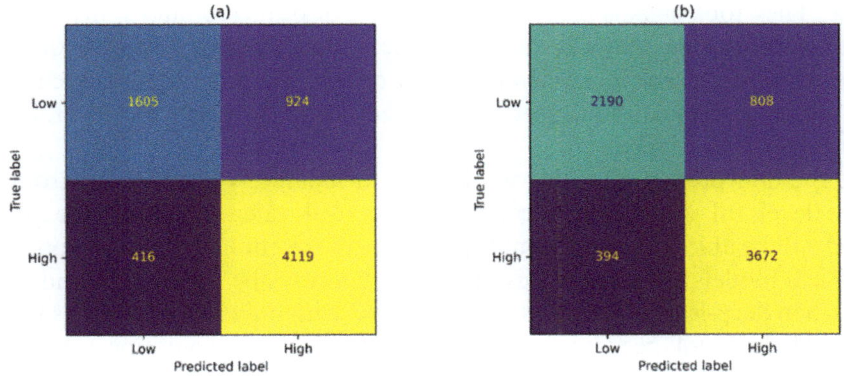

Figure 5.8. Confusion matrices for binary classification of (a) arousal, and (b) valence.

Table 5.4. Comparisons of classification accuracy and recognition intervals with previous studies utilising the DEAP database.

Authors	Year	Signal	Method	Windows length	Arousal (%)	Valence (%)
Lee *et al* [33]	2019	PPG	1D CNN	1.1 s	76.2	75.3
Lee *et al* [34]	2020	PPG	CNN	10 s	80.9	82.1
Lee *et al* [42]	2022	PPG and EMG	Sparse autoencoder	10 pulses	80.18	75.86
Proposed method	**2022**	**PPG**	**XGBoost**	**10 s**	**81.03**	**82.98**

negatives, respectively. In figure 5.8(b), a confusion matrix for the binary classification of valence is shown. For valence, the results contained 394 false negatives and 808 false positives. Furthermore, there were 3672 true positives and 2190 true negatives. In both cases, the models have a higher number of false positives compared to false negatives.

The use of different datasets and different choices of evaluation metrics makes a comparison between the reported performance of various research groups in the literature very difficult. In table 5.4, various works using the DEAP dataset are compared where they classified arousal and valence. Different research groups have utilised various physiological signals, which are all collected in the dataset.

Very few works have used PPG for emotion classification. Lee *et al* [33] used 1.1 s PPG signals for a fast emotion-recognition framework, whereas a CNN was used for emotion classification. They achieved a respectable accuracy of 76.2% and 75.3% for arousal and valence, respectively. In 2020, Lee *et al* [34] used a CNN with 10 s PPG signals to classify valence and arousal. Their work exhibited state-of-the-art performance for emotion classification using PPG, with an accuracy of 80.9% and 82.1% for arousal and valence, respectively. Lee *et al* [42] used a sparse autoencoder approach, where both PPG and EMG signals were inputted to classify arousal and valence. They took signals based on the number of beats (10 pulses) instead of time in seconds. With this, they were able to achieve an accuracy of 80.18% and 75.86% for arousal and valence, respectively. Our proposed method outperformed all these works utilising PPG, and attained an accuracy of 81.03% and 82.98% for arousal and valence, respectively.

The method presented in this work aims to separately classify the arousal and valence levels of a person. According to arousal–valence theory, the proposed method will be able to recognise multiple stages of the emotions of a person. The use of classical models means that this method will always be lightweight and easier to deploy then deep-learning models. Furthermore, with only PPG signals as the input, the model does not need any other data for emotion recognition. However, to further validate the method, additional data need to be collected. Subjects used should have variations in ethnicity, age, gender, etc. This will allow us to test the robustness of the model more rigorously.

5.4 Conclusion

In this chapter, the DEAP dataset was used to classify the emotions of 32 subjects. Arousal–valence space theory was used to formulate the emotion classification into the binary classification of arousal and valence. PPG signals were used for the classification tasks to leverage their availability and practicality in real-world applications. The signals were pre-processed, and features from the time domain, frequency domain, and statistical domain were extracted. Various ML models were trained in a fivefold cross-validation setting to ensure that a robust model was created. The trained models were examined using standard metrics, and the best model presented outperformed the state-of-the-art results in the literature. This work tries to emphasise the viability of using PPG signals for emotion classification, as PPG signals will allow easier implementation in wearable devices. Furthermore, by using classical ML models, the deployment package will be lightweight and hence will be less resource intensive. In our future work, a three-class approach could be used where emotions have low, medium and high levels instead of just low and high levels. This would allow us to explore more degrees of emotion in the subjects. Furthermore, a regression approach could also be used to predict the score for arousal and valence instead of just classifying them. The regression approach will allow us to get even more resolution in the degree of emotions. A multi-modal approach, wherein video data and PPG signals are combined, could also be used for emotion recognition. The variation in facial expression could provide another dimension for this classification task.

References

[1] Panksepp J 2004 *Affective Neuroscience: The Foundations of Human and Animal Emotions* (Oxford: Oxford University Press)

[2] Cabanac M 2002 What is emotion? *Behav. Process.* **60** 69–83

[3] Schacter D L, Gilbert D T and Wegner D M 2009 *Psychology* (London: Macmillan)

[4] Murugappan M, Baharuddin N Q I and Jerritta S 2012 DWT and MFCC based human emotional speech classification using LDA *2012 Int. Conf. on Biomedical Engineering (ICoBE) (Penang, Malaysia)* pp 203–6
[5] Lin Y-P *et al* 2010 EEG-based emotion recognition in music listening *IEEE Trans. Biomed. Eng.* **57** 1798–806
[6] Harms M B, Martin A and Wallace G L 2010 Facial emotion recognition in autism spectrum disorders: a review of behavioral and neuroimaging studies *Neuropsychol. Rev.* **20** 290–322
[7] Ali M *et al* 2018 Emotion recognition involving physiological and speech signals: a comprehensive review *Recent Advances in Nonlinear Dynamics and Synchronization Studies in Systems, Decision and Control* ed K Kyamakya, W Mathis, R Stoop, J Chedjou and Z Li (Cham: Springer) pp 287–302
[8] Wu C-H, Chuang Z-J and Lin Y-C 2006 Emotion recognition from text using semantic labels and separable mixture models *ACM Trans. Asian Lang. Inf. Process.* **5** 165–83
[9] Hönig F, Batliner A and Nöth E 2007 Real-time recognition of the affective user state with physiological signals *Affective Computing and Intelligent Interaction, Doctoral Consortium*, Lisbon, Portugal pp 1–8
[10] Cowie R *et al* 2001 Emotion recognition in human–computer interaction *IEEE Signal Process Mag.* **18** 32–80
[11] Lee C *et al* 2017 Soft robot review *Int. J. Control Autom. Syst.* **15** 3–15
[12] Russell J A 1980 A circumplex model of affect *J. Pers. Soc. Psychol.* **39** 1161
[13] Maruthapillai V and Murugappan M 2016 Optimal geometrical set for automated marker placement to virtualized real-time facial emotions *PLoS One* **11** e0149003
[14] Yoo G *et al* 2018 Emotion extraction based on multi bio-signal using back-propagation neural network *Multimed. Tools Appl.* **77** 4925–37
[15] Jerritta S *et al* 2013 Emotion detection from QRS complex of ECG signals using Hurst exponent for different age groups *2013 Humaine Association Conf. on Affective Computing and Intelligent Interaction, Geneva, Switzerland* pp 849–54
[16] Sim H, Lee W-H and Kim J-Y 2015 A study on emotion classification utilizing bio-signal (PPG, GSR, RESP) *Advanced Science and Technology Letters* 87 pp 73–7
[17] Domínguez-Jiménez J A *et al* 2020 A machine learning model for emotion recognition from physiological signals *Biomed. Signal Process. Control* **55** 101646
[18] Ibtehaz N and Japa Rahman M S 2020 PPG2ABP: translating photoplethysmogram (PPG) signals to arterial blood pressure (ABP) waveforms using fully convolutional neural networks *Bioeng. (Basel)* **15** 692
[19] Mahmud S *et al* 2022 A shallow U-Net architecture for reliably predicting blood pressure (BP) from photoplethysmogram (PPG) and electrocardiogram (ECG) signals *Sensors* **22** 919
[20] Wagner J, Kim J and André E 2005 From physiological signals to emotions: implementing and comparing selected methods for feature extraction and classification *2005 IEEE Int. Conf. on Multimedia and Expo. (Piscataway, NJ)* (IEEE) pp 940–43
[21] Jerritta S *et al* 2011 Physiological signals based human emotion recognition: a review *2011 IEEE 7th Int. Coll. on Signal Processing and Its Applications (Piscataway, NJ)* (IEEE) pp 410–15
[22] Maithri M *et al* 2022 Automated emotion recognition: current trends and future perspectives *Computer Methods and Programs in Biomedicine* **215** 106646
[23] Liu Y, Sourina O and Nguyen M K 2011 Real-time EEG-based emotion recognition and its applications *Trans. on Computational Science XII* (Berlin: Springer) pp 256–77

[24] S. Jerritta M *et al* 2014 Emotion recognition from facial EMG signals using higher order statistics and principal component analysis *J. Chin. Inst. Eng.* **37** 385–94

[25] Li C, Xu C and Feng Z 2016 Analysis of physiological for emotion recognition with the IRS model *Neurocomputing* **178** 103–11

[26] Kim J and André E 2008 Emotion recognition based on physiological changes in music listening *IEEE Trans. Pattern Anal. Mach. Intell.* **30** 2067–83

[27] Giakoumis D *et al* 2011 Automatic recognition of boredom in video games using novel biosignal moment-based features *IEEE Trans. Affect. Comput.* **2** 119–33

[28] Wang X-W, Nie D and Lu B-L 2014 Emotional state classification from EEG data using machine learning approach *Neurocomputing* **129** 94–106

[29] Jenke R, Peer A and Buss M 2014 Feature extraction and selection for emotion recognition from EEG *IEEE Trans. Affect. Comput.* **5** 327–39

[30] Mert A and Akan A 2018 Emotion recognition from EEG signals by using multivariate empirical mode decomposition *Pattern Anal. Appl.* **21** 81–9

[31] Hassan M M *et al* 2019 Human emotion recognition using deep belief network architecture *Inf. Fusion* **51** 10–8

[32] Dar M N *et al* 2022 EEG-based emotion charting for Parkinson's disease patients using convolutional recurrent neural networks and cross dataset learning *Comput. Biol. Med.* **144** 105327

[33] Lee M S *et al* 2019 Fast emotion recognition based on single pulse PPG signal with convolutional neural network *Appl. Sci.* **9** 3355

[34] Lee M *et al* 2020 Emotion recognition using convolutional neural network with selected statistical photoplethysmogram features *Appl. Sci.* **10** 3501

[35] Rakshit R, Reddy V R and Deshpande P 2016 Emotion detection and recognition using HRV features derived from photoplethysmogram signals *Proc. 2nd Workshop on Emotion Representations and Modelling for Companion Systems* pp 1–6

[36] Lazarus R S, Speisman J C and Mordkoff A M 1963 The relationship between autonomic indicators of psychological stress: heart rate and skin conductance *Psychosom. Med.* **25** 19–30

[37] Park M W *et al* 2013 Individual emotion classification between happiness and sadness by analyzing photoplethysmography and skin temperature *2013 4th World Congress on Software Engineering (Piscataway, NJ)* (IEEE)

[38] Li F *et al* 2017 Differences in photoplethysmography morphological features and feature time series between two opposite emotions: happiness and sadness**18** 7–13

[39] Goshvarpour A and Goshvarpour A 2020 Evaluation of novel entropy-based complex wavelet sub-bands measures of PPG in an emotion recognition system *J. Med. Biol. Eng.* **40** 451–61

[40] Goshvarpour A and Goshvarpour A 2018 Poincaré's section analysis for PPG-based automatic emotion recognition *Chaos Solitons Fractals* **114** 400–7

[41] Wang S-W and Yu S-N 2021 Emotion recognition based on photoplethysmography using ResNet and BiLSTM networks *2021 Int. Conf. on e-Health and Bioengineering (EHB) (Piscataway, NJ)* (IEEE)

[42] Lee Y K *et al* 2022 Emotion recognition with short-period physiological signals using bimodal sparse autoencoders *Intelligent Automation & Soft Computing* **32** 657–73

[43] Koelstra S *et al* 2011 DEAP: a database for emotion analysis; using physiological signals *IEEE Trans. on Affective Computing* **3** 18–31

[44] Chatterjee A and Roy U K 2018 PPG based heart rate algorithm improvement with Butterworth IIR filter and Savitzky–Golay FIR filter *2018 2nd Int. Conf. on Electronics, Materials Engineering and Nano-Technology (IEMENTech) (Piscataway, NJ)* (IEEE) pp 1–6

[45] Wang Y and Markert R J S P 2016 Filter bank property of variational mode decomposition and its applications *Signal Processing* **120** 509–21

[46] Shuzan M N I *et al* 2021 A novel non-invasive estimation of respiration rate from motion corrupted photoplethysmograph signal using machine learning model *IEEE Access* **9** 96775–90

[47] Hossain M S *et al* 2022 Motion artifacts correction from EEG and fNIRS signals using novel multiresolution analysis *IEEE Access* **10** 29760–77

[48] Hossain M S *et al* 2022 Motion artifacts correction from single-channel EEG and fNIRS signals using novel wavelet packet decomposition in combination with canonical correlation analysis *Sensors* **22** 3169

[49] Chowdhury M E *et al* 2019 Real-time smart-digital stethoscope system for heart diseases monitoring *Sensors* **19** 2781

[50] Chowdhury M H *et al* 2020 Estimating blood pressure from the photoplethysmogram signal and demographic features using machine learning techniques *Sensors* **20** 3127

[51] Chowdhury M E *et al* 2019 Wearable real-time heart attack detection and warning system to reduce road accidents *Sensors* **19** 2780

[52] Velliangiri S and Alagumuthukrishnan S J P C S 2019 A review of dimensionality reduction techniques for efficient computation *Procedia Computer Science* **165** 104–11

[53] Chawla N V *et al* 2002 SMOTE: synthetic minority over-sampling technique *J. Artificial Intelligence Research* **16** 321–57

[54] Haque F *et al* 2022 Evaluating performance of machine learning models for diabetic sensorimotor polyneuropathy severity classification using biomechanical signals during gait arXiv:2205.10581

Chapter 6

EEG-based human emotion classification from channel-wise feature extraction and feature selection

Lucky Odirile Mohutsiwa and Rodrigo S Jamisola Jr

This chapter focuses on the use of electroencephalogram (EEG) signals to classify human emotions by performing both feature extraction and feature selection for each channel of an Emotiv Epoc+ headset. For feature extraction, we use Shannon entropy, log energy entropy, differential asymmetry, and rational asymmetry. For feature selection, we only use one method, that is, a minimum redundancy and maximum relevance algorithm. The features for each channel give higher emotion classification accuracy (CA) compared to multi-channel features (MCFs) because they give more information per channel. We classify five emotions, namely, amused, sad, neutral, scared, and anger, using two supervised machine-learning algorithms, a random forest (RF) and a long short-term recurrent neural network (LSTM RNN). We perform a 14-channel EEG brain signal experiment with six subjects, four males and two females, aged 19–35, using a 12 min video stimulus to elicit the desired five human emotions. We process the signal data in terms of channel-wise features (CWFs) and compare them against the MCFs. We achieve a maximum CA for the LSTM RNN of 83.80% (CWF) and 36.00% (MCF), and for the RF of 54.90% (CWF) and 39.90% (MCF). Next, we repeat the same process to verify our proposed approach using a publicly available human emotion dataset, SEED-IV. In this dataset, we achieve a maximum CA for the LSTM RNN of 99.80% (CWF and MCF), and for the RF of 48.0% (CWF) and 46.1% (MCF). The results show that using channel-wise signal data processing retained feature information per channel necessary for achieving better accuracy. We conclude that this approach can be used in healthcare facilities to more accurately and quickly diagnose the emotional status of patients using their biophysical signals, and thereby deter any health problems that undetected emotions would have caused.

doi:10.1088/978-0-7503-5182-9ch6

6.1 Introduction

Affective computing is described as the process of developing systems and devices that can detect and respond to various human emotions. The application of such devices in healthcare can be instrumental to medical practitioners, who need to diagnose the emotional states of their patients accurately. In such cases, some patients may be unable to verbally express their true emotions or may provide misleading information. It is imperative to diagnose the emotional status of patients, as studies have shown that some emotions, such as stress, can cause physical and mental health problems (Dalton and Hammen 2018). It is particularly important to diagnose the emotions of members of the armed forces, serving in the military, due to their stressful work environment, which can lead soldiers to develop depression due to chronic stress, and which may also be detrimental to their physical health; some may even develop suicidal thoughts (Tokuno *et al* 2011). In recent times, the so-called affective brain–computer interface (ABCI) has received increasing amounts of attention, which entails building machines or robots that can detect and respond to human feelings (Mühl *et al* 2014). The technology is inspired by a sudden rise of humanoid robots that serve as home assistants. ABCI intends to give such robots the ability to discern human emotions and respond accordingly without the person's instruction or interference. A possible example of such is when a person is stressed, a humanoid assistant robot can make them a cup of coffee or bring them some medication to avoid any health consequences. Many types of research have been conducted to advance affective computing and the ABCI to make it a reality. However, there are still many problems concerning the ethics of the ABCI (Steinert and Friedrich 2020), and even the methods of processing affective data have not been agreed upon by researchers (Hu *et al* 2019). Some researchers, such as Sarkar and Etemad (2020) and Dissanayake *et al* (2019), have used electrocardiograph (ECG) data to estimate human affects, while most other researchers propose using electroencephalographic data (EEG) (Zheng *et al* 2015, Suhaimi *et al* 2020). Furthermore, these biophysical signals are prone to noise, interference, and artefacts from other biophysical signals. To this effect, researchers have proposed various methods to denoise these signals and remove artefacts. The extraction of informative and salient features has also posed a major challenge to estimating human affects using biophysical signals. In the case of using EEG signals of brain activity to infer human affects, the features can either be extracted from individual channels or a data segment with multiple channels. The difference between these feature-extraction approaches has not been well explored in terms of their comparison and how they affect the classification accuracies (CAs) of machine-learning models. Furthermore, there is a need to use a limited number of EEG channels in the acquisition of the necessary information in order to classify the different human emotions. This is important because it reduces computational time and enhances the performance of real-time classification of human emotions.

In this chapter, we make two contributions to the classification of human emotions using EEG data. The first contribution is a quantitative comparison between channel-wise features (CWFs) and multi-channel features (MCFs). We claim this contribution because, according to our research, no work yet has experimentally compared the performance of CWFs and MCFs. In this study, we have experimented to investigate the difference between adopting CWFs and MCFs when inferring human emotions from EEG signals. Our second claim of contribution is towards the selection of a good combination of off-the-shelf feature-extraction and feature-selection tools, which results in improved CAs for the CWFs. These carefully selected tools entail Shannon entropy, log energy entropy, differential asymmetry (DASM), rational asymmetry (RASM), and the minimum redundancy and maximum relevance (mRMR) algorithm. In the classification step, we used two supervised machine-learning classifiers, namely, a long short-term memory recurrent neural network (LSTM RNN) at 83.80% (CWF) and 36.00% (MCF) accuracy, and a random forest (RF) at 54.90% (CWF) and 39.90% (MCF) accuracy. The previous studies that are closest to our work are those of Jin and Kim (2020) and Chao *et al* (2020), who used EEG signals to classify human emotions. In the former study, the authors achieved a maximum accuracy of 99.63% from CWFs using the DEAP and SEED datasets. In our study, we achieved a maximum accuracy of 99.80% from CWFs using a public database, SEED-IV. The authors in Chao *et al* (2020) used MCFs, and achieved a maximum accuracy of 71.70% in the arousal dimension and 69.96% for the valence dimension using their experimental dataset, while we achieved an accuracy of 83.80% using our experimental dataset with CWFs. This further supports our claim that CWFs yield higher EEG-based human emotions CAs than MCFs.

Historically, entropy has proved to be more effective in tracing informative patterns in EEG data that result in higher CAs, as shown by the well-cited study of Kannathal *et al* (2005). Entropy is concerned with the measure of diversity/uniformity that is available in a dataset and can help to give more information about an EEG dataset. Studies have also shown that entropy truly reflects the intra-cortical information flow in an EEG dataset. mRMR methods select prominent features from the entire feature set that have a strong correlation with the classification variable. The selected features are mutually different from each other whilst contributing maximally to the classification variable. This method has been proven to be very effective in selecting both EEG and non-EEG features, as shown by the authors in Peng *et al* (2005). Similarly, a LSTM RNN has been used by many researchers in EEG classification and has proven better able to yield higher accuracies in both motor imagery brain–computer interface (MI-BCI) applications and emotion recognition. This method solves the problem of long-term dependence by using gated LSTM cells that control which information must be remembered and which forgotten. The effectiveness of LSTM RNNs for EEG-based human emotion recognition is well attested to in another well-cited work (Alhagry *et al* 2017). These findings from the related literature serve as our justification for selecting these tools for feature extraction (Shannon entropy, log energy entropy, DASM, and RASM), feature selection (mRMR), and classification (LSTM RNN).

6.2 Related literature

6.2.1 Affective computing

Affective computing is a field of study that is concerned with the development of systems or devices that are capable of eliciting, recognising, and classifying various human affects. Researchers have investigated the use of affective computing and the BCI in the combined field of the ABCI (Steinert and Friedrich 2020). This field of study has received increasing attention in recent years as more researchers gravitate towards building machines or robots that can discern human emotions and respond accordingly. Many studies have been conducted around the topic of affective computing, and they mostly agree that it is key to understanding human behaviour and might have an influence on human intelligence (Tao and Tan 2005). Other researchers, such as Kaliouby *et al* (2006), have studied the possibilities of using affective computing to assist people with autism by modifying technology such that they would have a better socio-emotional experience. Researchers have explored various biophysical signals, such as ECGs and EEGs, to accurately detect and distinguish different human affects (Assabumrungrat *et al* 2022, Alqahtani *et al* 2019, Siddharth *et al* 2019).

6.2.2 Brain–computer interface devices

In this subsection, we review various brain–computer devices that have been used to harness EEG signals classifying human affects. Since the emergence of non-invasive dry electrodes, EEG headsets have been mostly used to record signals of brain activity from the person's scalp (Kam *et al* 2019). Many commercial consumer-grade EEG headsets are affordable and specifically designed for research purposes. Emotiv is one of the leading producers of brain data recording hardware. They specialised in manufacturing portable, easy-to-use, and high-quality non-invasive EEG headsets that are used for research purposes (Gao *et al* 2020). Some studies have used the five-channel Emotiv insight headset in their human emotion study experiments (González-Hernández *et al* 2018). The five channels are AF3, AF4, T7, T8, and Pz, recording EEG signals at a 128 Hz sampling frequency. A nine-axis inertial measurement unit (IMU) records the movement of the head on the x-axis, y-axis, and z-axis, sampled at 32 Hz. An advanced version of this headset, which has additional useful features such as improved battery life, radio connectivity, and others, is priced at $499.00.

A 14-channel Emotiv headset is widely used in human emotions and MI-BCI studies (Mohutsiwa and Jamisola 2021, Chowdhury *et al* 2014, Malete *et al* 2019, Jatupaiboon *et al* 2013). The 14 channels are AF3, F7, F3, FC5, T7, P7, O1, O2, P8, T8, FC6, F4, F8, and AF4, which are arranged in a 10–20 standard. This headset records EEG signals at a 128 Hz sampling frequency and possesses a nine-axis IMU, operating at 32 Hz. Work carried out by Stytsenko *et al* (2011) evaluated the performance and quality of the 14-channel Emotiv epoc neuro-headset, and they found that it acquires high-quality EEG data. Currently, the headset is priced at $849.00.

The last product from Emotiv is a wireless epoc+ flex neuro-headset with 32 electrode sensors, which can either be saline sensors or gel sensors. This headset is mostly used in MI-BCI and makes use of the EasyCap system, which is configurable according to the 10–20 standard (Williams *et al* 2020). In MI-BCI, most of the electrodes are centred around the sensory-motor cortex of the brain to effectively record motor imagery signals, while the other electrodes can optionally be removed. The 32 channels are Cz, Fz, Fp1, F7, F3, FC1, C3, FC5, FT9, T7, CP5, CP1, P3, P7, PO9, O1, Pz, Oz, O2, PO10, P8, P4, CP2, CP6, and T8, which record EEG signals at 128 Hz sampling frequency. The headsets are priced at $1699.00 for the saline sensor and $2099.00 for the gel sensor headset. All three consumer-grade Emotiv headsets use the EmotivPro software as a recording medium and for storing raw EEG signals.

Other studies have used research-grade neuro-headsets to record brain signals for human emotion studies. Here, we review EEG headsets used to record high-quality EEG data for the two most used public databases for human emotion, the DEAP and SEED-IV datasets. For the DEAP dataset, a 48-channel BioSemi headset was used to record EEG signals at a 512 Hz sampling frequency (Koelstra *et al* 2011). A 62-channel ESI Neuroscan system was used to record human emotion signals for the SEED-IV dataset (Zheng *et al* 2018, Zheng *et al* 2015).

6.2.3 Elicitation of human emotions

According to studies, basic human emotions can be categorised according to a two-dimensional model or a three-dimensional model, as shown in figures 6.1 and 6.2. In the former, emotions are represented in terms of valence and arousal. The valence dimension distinguishes positive emotions and negative emotions, while the arousal dimension scales emotions from low arousal to high arousal (Sokolov 2018). The three-dimensional model categorises emotions in terms of valence, arousal, and dominance, where the dominance dimension quantifies the amount of control a person has on those emotions (Torres *et al* 2020). The dominance dimension ranges from submissive (no control) to dominant (in full control). To elicit these emotions, the most commonly used stimuli are video clips (Koelstra *et al* 2011), music (Er *et al* 2021), and pictures (Croy *et al* 2011). Other researchers have explored the use of

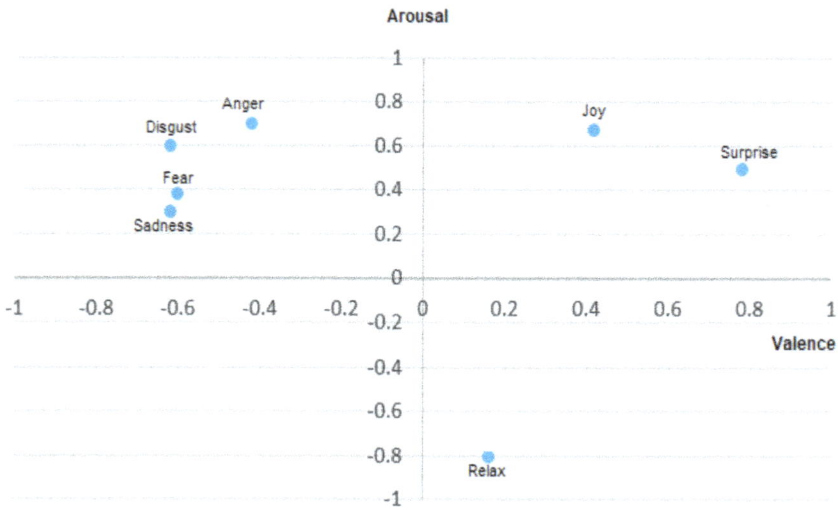

Figure 6.1. A two-dimensional human emotion model. This model categorises human emotions into valence and arousal. Reproduced from Torres *et al* (2020). CC BY 4.0.

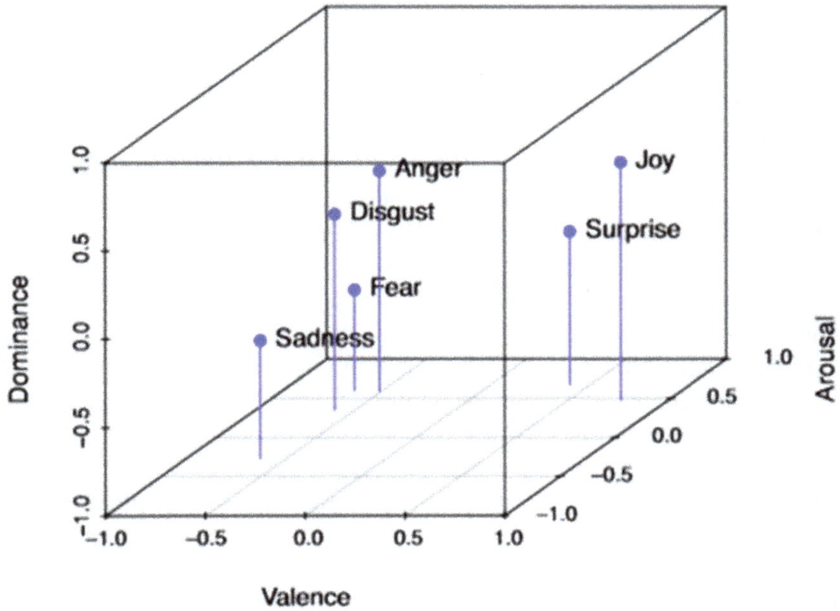

Figure 6.2. A three-dimensional human emotion model. In addition to the two-dimensional model shown in figure 6.1, this model adds a third dimension, dominance, which entails the amount of control that a person has on a particular emotion. Reproduced from Torres *et al* (2020). CC BY 4.0.

imagination, where subjects are asked to recall their experiences that had elicited certain emotions (Iacoviello *et al* 2015). Studies such as Marín-Morales *et al* (2018) have explored the use of virtual reality stimuli to evoke emotions in subjects (Zhang *et al* 2017). However, studies have shown that video stimuli are more effective than others since they engage the sense of hearing, seeing, and in some cases imagination.

6.2.4 Pre-processing methods

Pre-processing is the first step after the data have been recorded in the experimental setting. Usually, the data are band-pass filtered to attenuate any data that is outside the desired frequencies (Rahman *et al* 2021). The data can then be downsampled into low and workable frequencies such as 128 Hz. They are then segmented into small manageable chunks, or data pockets, with the desired window size. Each epoc + that is recorded during human emotion experiments contains low-power noise from power line interference, instrumental noise, head movements, and artefacts such as electromyogram, electrooculogram, and ECG artefacts, among others. Therefore, there is a huge need to filter this data. The most used method for artefact removal is independent component analysis, as used by the authors in (Bhardwaj *et al* 2015). Other methods, such as common average reference (Yazdani *et al* 2009), Laplacian (Khalili and Moradi 2009), and average mean referencem, are additionally often used as part of pre-processing pipelines (Alarcão and Fonseca 2019).

6.2.5 Feature extraction

Researchers have typically extracted either time-domain, frequency-domain, time–frequency, or entropy features during the analysis of human emotions using EEG signals (Rahman *et al* 2021, Jenke *et al* 2014, Chawla *et al* 2023). In the time domain, authors have explored event-related potentials (Ding *et al* 2017), Hjorth parameters (activity, mobility, and complexity) (Yuen *et al* 2009), statistical parameters (mean, skewness, kurtosis, and others) (Yuen *et al* 2009), and high-order crossings (Bastos-Filho *et al* 2012, Ackermann *et al* 2016). In the frequency domain, methods such as power spectral density, common spatial pattern, and band power have been used to extract informative features; in addition, some authors have explored DASM and RASM, in which they find the difference and ratio of the powers of asymmetrical channels (Nawaz *et al* 2020). Time–frequency methods include wavelet transform, as explored by the authors in Murugappan *et al* (2009). Entropy features include Shannon entropy, sample entropy, log energy entropy, permutation entropy, spectral entropy, and single-value decomposition entropy (Nawaz *et al* 2020, Chen *et al* 2018).

6.2.6 Feature selection

Feature selection involves selecting the most important features while discarding the least important and redundant ones from a high-dimensional feature set (Jenke *et al* 2014). This process helps to address issues of overfitting machine-learning models during classification, hence maximising the CAs of the machine-learning models. Researchers have used feature-selection algorithms such as mRMR in multi-classification (Peng *et al* 2005), while ReliefF (Zhang *et al* 2017) has been used for binary classification. Principal component analysis was used by previous researchers (Zheng *et al* 2017) to reduce the dimensions of a given feature set.

6.2.7 Machine-learning classification

After feature selection, the last step is to train a machine-learning model that can classify the different emotions from an unseen dataset. Researchers have used traditional supervised machine-learning models such as support vector machines (Gupta *et al* 2018), decision trees (Qing *et al* 2019), naïve Bayes classifiers, logistic regression, *K*-nearest neighbours (Liu *et al* 2018), and RFs (Gupta *et al* 2018), as well as neural network models such as RNNs, convolutional recurrent neural network (CRNN) (Yang *et al* 2018), LSTM RNNs (Acharya *et al* 2020), deep belief networks (Hassan *et al* 2019), and dynamical graph neural networks (Song *et al* 2018).

6.3 Methodology

In this work, we propose a method of classifying human affects using EEG signals by using channel-wise or single-channel feature extraction. Figure 6.3 illustrates the steps in our methodology. The first step in our methodology is to prepare our input datasets, for which we used experimental data and the publicly available SEED-IV human emotions dataset. The data are pre-processed by filtering with a notch filter

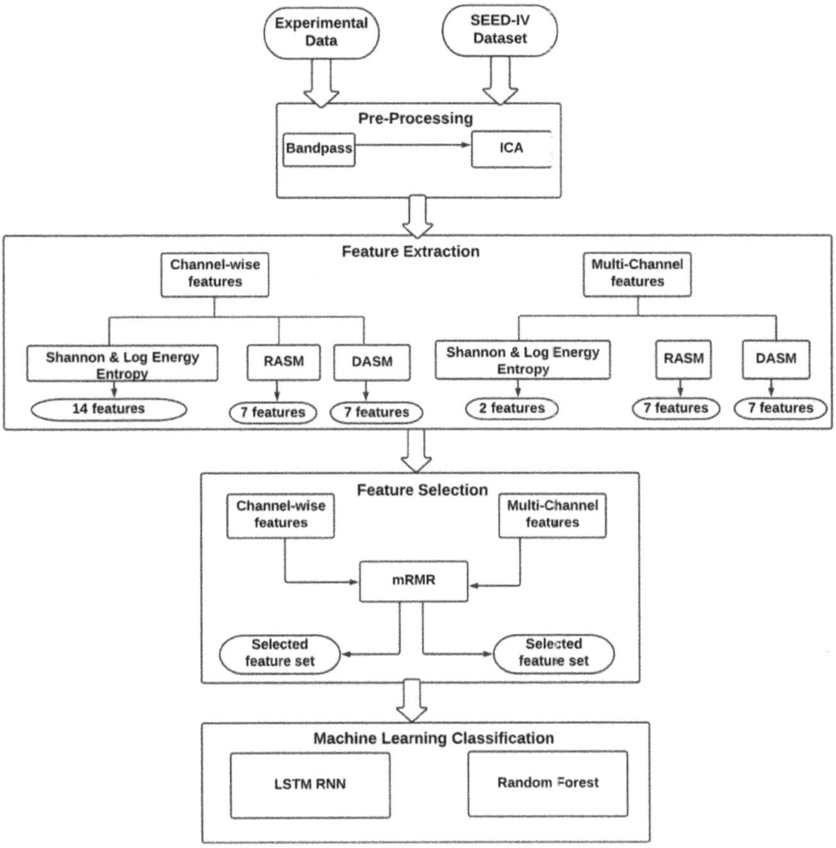

Figure 6.3. Flow chart showing detailed flow of the steps taken in our methodology.

and artefacts removed using independent component analysis (ICA). The filtered data is put through a processing pipeline, where the salient features are extracted. We extract features from individual EEG channels (CWF extraction) and from a data segment with all channels (MCFs). Next, the mRMR algorithm is used to select the most important features from the CWFs and MCFs. Lastly, we use the trained and tested LSTM RNN and RF supervised machine-learning models to classify five human emotions from our experimental data and four emotions from the SEED-IV dataset.

6.3.1 The experiment and experimental data

Our experimental setting consisted of three major components: a stimulus, a brain–computer interface device (BCI), and human subjects. We here used a video as our stimulus to elicit emotions of interest from our subjects. Various video clips from movie scenes and YouTube videos were put together strategically to elicit amused, sad, scared, neutral, and disgusted human emotions. Figure 6.4 shows how the emotion-eliciting video clips were arranged throughout their duration. The video starts with a relaxing clip of flowing water in a stream, which attempts to put the

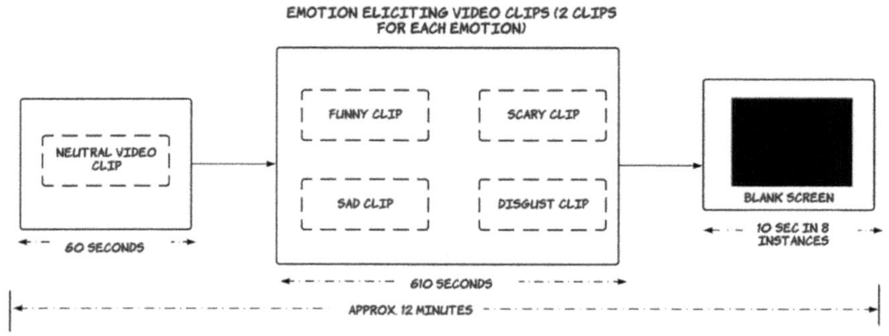

Figure 6.4. Flow chart showing the arrangement of scenes in the stimulus video clip. The emotion-eliciting scenes appeared on the screen in random order.

subject into a neutral state. After 20 s, another potential emotion-eliciting video clip appears on the screen. There is a 10 s break in between the clips, represented by a blank screen. The process repeats for sad, scared, amused, and disgusted emotions for 610 s in total, including the breaks.

We used a 14-channel Emotiv headset as a BCI device to harness EEG signals of brain activity from our subjects. The headset was configured at a 128 Hz sampling rate. The 14 channels are AF3, AF4, F3, F4, F7, F8, FC5, FC6, P7, P8, T7, T8, O1, and O2, arranged in a 10–20 standard. Six (four males and two females) healthy subjects with no reported history of any brain disease volunteered in our experiment. They were aged between 19 and 35 years old. We clearly explained the mission of the experiment to them, and they signed a consent form to agree with the terms of the experiment.

At the beginning of the experiment, a subject was set on a comfortable chair in front of a monitor. We placed a BCI headset on their head and achieved a good contact quality of 80% between the electrodes and the scalp. We recorded raw EEG data using the EmotivPro software whilst the subject watched the emotion-eliciting video clips.

6.3.1.1 Experimental data

At the end of the experiment, we obtained a raw EEG dataset for six subjects. For each subject, we obtained 85 760 samples (670 × 128, sampling rate) and a total of 514 569 data samples for all six subjects. Because we used a headset with 14 channels, the final dataset formed a matrix of 514 569 (samples) and 14 (channels), and each value in the matrix indicated the voltage fluctuations, in microvolts, that were recorded on the subjects' scalp. We used a 4 s Hanning window to segment the data into 1000 small portions. The durations of the emotion-eliciting clips in our stimulus video were used as event markers to label the segments into corresponding emotions.

6.3.1.2 SEED-IV dataset

In addition, we used a public multi-modal human emotion dataset, known as SEED-IV. In this dataset, 72 film clips from Chinese movies were carefully selected to elicit four emotions, which were happy, neutral, fear, and sad. In their experiment, each subject participated in three sessions with 24 trials for each session, which were conducted on different days. Figure 6.5 shows the schedule diagram of each trial.

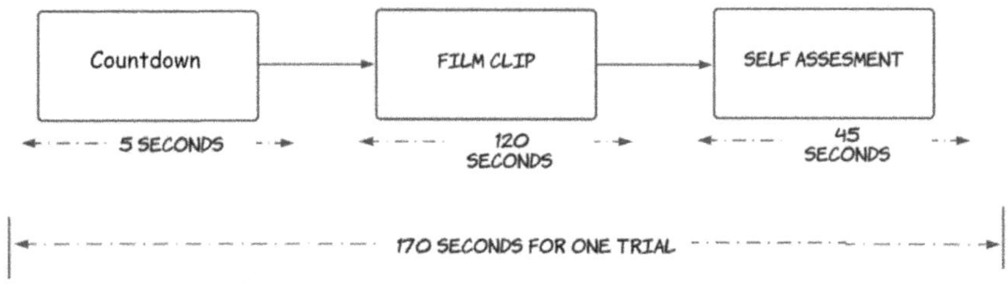

Figure 6.5. Flow chart showing the procedure to elicit human emotions in a single trial of the SEED-IV experiment.

In each trial, the experiment began with a 5 s countdown displayed on the monitor, followed by a 2 min emotion-eliciting video clip, and ending with a 45 s self-assessment, which served as feedback information. In our study, we only used data acquired in session one. Similarly, we divided the data into 4 s segments to ease processing. The SEED-IV dataset utilised a 62-channel ESI NeuroScan System. It It is composed of 15 subjects (seven males and eight females) with no reported history of any neurological disorder.

6.3.2 Pre-processing

Frequencies between 0.1 Hz and 60 Hz were extracted from raw EEG segments using a band-pass filter in MATLAB. We attenuated the signals that were below or above the band-pass cut-off frequencies. In addition, we used ICA to remove biophysical artefacts generated by eye blinks, muscle movement, heartbeats, and others. ICA is a solution to the blind-source separation problem, whereby useful information is extracted from a mix of source data and noisy data with little information about the nature of the source data. The ICA formula is defined by

$$S = Wx, \tag{6.1}$$

where W is an unmixing matrix that separates source data from a mixture of signals, and S and x represent the source and the mixed data, respectively. In our application, x represents the raw EEG signals containing many biophysical artefacts. We used the ICA algorithm in the EEGLAB software to find the unmixing matrix W and consequently computed the source or original EEG signal S using the equation. In addition, the implementation of ICA in the EEGLAB software allows the mapping of independent components into a human scalp for further analysis. Each independent component can be assessed depending on the quantity of data that was measured coming from the brain. Those independent components whose majority of data comes from other parts of the human body can be marked as artefacts to be rejected, as shown in figure 6.6.

6.3.3 Feature extraction

In the feature-extraction step, we used methods that would trace salient and informative traits in the data. We extracted these features from individual EEG channels to form a

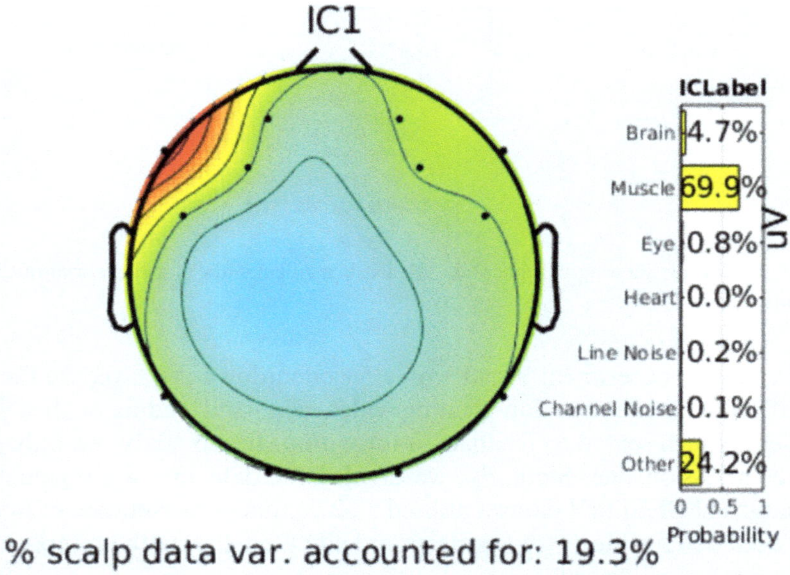

Figure 6.6. Independent component analysis (IC1) showing the quantities of data that are coming from the brain and other parts of the body. Since most of the data originate from the muscles, this independent component can be marked as an artefact to be rejected.

feature set with 14 CWFs. At the same time, we also extracted the features from the entire data segment to form a MCF set. We employed Shannon entropy, log energy entropy, DASM, and RASM as feature-extraction methods. Due to the complexity and non-stationary nature of EEG signals when the subject is awake, Shannon entropy is ideal to quantify the degree of complexity in the time-series EEG data by measuring the uncertainty of a probability distribution. Log energy entropy is also proven to be very effective in tracing information in EEG signals, as shown in well-cited literature (Das and Bhuiyan 2016). For DASM and RASM, studies have shown that the left and right symmetries of the human brain have a relation to positive and negative emotions, respectively (Davidson and Fox 1982).

6.3.3.1 *Entropy features*

Entropy is a measure of the disorder in the dataset, and hence it can give an insight into how much information is available within that dataset. Shannon entropy is a measure of the uncertainty of a probability distribution. It is given by formula (6.2):

$$E_{\text{sh}}(x) = -\sum_{i=0}^{N-1} (p_i(x))^2 \left(\log_2(p_i(x))\right)^2, \tag{6.2}$$

where p_i is the probability distribution, and x is a discrete data source of interest with N samples. In addition, we also extracted the log energy entropy using formula (6.3):

$$E_{\text{Log Energy}} = -\sum_{i=0}^{N-1}\left(\log_2(p_i(x))\right)^2. \tag{6.3}$$

6.3.3.2 Entropy asymmetry features

In addition to entropy features, we also extracted DASM features and RASM features. These features are measured with the difference and ratio of the differential entropy (DE) of a symmetrical pair of channels, respectively. For a continuous random dataset X, the DE, $h(X)$, is given by (6.4)

$$\text{DE} = h(X) = \int_{-\infty}^{\infty} f(x)\log\left(\frac{1}{f(x)}\right)\mathrm{d}x, \tag{6.4}$$

where $f(x)$ is a probability density function. If X is time-domain data that obey a Gaussian distribution $N(\mu, \sigma^2)$, the DE becomes (6.5)

$$\text{DE}_{\text{time domain}} = h(X) = \frac{1}{2}\log(2\pi e\sigma 2). \tag{6.5}$$

In DASM, we calculated the difference in the absolute DE of an asymmetrical pair of channels. For our 14-channel Emotiv Epoc headset, we obtained seven DASM features from the pairs AF3-AF4, F3-F4, F7-F8, FC5-FC6, T7-T8, P7-P8, and O1-O2. Similarly, for RASM we calculated the DE of the ratio of these pairs, e.g., the ratio of the DE of AF3 and AF4, the DE of the ratio of the F3 and F4, and so on. These are illustrated by the equations below:

$$\text{DASM}_j = h\left(X_{j-}{}^{\text{left}}\right) - h\left(X_{j+}{}^{\text{right}}\right), \tag{6.6}$$

$$\text{RASM}_j = \frac{h\left(X_{j-}{}^{\text{left}}\right)}{h\left(X_{j+}{}^{\text{right}}\right)}, \tag{6.7}$$

where j^- and j^+ are the left and the right channels in a single pair, for instance the pair of AF3 (j^-) and AF4 (j^+). The variable j represents the number of channel pairs; in our case, with a 14-channel headset, this variable ranges from 1 to 7.

6.3.3.3 Channel-wise vs multi-channel feature extraction

In the CWF extraction method, we extracted all these features from individual channels to obtain a feature set with dimensions m by n, where m represents the total number of samples for all data segments and n signifies the channels that serve as the columns or features for our feature set. Figure 6.7 shows an illustration of the CWFs table. Each entity represents the entropy calculated at each channel in the raw data segment. In addition to the channel features, we extended the dimension of our feature set to include DASM and RASM features. For our experimental dataset and single features, we obtained a feature set with 28 features. In the case of the SEED-IV dataset, which had 62 channels, we obtained 124 features. In the case of MCFs, we extracted two entropy features, Shannon entropy and log energy entropy, from

Data segments		Chan 1	...	Chan 14
seg. 1	Shan. Entropy			
	Log En. Entropy			
seg. 2	Shan. Entropy			
	Log En. Entropy			
...	...			
	...			
seg. n	Shan. Entropy			
	Log En. Entropy			

Figure 6.7. Illustration of the features table in the CWF extraction method. Each cell entity represents a feature value of a particular channel in a particular data segment.

Data segments	Shan.Entropy	Log En. Entropy
seg. 1		
seg. 2		
...		
seg. n		

Figure 6.8. Illustration of the features table in the MCF extraction method. Each cell entity represents a feature value for the entire data segment.

the entire data segment, as shown in figure 6.8. In addition to these two features, we also added DASM and RASM features. We obtained 16 features for our experimental dataset and 64 for the SEED-IV dataset.

6.3.4 Feature selection

In the feature-selection step, we intended to select prominent features that would largely contribute to a good classification of human emotion. We used the mRMR method, whose objective is to rank features according to their relevance to a class. The algorithm also considers the redundancy factor of a feature, whereby the least redundant features are more highly ranked than the more redundant features (figure 6.9). Figure 6.10 shows a graph of this feature ranking using the mRMR algorithm in MATLAB. A certain threshold importance score can be set such that features above the set threshold are selected while the rest are discarded. We performed feature selection on both the CWFs and MCFs.

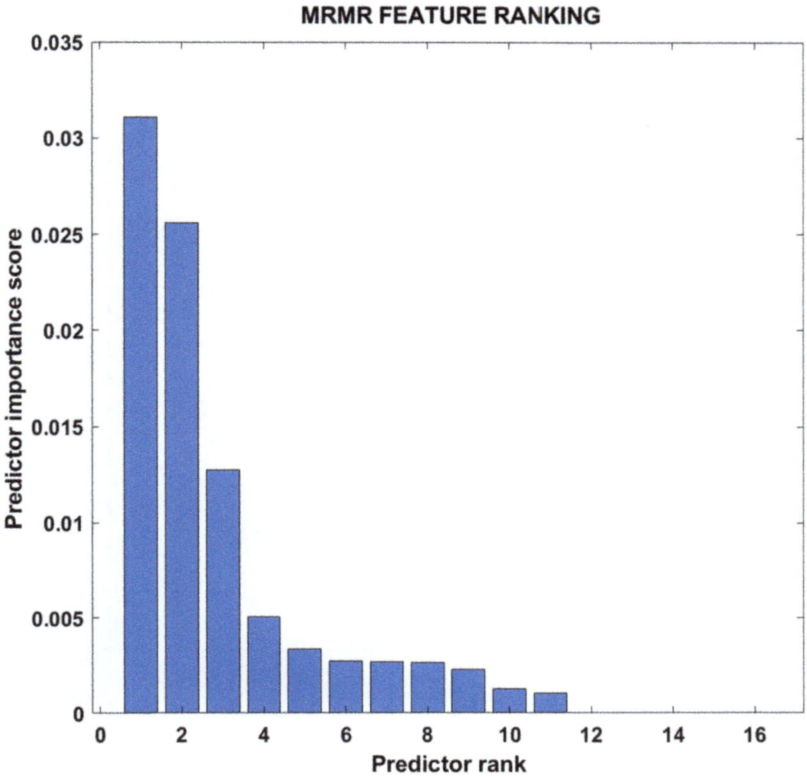

Figure 6.9. Features ranking using the mRMR feature-ranking method. Here, features 12–16 have been ranked with zero importance scores while the highest feature had a score of above 0.03.

6.3.5 Machine-learning classification

In the final step of our approach, we employed two supervised machine-learning models, LSTM RNN and RF, to classify different human emotions from the prepared feature sets.

6.3.5.1 Long short-term memory recurrent neural network

A LSTM network is a type of recurrent neural network used to classify sequential data and to solve the problem of memory loss in recurrent neural networks by learning long-term dependencies in the data sequence. The architecture of our LSTM network consisted of an input layer with the size of our feature set (number of features), a fully connected bidirectional LSTM layer with 150 units, a softmax layer, and a classification layer.

6.3.5.2 Random forest

A RF is a supervised ensemble method that works by building several samples of the data as training subsets and employing decision trees to perform classification on each sample. The overall CA is decided based on the majority of samples with

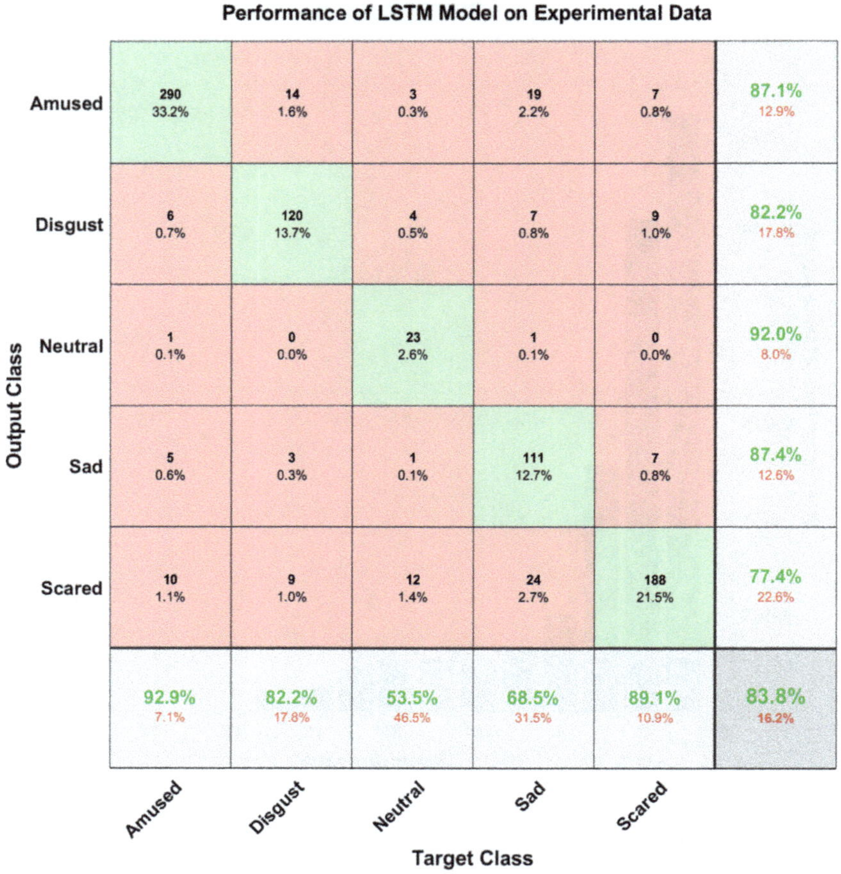

Figure 6.10. A confusion matrix for the LSTM model showing the classification of five human emotions from our experimental data.

similar classification results. In our case, we implemented a RF in MATLAB with the help of the classification learner application.

6.4 Results and analysis

In this section, we present the results of the performance of the LSTM and RF classifiers of various feature sets. First, we present a table showing the performance of the LSTM and RF on our experimental data before and after pre-processing. The results show how these models performed for CWFs and MCFs. In addition, we show the results of the performance of the classifiers on the mRMR-selected feature set. Second, we repeat and verify the same process using the SEED-IV dataset.

6.4.1 Experimental results

Table 6.1 shows the experimental results for the performance of the LSTM classifier. The model was trained using an adaptive moment estimation optimisation

Table 6.1. Classification results of the LSTM RNN using experimental data.

	Experimental data			
	Raw (%)		Filtered (%)	
Feature sets	Channel-wise features	Multi-channel features	Channel-wise features	Multi-channel features
All features	42.00	26.00	**83.80**	35.80
mRMR-selected features	43.00	36.00	68.40	34.20

The bold value indicates the highest accuracy recorded in the table.

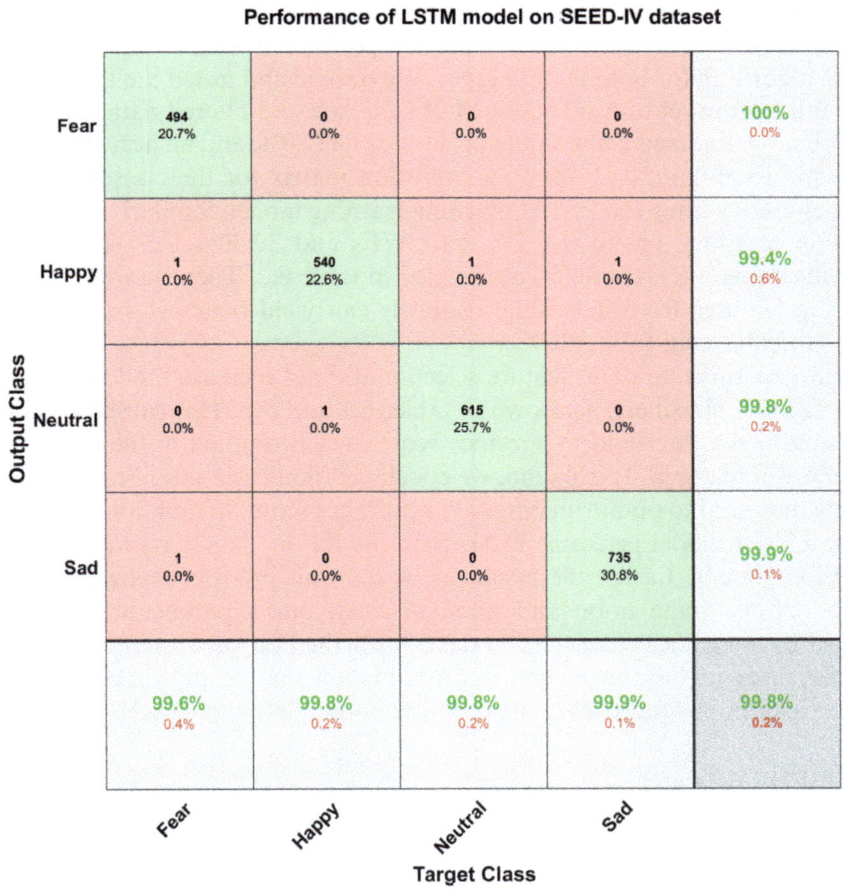

Figure 6.11. A confusion matrix for the LSTM model showing the classification of four human emotions from the SEED-IV dataset.

Table 6.2. Classification results of the RF using experimental data.

Feature sets	Experimental data			
	Raw (%)		Filtered (%)	
	Channel-wise features	Multi-channel features	Channel-wise features	Multi-channel features
All features	**54.90**	26.00	39.93	39.50
mRMR-selected features	50.60	36.00	40.12	39.90

The bold value indicates the highest accuracy recorded in the table.

algorithm, an initial learning rate of 0.01, a gradient decay factor of 0.9, a squared gradient decay factor of 0.9990, and an L2 regularisation factor of 0.0001. The experimental data were divided into raw data and filtered data. In each dataset, both CWFs and MCFs were extracted. We then performed feature selection using the mRMR algorithm for both feature types. We trained and tested the LSTM classifier on the full feature set of CWFs and MCFs for raw and filtered data. In the case of the CWFs, we obtained a maximum accuracy of 83.80%, and an accuracy of 36.00% for the MCFs. Figure 6.11 shows a confusion matrix for the classification of five human emotions using the LSTM machine-learning model. Similarly, we obtained a maximum accuracy of 54.90% for the CWFs and 39.50% for the MCFs when classifying using a RF classifier, as detailed in table 6.2. These results indicate that extracting features from individual channels can yield better classification results than when extracting from MCFs.

In our experimental data, feature selection did not increase the CAs of both the LSTM and RF classifiers, as shown in tables 6.1 and 6.2. This can be attributed to the setting of the threshold importance score, which resulted in the attenuation of some relevant features. To this end, we concluded that there is a need to thoroughly tune this threshold to obtain an optimal importance score. In addition, we concluded that the LSTM model performs better than the RF in classifying human emotions using EEG signals. Lastly, the results show that our pre-processing methods were able to remove some noise and artefacts from our experimental data. This is indicated by a significant increase in the CA for the best-performing LSTM model. However, there are instances where our results show that the pre-processing methods did not yield an improved CA.

6.4.2 SEED-IV dataset

To verify our experimental results, we used a multi-modal public dataset for human emotion, SEED-IV. Tables 6.3 and 6.4 show the performance of the LSTM and RF models, respectively, on the raw and filtered dataset. Similarly, we extracted CWFs and MCFs and performed feature selection with the mRMR algorithm on each feature set. For LSTM we obtained a maximum accuracy of 99.8% for the CWFs and MCFs extracted from the raw dataset, as shown in the confusion matrix in

Table 6.3. Classification results of the LSTM RNN using the SEED-IV dataset.

	SEED-IV dataset			
	Raw (%)		Filtered (%)	
Feature sets	Channel-wise features	Multi-channel features	Channel-wise features	Multi-channel features
All features	99.60	30.80	72 40	41.90
mRMR-selected features	**99.80**	**99.80**	77.90	41.92

The bold value indicates the highest accuracy recorded in the table.

Table 6.4. Classification results of the RF using the SEED-IV dataset.

	SEED-IV dataset			
	Raw (%)		Filtered (%)	
Feature sets	Channel-wise features	Multi-channel features	Channel-wise features	Multi-channel features
All features	**48.00**	46.10	29.30	26.70
MRMR-selected features	43.60	42.90	29.80	26.20

The bold value indicates the highest accuracy recorded in the table.

figure 6.11. This accuracy was obtained using a full feature set of CWFs and after performing feature selection using mRMR on a MCF set. Since the MCF set contains both DASM and RASM, mRMR was able to select only these features while discarding the Shannon and log energy entropy features. The resulting feature sets become similar to the selected feature set for CWFs, hence the identical CAs.

It is quite evident that using raw data resulted in better CAs than filtered data. This can be attributed to the selection of independent components during artefact removal using ICA. The manual analysis of the independent components might have resulted in a loss of important data, and hence the raw SEED-IV dataset yielded better results than the filtered data for both LSTM and RF. To this end, we conclude that more care has to be taken during the selection of independent components in the application of ICA to avoid the loss of important information, wherein some independent components are wrongly rejected. Lastly, the results maintain that CWFs are better than MCFs and that the LSTM yields better performance than the RF classifier for the classification of human emotions.

6.4.3 Application to healthcare

Inferring human affects using EEG signals is one of the safest and cheapest ways of accurately determining the emotional status of patients. In this study, we have shown that when using EEG biophysical signals, it is more accurate and effective to perform feature extraction from individual channels as opposed to a multi-channel approaches. Moreover, we showed that when using the Emotiv Epoc+ headset the channels AF3, F7, F3, O1, O2, P8, FC6, F4, and AF4 proved able to carry more information than others. This solution can be applied in healthcare to build a less computationally intensive and real-time system for diagnosing different human emotions in patients, so that they can receive the help that their situation requires.

6.5 Discussion and conclusions

EEG-based human emotion classification methods are used to recognise the emotional states of people using signals of their brain activity and not verbal expression. This approach has been hypothesised to be more precise and reliable rather than depending on subjects' ways of expressing their emotional status (Bos 2006). An effective algorithm that can execute this emotion inference from EEG signals has not yet been established with certainty. Historically, authors have proposed the use of machine-learning classification algorithms as the only means to recognise human emotion, where raw EEG signals are used as the input. In recent times, many authors have followed a convention of adopting some pre-processing, feature extraction and selection before then executing the machine-learning classification as their signal-processing pipeline to infer human emotions. However, a range of authors have proposed a variety of dissimilar tools or methods for each step in this pipeline. In particular, the methods applied to extract informative features have proved the most controversial. The authors in Tao *et al* (2020) show that spatial information in EEG signals can be traced from individual channels while temporal information can be traced from time-based channel slices. The study, however, does not quantitatively compare the information contained in the entire data segment with that in individual channels to establish that the channel-wise approach is more informative. In addition, the study proposed a new method, an attention-based convolutional recurrent neural network, and used two sets of publicly available human emotion datasets, DREAMER and DEAP, achieving a maximum accuracy of 97.98%. Our study builds on the work of these authors to quantitatively prove the efficacy of CWF extraction by using the conventional EEG signal-processing pipeline as compared to extracting features from data segments. In addition, we used our own experimental dataset and a publicly available human emotion dataset, SEED-IV, to verify the proposed method. From our study, we can conclude that CWF extraction leads to a better classification of human emotions than the MCF extraction method. We also show that, when using a 14-channel Emotiv headset, there are specific channels that carry more information than others. Log energy entropy, Shannon entropy, DASM, and RASM have proved to be reliable feature-extraction methods when applied to each channel. As shown in this study and as previously demonstrated by other researchers, mRMR (feature selection) and ICA (pre-processing) show superior performance as off-the-shelf tools to be used in human emotion recognition using EEG signals. Our proposed method yielded a maximum CA of 99.8% from the SEED-IV dataset and 83.80% from our experimental dataset when using the LSTM classification method. However, we acknowledge that there remains room for improvement, especially with respect to ensuring that this emotion classification process can run in as near real time as possible.

6.6 Challenges and future works

The total removal of artefacts has remained a persistent challenge when using physiological signals to infer human emotions. For EEG signals, this problem is particularly daunting because the collected signals are usually contaminated with noise recorded by the electrodes. Even though our pre-processing techniques significantly reduce these noise and artefacts, they cannot remove them completely. Hence, they are included in the next stages of the signal-processing pipeline and consequently affect the generalisation of the machine-learning models. In the future, we propose to use only the most relevant and a minimal number of EEG channels to provide the EEG data necessary for emotion recognition. In doing so, redundant and noisy EEG channels will be removed, which will further reduce the overall noise or artefacts present in the dataset. Another challenge encountered in this work is the lack of a real-time implementation of our emotion recognition method. We learned that the time it takes to record EEG signals from human subjects in order to classify their emotions is longer than anticipated. This is a result of the computationally intensive methods involved in the pre-processing and feature-extraction and feature-selection steps. To address this, in future we intend to use the Lab Stream Layer support software, which will allow us to stream live time-series brain signals and to process them in real time. Furthermore, the reduction of EEG channels can also reduce the computational load in the signal-processing pipeline, and therefore enhance real-time computation (Maithri *et al* 2022).

References

Acharya D, Goel S, Bhardwaj H, Sakalle A and Bhardwaj A 2020 A long short term memory deep learning network for the classification of negative emotions using EEG signals *2020 Int. Joint Conf. on Neural Networks (IJCNN)* pp 1–8

Ackermann P, Kohlschein C, Bitsch J A, Wehrle K and Jeschke S 2016 EEG-based automatic emotion recognition: feature extraction, selection and classification methods *2016 IEEE 18th Int. Conf. on E-Health Networking, Applications and Services (Healthcom)* pp 1–6

Alarcão S M and Fonseca M J 2019 Emotions recognition using EEG signals: a survey *IEEE Trans. Affect. Comput.* **10** 374–93

Alhagry S, Fahmy A A and El-Khoribi R A 2017 Emotion recognition based on EEG using LSTM recurrent neural network *Int. J. Adv. Comput. Sci. Appl.* **8**

Alqahtani F, Katsigiannis S and Ramzan N 2019 ECG-based affective computing for difficulty level prediction in intelligent tutoring systems *2019 UK/China Emerging Technologies (UCET)* pp 1–4

Assabumrungrat R, Sangnark S, Charoenpattarawut T, Polpakdee W, Sudhawiyangkul T, Boonchieng E and Wilaiprasitporn T 2022 Ubiquitous affective computing: a review *IEEE Sens. J.* **22** 1867–81

Bastos-Filho T F, Ferreira A, Atencio A C, Arjunan S and Kumar D 2012 Evaluation of feature extraction techniques in emotional state recognition *2012 4th Int. Conf. on Intelligent Human–Computer Interaction (IHCI)* pp 1–6

Bhardwaj A, Gupta A, Jain P, Rani A and Yadav J 2015 Classification of human emotions from EEG signals using SVM and LDA Classifiers *2015 2nd Int. Conf. on Signal Processing and Integrated Networks (SPIN)* pp 180–5

Bos D O 2006 *EEG-based emotion recognition: the influence of visual and auditory stimuli* http://hmi.ewi.utwente.nl/verslagen/capitaselecta/CS-Oude_Bos-Danny.pdf

Chao H, Dong L, Liu Y and Lu B 2020 Improved deep feature learning by synchronization measurements for multi-channel EEG emotion recognition *Complexity* **2020** 6816502

Chawla P, Rana S B, Kaur H, Singh K, Yuvaraj R and Murugappan M 2023 A decision support system for automated diagnosis of Parkinson's disease from EEG using FAWT and entropy features *Biomed. Signal Process. Control* **79** 104116

Chen T, Ju S, Yuan X, Elhoseny M, Ren F, Fan M and Chen Z 2018 Emotion recognition using empirical mode decomposition and approximation entropy *Comput. Electr. Eng.* **72** 383–92

Chowdhury P, Shakim S S K, Karim M R and Rhaman M K 2014 Cognitive efficiency in robot control by Emotiv EPOC *2014 Int. Conf. on Informatics, Electronics and Vision (ICIEV)* pp 1–6

Croy I, Olgun S and Joraschky P 2011 Basic emotions elicited by odors and pictures *Emotion* **11** 1331

Dalton E D and Hammen C L 2018 Independent and relative effects of stress, depressive symptoms, and affect on college students' daily health behaviors *J. Behav. Med.* **41** 863–74

Das A B and Bhuiyan M I H 2016 Discrimination and classification of focal and non-focal EEG signals using entropy-based features in the EMD-DWT domain *Biomed. Signal Process. Control* **29** 11–21

Davidson R J and Fox N A 1982 Asymmetrical brain activity discriminates between positive and negative affective stimuli in human infants *Science* **218** 1235–7

Ding R, Li P, Wang W and Luo W 2017 Emotion processing by ERP combined with development and plasticity *Neural Plast.* **2017** 5282670

Dissanayake T, Rajapaksha Y, Ragel R and Nawinne I 2019 An ensemble learning approach for electrocardiogram sensor based human emotion recognition *Sensors* **19** 4495

Er M B, Çiğ H and Aydilek İ B 2021 A new approach to recognition of human emotions using brain signals and music stimuli *Appl. Acoust.* **175** 107840

Gao Q, Wang C, Wang Z, Song X, Dong E and Song Y 2020 EEG based emotion recognition using fusion feature extraction method *Multimed. Tools Appl.* **79** 27057–74

González-Hernández F, Zatarain-Cabada R, Barrón-Estrada M L and Rodríguez-Rangel H 2018 Recognition of learning-centered emotions using a convolutional neural network *J. Intell. Fuzzy Syst.* **34** 3325–36

Gupta V, Chopda M D and Pachori R B 2018 Cross-subject emotion recognition using flexible analytic wavelet transform from EEG signals *IEEE Sens. J.* **19** 2266–74

Hassan M M, Alam M G R, Uddin M Z, Huda S, Almogren A and Fortino G 2019 Human emotion recognition using deep belief network architecture *Inf. Fusion* **51** 10–8

Hu X, Chen J, Wang F and Zhang D 2019 Ten challenges for EEG-based affective computing *Brain Sci. Adv.* **5** 1–20

Iacoviello D, Petracca A, Spezialetti M and Placidi G 2015 A real-time classification algorithm for EEG-based BCI driven by self-induced emotions *Comput. Methods Programs Biomed.* **122** 293–303

Jatupaiboon N, Pan-ngum S and Israsena P 2013 Emotion classification using minimal EEG channels and frequency bands *The 2013 10th Int. Joint Conf. on Computer Science and Software Engineering (JCSSE)* pp 21–4

Jenke R, Peer A and Buss M 2014 Feature extraction and selection for emotion recognition from EEG *IEEE Trans. Affect. Comput.* **5** 327–39

Jin L and Kim E Y 2020 Interpretable cross-subject EEG-based emotion recognition using channel-wise features *Sensors* **20** 6719

Kaliouby R E, Picard R and Baron-Cohen S 2006 Affective computing and autism *Ann. N.Y. Acad. Sci.* **1093** 228–48

Kam J W Y, Griffin S, Shen A, Patel S, Hinrichs H, Heinze H-J, Deouell L Y and Knight R T 2019 Systematic comparison between a wireless EEG system with dry electrodes and a wired EEG system with wet electrodes *Neuroimage* **184** 119–29

Kannathal N, Choo M L, Acharya U R and Sadasivan P K 2005 Entropies for detection of epilepsy in EEG *Comput. Methods Programs Biomed.* **80** 187–94

Khalili Z and Moradi M H 2009 Emotion recognition system using brain and peripheral signals: using correlation dimension to improve the results of EEG *2009 Int. Joint Conf. on Neural Networks* pp 1571–5

Koelstra S, Muhl C, Soleymani M, Lee J-S, Yazdani A, Ebrahimi T, Pun T, Nijholt A and Patras I 2011 Deap: a database for emotion analysis using physiological signals *IEEE Trans. Affect. Comput.* **3** 18–31

Liu N, Fang Y, Li L, Hou L, Yang F and Guo Y 2018 Multiple feature fusion for automatic emotion recognition using EEG signals *2018 IEEE Int. Conf. on Acoustics, Speech and Signal Processing (ICASSP)* pp 896–900

Maithri M, Raghavendra U, Gudigar A, Samanth J, Barua P D, Murugappan M and Acharya U R 2022 Automated emotion recognition: current trends and future perspectives *Comput. Methods Programs Biomed.* **215** 106646

Malete T N, Moruti K, Thapelo T S and Jamisola R S 2019 EEG-based control of a 3D game using 14-channel Emotiv epoc+ *2019 IEEE Int. Conf. on Cybernetics and Intelligent Systems (CIS) and IEEE Conf. on Robotics, Automation and Mechatronics (RAM)* pp 463–8

Marín-Morales J, Higuera-Trujillo J L, Greco A, Guixeres J, Llinares C, Scilingo E P, Alcañiz M and Valenza G 2018 Affective computing in virtual reality: emotion recognition from brain and heartbeat dynamics using wearable sensors *Sci. Rep.* **8** 1–15

Mohutsiwa L O and Jamisola R S 2021 EEG-based human emotion classification using combined computational techniques for feature extraction and selection in six machine learning models *2021 5th Int. Conf. on Intelligent Computing and Control Systems (ICICCS)* 1095–102

Mühl C, Allison B, Nijholt A and Chanel G 2014 A survey of affective brain computer interfaces: principles, state-of-the-art, and challenges *Brain–Comput. Interfaces* **1** 66–84

Murugappan M, Juhari M R B M, Nagarajan R and Yaacob S 2009 An investigation on visual and audiovisual stimulus-based emotion recognition using EEG *Int. J. Med. Eng. Inf.* **1** 342

Nawaz R, Cheah K H, Nisar H and Yap V V 2020 Comparison of different feature extraction methods for EEG-based emotion recognition *Biocybern. Biomed. Eng.* **40** 910–26

Peng H, Long F and Ding C 2005 Feature selection based on mutual information criteria of max-dependency, max-relevance, and min-redundancy *IEEE Trans. Pattern Anal. Mach. Intell.* **27** 1226–38

Qing C, Qiao R, Xu X and Cheng Y 2019 Interpretable emotion recognition using EEG signals *IEEE Access* **7** 94160–70

Rahman M M, Sarkar A K, Hossain M A, Hossain M S, Islam M R, Hossain M B, Quinn J M W and Moni M A 2021 Recognition of human emotions using EEG signals: a review *Comput. Biol. Med.* **136** 104696

Sarkar P and Etemad A 2020 Self-supervised ECG representation learning for emotion recognition *IEEE Trans. Affect. Comput.* **13** 1541–54

Siddharth S, Jung T-P and Sejnowski T J 2019 Utilizing deep learning towards multi-modal bio-sensing and vision-based affective computing *IEEE Trans. Affect. Comput.* **13** 96–107

Sokolov S 2018 Neural network based multimodal emotion estimation *ICAS* **2018** 4–7

Song T, Zheng W, Song P and Cui Z 2018 EEG emotion recognition using dynamical graph convolutional neural networks *IEEE Trans. Affect. Comput.* **11** 532–41

Steinert S and Friedrich O 2020 Wired emotions: ethical issues of affective brain–computer interfaces *Sci. Eng. Ethics* **26** 351–67

Stytsenko K, Jablonskis E and Prahm C 2011 Evaluation of consumer EEG device Emotiv EPOC *MEi: CogSci Conf.* p 99

Suhaimi N S, Mountstephens J and Teo J 2020 EEG-based emotion recognition: a state-of-the-art review of current trends and opportunities *Comput. Intell. Neurosci.* **2020** 8875426

Tao J and Tan T 2005 Affective computing: a review *Affective Computing and Intelligent Interaction Lecture Notes in Computer Science* ed J Tao, T Tan and R W Picard vol 3784 (Berlin: Springer) pp 981–95

Tao W, Li C, Song R, Cheng J, Liu Y, Wan F and Chen X 2020 EEG-based emotion recognition via channel-wise attention and self attention *IEEE Trans. Affect. Comput.* **14** 382–93

Tokuno S, Tsumatori G, Shono S, Takei E, Yamamoto T, Suzuki G, Mituyoshi S and Shimura M 2011 Usage of emotion recognition in military health care *2011 Defense Science Research Conf. and Expo (DSR)* pp 1–5

Torres E P, Torres E A, Hernández-Álvarez M and Yoo S G 2020 EEG-based BCI emotion recognition: a survey *Sensors* **20** 5083

Williams N S, McArthur G M, de Wit B, Ibrahim G and Badcock N A 2020 A validation of Emotiv EPOC flex saline for EEG and ERP research *PeerJ* **8** e9713

Yang Y, Wu Q, Qiu M, Wang Y and Chen X 2018 Emotion recognition from multi-channel EEG through parallel convolutional recurrent neural network *2018 Int. Joint Conf. on Neural Networks (IJCNN)* pp 1–7

Yazdani A, Lee J-S and Ebrahimi T 2009 Implicit emotional tagging of multimedia using EEG signals and brain computer interface *Proc. 1st SIGMM Workshop on Social Media* 81–8 pp

Yuen C T, San San W, Seong T C and Rizon M 2009 Classification of human emotions from EEG signals using statistical features and neural network *Int. J. Integr. Eng.* **1**

Zhang W, Shu L, Xu X and Liao D 2017 Affective virtual reality system (AVRS): design and ratings of affective VR scenes *2017 Int. Conf. on Virtual Reality and Visualization (ICVRV)* pp 311–4

Zheng W-L, Guo H-T and Lu B-L 2015 Revealing critical channels and frequency bands for emotion recognition from EEG with deep belief network *7th Int. IEEE/EMBS Conf. on Neural Engineering (NER)* pp 154–7

Zheng W-L, Liu W, Lu Y, Lu B L and Cichocki A 2018 Emotionmeter: A multimodal framework for recognizing human emotions *IEEE Trans. Cybernet.* **49** 1110–22

Zheng W-L, Zhu J-Y and Lu B-L 2017 Identifying stable patterns over time for emotion recognition from EEG *IEEE Trans. Affect. Comput.* **10** 417–29

IOP Publishing

Affective Computing in Healthcare
Applications based on biosignals and artificial intelligence
M Murugappan

Chapter 7

Detection of physiological body movements in affective disorder patients using EEG signals and deep neural networks

Jason Elroy Martis, M S Sannidhan, Sunil Kumar Aithal, R Balasubramani and K B Sudeepa

Studies from as far back as medieval times have proved that the human brain is an exceedingly vital and complex organ responsible for the comprehensive monitoring and autonomous control of physiological movements through neural signals. Today, with the advancement of modern technology, we can track neurological signals from brain activities using dedicated electroencephalogram sensors mounted on an individual's head using a method known as electroencephalography (EEG). Traditionally many forms of this technique has been utilised, but nowadays they are inefficient and obsolete. The tracing and tracking of neurological signals are highly beneficial in medical sciences for treating diseases such as dysplasia and epilepsy. Current methodologies propose manual feature-extraction and feature-classification systems that map the signals to bodily movements in order to trace the neurological signals. However, the existing systems have suffered a lot in achieving high accuracy. Hence, to overcome the issues with current systems, we propose analysing brain activity through EEG sensor data series to detect and classify different physiological body movements using deep neural networks. We have also taken advantage of three different strategies adopted for the assessment model to further increase classification accuracy. Experimental investigations were carried out using standard datasets, and their outcomes were compared with other traditional classification techniques. The results reveal that the proposed system outperforms the various traditional approaches by achieving an average classification accuracy of 68% using transformer networks for body movement analysis.

doi:10.1088/978-0-7503-5182-9ch7

7.1 Introduction

The human brain is the most complex organ in the human body. Its composition consists of white matter and grey matter. Grey matter recognises and interprets information, whereas white matter transmits data. Similarly, the human brain is divided into three main parts: the cerebrum; the cerebellum. The cerebrum is the most significant part of the brain, which induces body movement, regulates temperature, and so on. The cerebellum and brainstem do not possess cognitive abilities but serve as storage areas, with a more significant number of folds. Many neuronal pathways are excited to and fro whenever the brain processes any information, causing enormous induction of sodium ions [1]. This effect causes electric waves to be released, thereby creating a weak magnetic field in the vicinity of the brain. The magnetic field passes through the skull, creating various waves with different frequencies called brain signals, more technically known as electroencephalogram signals (EEG signals) [2, 3].

Consequently, a particular pattern of signal emission occurs for every body movement and brain processing activity. People incapable of this body movement still have these residual signals processed in the brain. Significant modern research involves capturing EEG waves for further information processing in the medical field. Several approaches to recognising and processing body movements exist, but EEG is an efficient and popular technique since real-time electric signals originate and are recorded directly from the brain area itself. EEG signal sequences are broadly categorised into different wave bands, e.g., alpha, beta, theta, and delta, based on their frequency. Several ranges of frequencies originate from other body signals, causing an amalgam of waves for each cognitive and kinetic ability. Traditional approaches intend to identify specific patterns in these waves and relate them to bodily movements. Several techniques based on body sensing using camera devices, to detect human activities and help patients overcome kinaesthetic problems, exist and exhibit efficient performance in aiding people lacking mobility. Another class of techniques involves using the electric signals generated by human muscles, also known as muscle movement recognition [4]. These electrical impulses accurately track bodily movement since they are based on direct measurement and targeted to a specific strength for action. Several challenges still exist while considering only the impulse-based sources, leading to limited research viability for physiological body movements and insufficient treatments for motor diseases like epilepsy and dysplasia. Despite their abilities and decent performance, these existing techniques involve a general interpretive aspect and are not specific to certain actions. Modern-day processing technologies employ the capabilities of deep neural networks to efficiently identify patterns by isolating mixed parameters. Our proposed system attempts to efficiently harness the power of a deep neural network for proper pattern recognition. Since no dedicated neural network can currently accomplish this task, we employ a hybrid strategy utilising three different neural networks that can isolate patterns from sequences. The proposed design helps us to determine the best deep neural approach for isolating several types of bodily movements from EEG signals.

7.1.1 Chapter organisation

The rest of the chapter is organised into four sections. Each section is described in detail corresponding to the achievement of the objectives of the chapter. Section 7.2 provides a detailed insight into the existing literature relating to the techniques and technologies required to implement the proposed methodology. After detailing this sufficient literature background, section 7.3 presents a well-organised description of the proposed system. Each subsection of the proposed approach gives a detailed explanation of each module involved in the proposed method. Experimental trials and their related outcomes are given under section 7.4, which offers a thorough investigation of the proposed system and also highlights its strengths and advantages. Finally, section 7.5 reveals the conclusion and recommended future directions of the research.

7.2 Literature survey

We have conducted an exhaustive literature review focusing on the utilisation of signals to track brain waves and map them to specific sets of activities corresponding to bodily movements. Further, we have referred to abundant research work concentrating on the classification and mapping of bodily movements via features extracted from brain signals. Different classification techniques from standard sets of research works were examined to design our proposed system involving mapping of brain signals to a set of body movements, involving fine movements also. In order to improve the feature-extraction process, leading to higher accuracy of classification, we have also investigated different techniques that could possibly improve the quality of the collected brain signals.

Hallett *et al* [5] in their review article performed a comparative analysis of body movement tracking using different signal forms such as EEG, electromyography (EMG), and magnetoencephalography. A set of experiments was performed by collecting different forms of signals from a set of individuals to track different bodily movements involving different parts of the hands and legs. The tracking was done by manual analysis of signals connected over a set of sensors corresponding to different bodily movements. In their analysis, combining several systems with EEG yields significantly improved accuracy in body movement tracking.

Abtahi *et al* [6] demonstrated an efficient support vector machine (SVM)-based classification model for neurological disorders corresponding to the characterisation of Parkinson's disease disorders. In their research work, they used both EEG and EMG signals for automatic classification of the signals into different classes of bodily movement relating to Parkinson's disease. On comparing the obtained results, the authors were able to attain a higher accuracy of 93% by using EEG data. However, their work also exhibited the detection of limited bodily movement narrowed down to Parkinson's disease due to the involvement of cluster-based classification technique.

Moreira *et al* [7] conducted research in connection with the identification of bodily movements through the collection of EEG signals. In their work, researchers trained two machine-learning models, a SVM and a *k*-nearest neighbour (*K*-NN) algorithm, to map physical movement with the imagination of the individual. Limited EEG signals from the brain were mapped to a limited number of movements, with an observed accuracy of 30% for *K*-NN and 57% for SVM. Upon analysis of their work, it was observed that the system was not trained for many of the finer bodily movements and predicted the wrong movement when tested. The reason behind this failure was due to limitations in its training and the incapability of machine-learning models to discriminate finer feature levels extracted from EEG signals.

Suhaimi *et al* [8] in their article highlighted the potential of virtual reality technology for emotion stimuli, and current practices for emotion recognition based on EEG signals were discussed. The significant impact of EEG for emotion classification was witnessed using portable, wireless, cost-effective EEG devices in the form of headsets that can be utilised for recording and recognising bodily movements and emotional activities. In their research efforts, the authors proved that the classification of EEG signals was better acheived using deep-learning models, which are more suitable for EEG-based brain activity recognition and classification. Their study did not cover the tracking of bodily movements through the collected EEG signals. However, application of the proposed technique for tracking the body movement through the collected EEG signals yielded very less accuracy rate of below 30% due to the degradation in the quality of collected EEG signals producing irrelevant results.

Jeon *et al* [9] proposed a methodology for detecting bodily movements restricted only to motion detection of the arms using EEG signals. From a set of EEG signals the brain signals only corresponding to movement of the arms were inferred for the classification left and right arm movements. SVM techniques and standard spatial pattern filtering were incorporated into their methodology for better performance and results. However, use of more sample datasets and a better noise-removal strategy still need to be addressed to overcome the study's drawbacks. After applying a common spatial pattern (CSP) filter, 91% accuracy was achieved, which can however be further improved by incorporating the best noise-reduction filters. The main drawback of this work is that it is restricted to identifying only arm movements with only a limited range of trained EEG signals. Apart from this, the brain signals are related to a stimulus in the muscle rather than the arms themselves. The work also failed to classify finer body movements such as in the fingers, wrists, etc.

Zhang *et al* [10] proposed another approach for hand-movement recognition based on long short-term memory (LSTM) deep neural networks using EEG signals. Frequency- and time-domain features were inferred from EEG signals, which together constitutes an attentive-neural-network-based methodology. Several existing state-of-the-art models were compared with the proposed technique, and various heterogeneous subjects were considered during performance evaluation for classifications. For their cross-validation scheme, an overall accuracy of 83% was reported, and for their intra-validation procedure, an overall accuracy of 98% was observed. Yet, the approach is complex and not robust in nature due to the incorporation of a hand-skill-based feature-extraction technique.

Leon-Urbano *et al* [11] in their research article proposed a time-series-based classification model for varying brain-waves recognition in EEG signals. The incorporation of a LSTM slowed the process but demonstrated a better performance in identifying different classes of waveforms and further achieved a higher accuracy when compared to traditional models. The work as implemented paves a way for using EEG signals in combination with LSTM-based deep-learning models in order to classify signals into different body movement identifications, also involving finer body parts.

Sun *et al* [12] demonstrated the significance of transformers for EEG signal classification in natural-language processing applications. Transformers can be combined with neural network models to improve overall accuracy in the classification process for sequential data processing. Spatial-based, temporal-based, convolutional neural network (CNN) with spatial, CNN with temporal, and transformer fusion models were compared, and the results showed that a CNN with a temporal-based transformer approach yielded 88% overall accuracy. Further, their work demonstrated that a positional embedding technique can be utilised to further increase the overall classification accuracy for large datasets. On investigating this work, there is a large scope to extend the proposed system for the classification of different bodily movements through EEG signals. The incorporation of transformers adds better accuracy, even to identify finer body movements.

Young-Eun Lee and Seo-Hyun Lee [13] proposed a transformer-based technique to recognise brain activities for imagination-oriented speech as compared to actual speech. The speech-realisation module incorporates an attention mechanism for classifying the several subjects considered. For medical purposes with less considered parameters using EEG signals, neural models exhibit enhanced performance in the classification aspects. Overall, there was still a need to improve the imagined speech recognition accuracy, where the model reported a less than 50% overall accuracy. The work proves, however, that transformers perform better in the classification of finer EEG signals, and it provides a motivation to extend the proposed methodology for the classification of bodily movements through EEG signals also involving fine movements as well as corresponding to individuals of different age groups.

Tao *et al* [14] proposed a modified gate-based transformer for experimenting with brain visuals through EEG signals and mapping them to bodily movements. In this research, the authors utilised a pre-trained ImageNet model consisting of a motor-imagery-based dataset. Further, the extracted features were classified by the utilisation of a gate-based transformer network. models for performance assessment. To verify the performance of the proposed system, the achieved outcomes were compared with other classification models. Analysis proved that the transformer network performed better in classifying EEG signals, with an accuracy rate of 52%. However, the work had a drawback in achieving a higher rate of accuracy due to the limited availability of samples in the dataset utilised for training.

In their thesis [15] Williams utilised transfer-learning techniques for EEG signal classification. The proposed research addresses subject variations, dataset scarcity, and time series based on several channels composed of data with shortcomings. Transfer learning can address multiple large heterogeneous datasets and classification activities for universal subjects. Traditional CNN-based approaches achieved less than 65% accuracy. In comparison, the transfer-based approach managed an overall 69% accuracy, which however still needs to be improved by choosing more efficient hyperparameters. In their work, it was noted that the classification could have been improved by pre-processing the signals to improve their quality in order to extract better features. Further, the work widens the scope to use the proposed model even to map different bodily movements.

In [16], Wang *et al* proposed a hybrid approach with a combination of unsupervised transfer learning along with a CSP model and Euclidean-based data alignment to effectively classify the abruptly varying nature of EEG signals. The authors observed an overall accuracy for a particular considered subject of 87%, which yielded a higher accuracy than compared to machine-learning and traditional CNN approaches. Their proposed system was extended by us in order to map EEG signals to bodily movements. However, we were only able to attain an accuracy of 54% for abstract movements and 29% for fine movements. Further, upon investigation, it was observed that due to abrupt variation in the signals based on time series, the accuracy rate was on the lower side for body movement identification. A possible solution to the problem is to use a time-series-based classification system.

Zheng *et al* in their research [17] addressed the limitations in classifying huge EEG signal datasets, which is time consuming, and insufficiently robust motor-imagery EEGs of existing commands. The work also highlighted the appearance of weak signals, leading to inaccurate predictions in classifying the brain signals. As a solution to the problem, their work recommends the application of transfer-learning techniques to enhance signal power for efficient new subject classifications by significantly reducing the measurement time during EEG signal recognition. However, though for limited sets of signals and limited classifications the system would perform better, it fails at predicting abruptly varying signals based on time series, as is required to classify different activities when mapping the signals. Hence, it fails to map EEG signals accurately to different movements corresponding to the individual's body.

Grana *et al* [18] suggested wireless-based EEG signal recognition considering wireless inertial-properties-based measurement units. Transfer-based learning and a random forest classification model resulted in the best results. A fusion-based approach yielded an overall accuracy of 0.9 on a small, considered dataset in a natural setting. The technique is highly suitable for tracking signals in a very small area corresponding to a few sensors. However, the strength the signal is on the weaker side and does not support accurate predictions for further classifications.

A research work [19] accomplished by Kumar *et al* proposed real-time classification of EEG signals using a novel predictive approach based on LSTM and CSP models. Depending on the dataset chosen, this novel approach results in an overall accuracy of 78.8%, which is an improvement over the CSP technique. A misclassification rate of around 3% was observed depending on the chosen hyperparameters, such as the size of the network, learning rates, etc. The main drawback of their work is that it focused on training and classification of a group of signals constrained to a particular set of EEG signals. A possible improvement could be made by utilising transformers for time-series-based classification.

On performing an exhaustive review of the existing literature, it can be seen that the majority of the extant work has focused on the utilisation of EEG signals due to their improved quality, thus supporting further classification with better accuracy. In addition, for classification, different techniques utilise a range of machine-learning and deep-learning systems to classify the EEG signals into bodily movements and other activities. Studies have proven that there is a higher amount of complexity involved when trying to classify EEG signals into bodily movements, especially with regards to fine movements. To this end, deep-learning systems are considered better than machine-learning and traditional classification models in yielding better rates of classification. Extended examination of the literature has highlighted that only a limited amount of work thus far has concentrated on classifying fine body movements. However, attempts have failed repeatedly due to insufficient training and abrupt variations in the signals based on time series. Hence, the literature review reveals scope to design a system that can accurately classify even fine body movements for a range of data samples involving a wide variety of signal forms.

7.3 Proposed system

We propose the following approach to address the reviewed literature and overcome the weaknesses present in the field. Figure 7.1 portrays the overall architecture of our proposed system. To explain our system's capability, we divide it into four stages, namely (i) data collection, (ii) pre-processing, (iii) training, and, finally, (iv) classification. The detailed architecture is explained in subsequent sections.

7.3.1 Data collection

Extracting EEG signals is done by attaching electrodes and measuring brain activity using EEG sensor modules placed at crucial locations on the head. Our implementation of sensors includes 64 sensors placed around the frontal, central, parietal, occipital, and temporal poles around the mastoid inion and nasion area [20]. Out of these, electrodes connected in the central area are ignored as they do not respond to our selected bodily movements. These sensors collect data in the form of micro- to millivolt signals ranging from 100 μV to 2 mV, which are then amplified and cleaned for further processing and stored in uncompressed waveform file format on a local storage drive. The areas mentioned above track alpha-wave activity, which tends to be around 8 to 13 Hz. Beta waves are categorised around the posterior region of the cortex, ranging from 13 to 30 Hz. Theta waves originate from the cortex's frontal area, which, in layman's terms, is the forehead. They range from 4 to 8 Hz and come in short burst activity. Delta waves originate from the thalamus area, a large part of the brain, with low frequencies of up to 4 Hz. In addition to these, there is another subset of waves, known as mu waves, which do not feature in the movements of the body. A combination of the first four wave ranges covers an individual's entire brain activity and can be used to determine what kind of task the person is performing. Table 7.1 gives a summary of the activities of individual brain waves.

Apart from the possible scenarios outlined in table 7.1, the human brain is also responsible for other bodily activities such as drawing, itching, waking up, yawning,

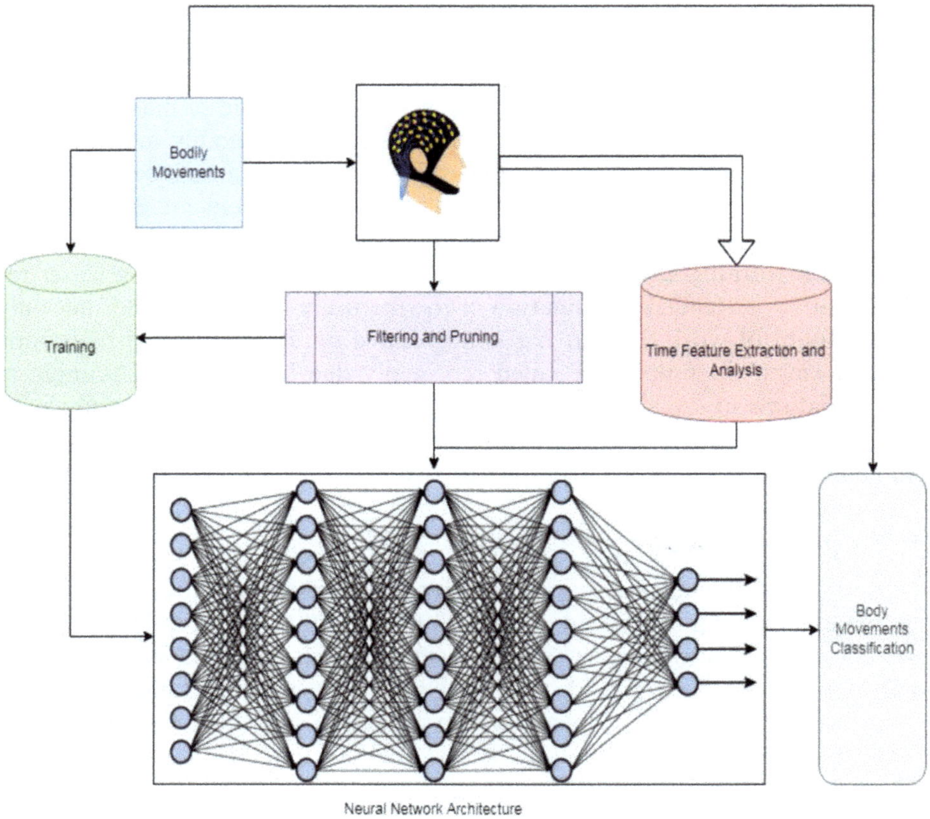

Figure 7.1. The overall architecture of our proposed system.

Table 7.1. Table portraying a summary of EEG behaviours.

Type of activity	Frequency range	Types of behaviour
Alpha	8–13 Hz	Calm and relaxed with less mental activity
Beta	13–30 Hz	An awake individual with high mental stimulation from the environment
Theta	4–8 Hz	A somnolent, sleepy individual experiencing only visual imagery
Delta	< 4 Hz	A sleepy individual with a dreamy scenario
Mu	9–11 Hz	Rest position (no body movement)

etc. These activities are all functionally dependent on the combined action of these aforementioned brain signals. Though there is an extensive interdependence between personality and bodily movements, we can safely assume that personality affects universally proper behaviour. These signals are then passed onto the next stage of model development for pattern recognition.

7.3.2 Pre-processing

In the pre-processing phase, we filter body movement data and read their corresponding EEG signals. Note that EEG signals work sequentially and can vary according to different thought patterns. As such, to perform this step, we use multiple iterations of a sequence for this approach. The series generated from this step contains a lot of noise, and hence must be filtered for training [2]. The filtering process involves low-pass filtering, negating higher frequencies. The data obtained from the EEG sensor are fragile and must be amplified to a suitable degree. Figure 7.2 shows the working of the amplification circuit.

The circuit accepts inputs from 64 gold-plated dry electrodes with a dimension of 10 × 4 × 3 cm, weighing about 100 g, and passes them through 64 different

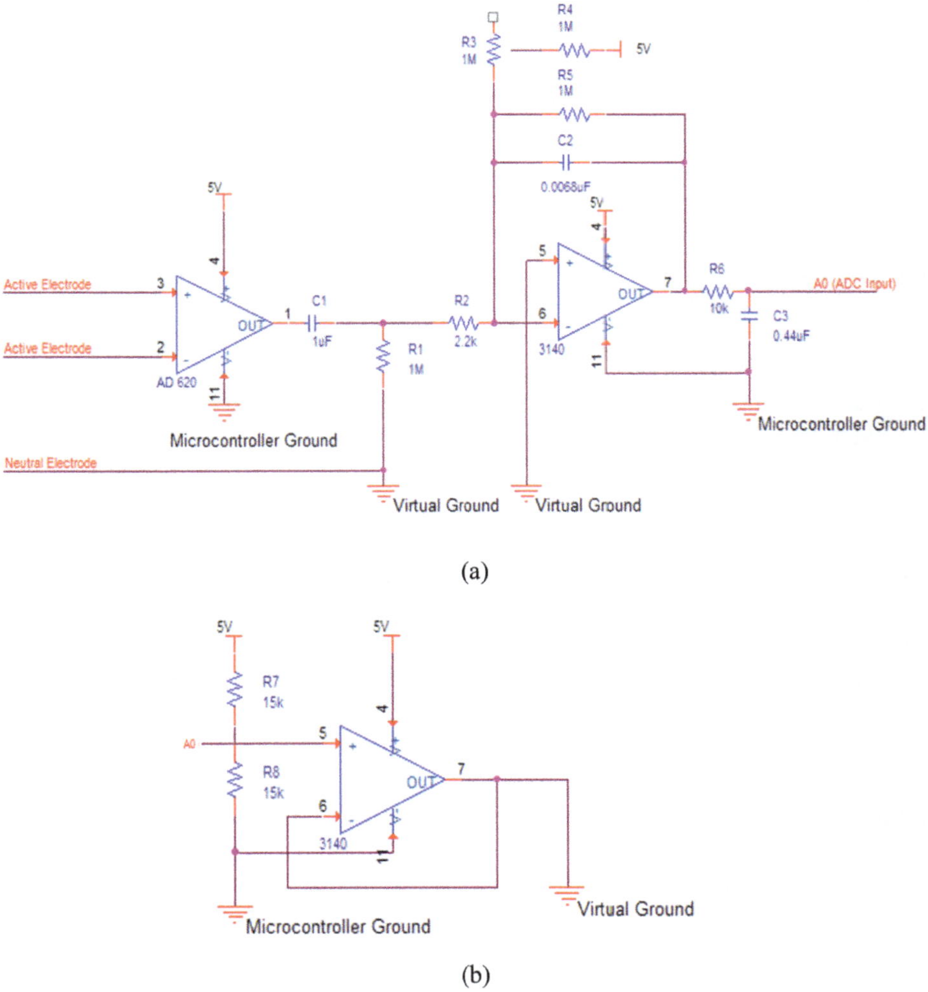

Figure 7.2. Schematic diagram of an EEG circuit: (a) amplification and filtering module, and (b) analogue-to-digital conversion module.

operational amplifiers, here selected as AD620. The main job of these amplifiers is to amplify the signals up to 5 V. The resistors and capacitors used in the schematic diagram prevent interference between the electrode signals and filter out noise signals. Our circuit uses a low-pass filter to remove unwanted signals by the process of moving out and etching away high-frequency signals. Further, boosting the low-voltage signals to higher voltages, ranging from 0 to 5 V is also essential, representing circuit gain. Equation (7.1) governs the mathematical representation of gain:

$$\text{Gain} = \frac{R_5^{-1} + R_3 + R_4}{R_2 + R_1^{-1}}. \tag{7.1}$$

Here, gain represents the total gain to be achieved from the circuit, and $R_{1,\ldots,5}$ represents the resistance values, with a tolerance level of ±5%. Since these signals obtain values ranging from 1 to 5 V, our neural network system cannot encode them properly due to high computational invalidity. Hence, to avoid this issue, we further normalise our voltage rating, ranging from 0 to 1. Equation (7.2) shows the normalisation formula used in this context:

$$\text{Value}_{\text{normalized}} = \frac{\text{value}_{\text{real}} - \text{value}_{\text{min}}}{\text{value}_{\text{max}} - \text{value}_{\text{min}}}. \tag{7.2}$$

As presented, figure 7.2(b) represents a microcontroller module that converts analogue wave signals into digital form. In the proposed system, we have used an Arduino Mega as our microcontroller, which has an inbuilt analogue-to-digital conversion (ADC) precision of 10 bits. To interface all the sensors with the ADC, we used four Arduino Mega controllers in parallel and stored the collected data in a local hard drive connected serially to a computer.

7.3.3 Data training

As aforementioned, the main aim of our present research is to map brain activity to bodily movements. Performing this task is tedious and requires many pattern-recognition techniques. Mathematically, the study seems feasible with an offset of many computations. To convert a possible real-world scenario into a model, we utilise an abstract mathematical model, depicted in equation (7.3):

$$\text{BodyMovement} = f(\text{Brain activity, time, samples, individual}), \tag{7.3}$$

where BodyMovement is a discrete element in the chain, classified into five basic actions as depicted in equation (7.4):

$$\text{BodyMovement} = \begin{cases} \text{Up} \\ \text{Handup} \\ \text{Down} \\ \text{HandDown} \\ \text{Bothlegsdown} \end{cases}. \tag{7.4}$$

We have chosen these movements for easiness's sake, with the possibility of further incorporating additional exercises. Coming back to equation (7.3), brain activity is recorded as an amalgam of the four types of brain wave spread across the entire frequency spectrum. The equation can be mathematically modelled as shown in equation (7.5):

$$\text{Brainactivity} = \theta\left(1|64\begin{Bmatrix}\text{Alpha}\\ \text{Beta}\\ \text{Theta}\\ \text{Delta}\end{Bmatrix}\right), \tag{7.5}$$

where θ is the brain activity mapper combining the interdependent alpha, beta, gamma, and delta brain frequencies categorised across the entire frequency band. The '64' indicates the presence of 64 sensors attached to the EEG cap. A total of 250 samples were used to extract valuable patterns across a time frame of 1 min. The individual parameter identifies the total number of people involved in the experiment.

7.3.4 Classification by neural networks

Neural networks have been proven to be highly effective at finding out patterns from unsorted data. The reason for using a neural network is that a given system will train until it reaches convergence. Though there are conflicting evaluations of neural networks, they are nonetheless proving to be an increasingly popular means of detecting patterns from nothingness [21]. However, neural networks require a great deal of computational time to reach convergence and its associated practices. In our proposal, we use the same concept from neural networks to tackle the present problem. Since brain waves occur in a sequence, adding sequential patterns is necessary. We employ different strategies of neural network classification and then assess the best-known solution for our objective. Figure 7.3 shows a flowchart of the strategy we deploy to fulfil this purpose.

As presented in figure 7.3, we employ three main strategies to classify bodily movements. The first stage involves mapping LSTM layers and organising time-based sequences into patterns. The second comprises a state-of-the-art system consisting of transformers, which are fast encoders-based sequencers. The final strategy involves a traditional transfer-learning approach to classification. Each designed process receives filtered EEG signals in common from a .wav file obtained via the EEG circuit presented in figure 7.2. These strategies are mainly intended because they serve as a standard benchmark for assessing classification-based networks. A detailed explanation of all three techniques is elucidated in the subsequent sections.

7.3.4.1 Strategy 1

The first strategy involves using sequence-based classification intervals by training the entire network from scratch. The network is straightforward and contains a

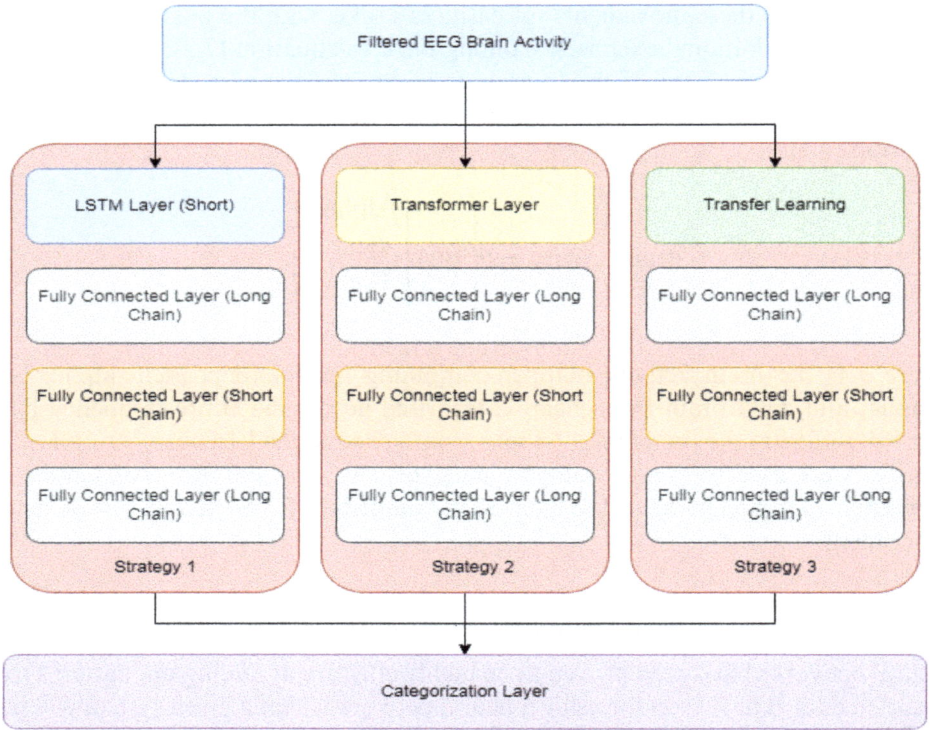

Figure 7.3. Strategy flowchart for classification task.

hidden layer dedicated to mapping sequences. The hidden layer includes a chain of long short-term lines padded with a layered flow of fully connected layers. Along with these fully connected layers, the padded long-short-long term structure ensures proper convergence. Figure 7.4 shows the structure of a LSTM neuron [22].

The LSTM neuron accepts sequences from the previous neuron, performs pattern analysis, and then passes it to the next neuron. In our case, we have used the tanh function for decision-making. Equations (7.6–7.9) give the mathematical formulation of the LSTM neuron:

$$z_i = \sigma(W_z \times [h_{i-1}, x_i]), \tag{7.6}$$

$$r_i = \sigma(W_r \times [h_{i-1}, x_i]), \tag{7.7}$$

$$\bar{h}_i = \tanh(W \times [r_i * h_{i-1}, x_i]), \tag{7.8}$$

$$h_i = (1 - z_i) * h_{i-1} + z_i * \bar{h}_i, \tag{7.9}$$

where i represents the current neuron, $i - 1$ the previous, and so on. The fully connected layer shown in strategy 1 of figure 7.3 consists of a dense set of neurons interconnected with each other, forming a more extensive collection of weight structures that together constitute a convergence of hyperparameters at the

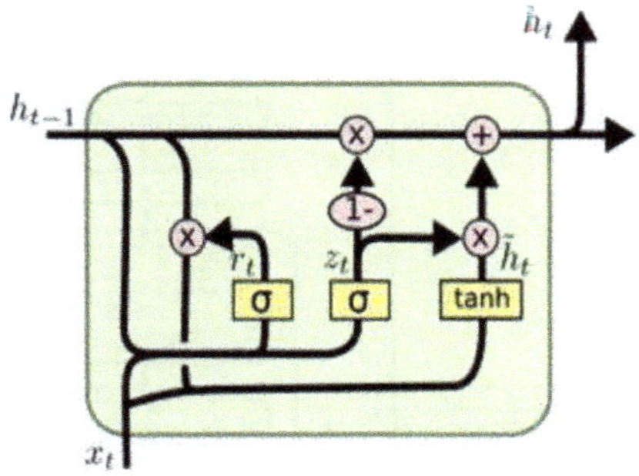

Figure 7.4. Structure of a LSTM neuron.

Table 7.2. The architecture of strategy 1.

Type of layer	Number of nodes/type	Hyperparameters
Input	Single node consisting of 64 channels × 250 samples spread across a three-dimensional array spectrum	64 × 250
Hidden layer	LSTM neurons with a total of 20 bidirectional nodes	236 353
	A fully connected layer consisting of 250 nodes	450 343 567
	A fully connected layer of 100 nodes	900 243 865
	A fully connected layer consisting of 250 nodes	1 300 243 945
Output layer	Categorisation into five body movements	5 400 567 123

classification layer. Table 7.2 provides a summary of the overall architecture of the network.

Our neural network consists of 5 400 567 123 interconnected hyperparameters. These hyperparameters are trained from scratch, assuming a standard random distribution of weights.

7.3.4.2 Strategy 2

In strategy 1, we have detailed the use of a hidden layer incorporating a pattern analysis layer that includes an LSTM node. However, in strategy 2, we use a more advanced type of structure called a transformer. A transformer is simply an encoder that accepts data from contextual knowledge in a sequence. The strategy of such transform encoders is entirely different from that of LSTM networks. Figure 7.5 gives an overview of the structure of a transformer network [23].

As seen in figure 7.5, our transformer layer includes multiple attention heads, shown in orange. The transformer's structure is similar to an LSTM neuron, distinguishing between addition and normalisation layers. These layers are necessary to limit the number of hyperparameters appearing in the encoder pool. Note that our network consists of three multi-head attention modules, which are structured in parallel and passed to the feed-forwarded normalisation layer. Equations (7.10) and (7.11) explain the mathematical model:

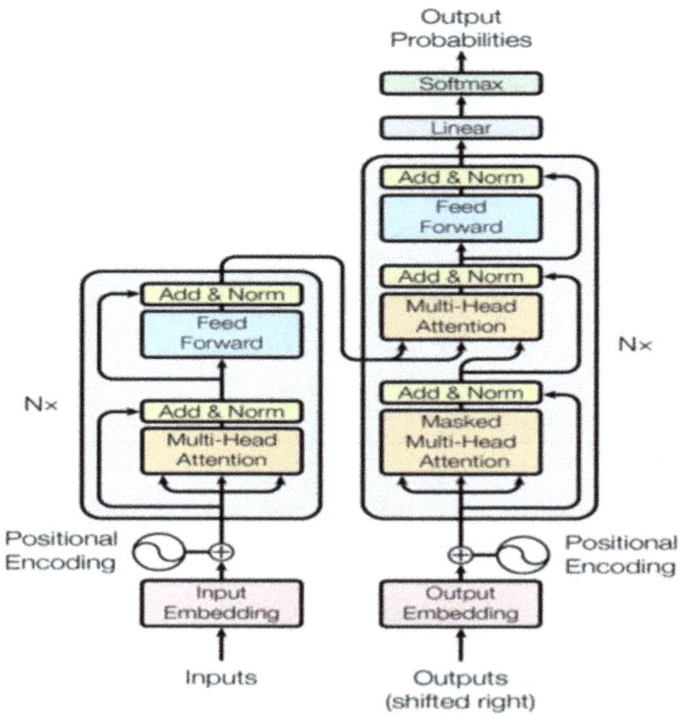

Figure 7.5. Transformer model used in strategy 2.

$$\text{Att}(q, k, v) = \delta\left(\frac{qK^i}{\sqrt{d_k}}\right)*v, \tag{7.10}$$

$$\delta(\text{val}) = \frac{1}{1 + e^{-\text{val}}}. \tag{7.11}$$

Here, q represents a matrix of sequences within the data, k represents the key vector representations for each subsequence within the entire series, and v denotes the values of the arrangement. The δ is the softmax operation, which allows easy classification to output the probabilities. Hence, the transformer layer is itself a classifier. We then embed a chain of dense layers of long-short-long sequences to increase the classification accuracy and impart convergence to the categorisation entity. As a last step, the network is then fit to the output layer, thereby completing our classification model. Table 7.3 portrays the overall architecture of the transformer model.

As seen in table 7.3, the output layer consists of 5 798 123 parameters used for classification. These hyperparameters are trained from scratch, assuming a standard random distribution of weights.

Table 7.3. The architecture of strategy 2.

Type of layer	Number of nodes/type	Hyperparameters
Input	Single node consisting of 64 channels × 250 samples spread across	64 × 250
Hidden layer	A transformer layer consisting of sequential embeddings of 64 channels among 250 channels	143 423
	A fully connected layer consisting of 250 nodes	567 324
	A fully connected layer of 100 nodes	932 123
	A fully connected layer consisting of 250 nodes	3 424 945
Output layer	Categorisation into five body movements	5 798 123

7.3.4.3 *Strategy 3*

The final strategy for our model utilises a completely new approach for classification. This model serves as a benchmark for resolving classification crises. The strategy assumes no prior knowledge of the model and trains only the final layer to attain convergence. Transfer learning is an approach that agrees upon a stored understanding to use it for an entirely new problem. It increases the efficiency of a learning agent because the learning convergence has already been reached for the previous problem, thereby reducing any heavy computations in the new issue. Transfer learning is a well-known approach that has gained a lot of importance in recent years. For our problem, we opt to use a similar network to classify the signals [24]. Though transfer learning has primarily been addressed to visual problems, there exists an existing network, known as YAMNet, that applies solely to audio classification. Since our problem deals with EEG signals, YAMNet perfectly suits our needs. The architecture of YAMNet is portrayed in figure 7.6.

From figure 3.6, we can infer that the input layer of YAMNet consists of M channels coded specifically for specific audio movements. We replace these M channels with our adopted value, which is 64. The next layer consists of a depth convolutional layer of size K, creating a $D_K{*}D_K$ network. In our case, we choose the value to be $K = 1$. This accelerates massive computations, creating a slight reduction in accuracy, which is acceptable. Equation (7.12) shows the depth convolution applied in YAMNet:

$$\hat{H}_{a,\,b,\,c} = \sum_{i,j} \hat{A}_{i,\,k,\,c} {*} \delta_{a+i-1,\,b+j-1,\,m}. \tag{7.12}$$

Here, $\hat{A}_{i,\,k,\,c}$ is the kernel value applied to a depth-wise convolutional filter creating a $D_K{*}D_K{*}64$ network. The YAMNet structure extracts feature vectors in a point-wise convolutional sequence, later applied to a MobileNet to further classify the type of signals. Figure 7.7 shows the overall working principle of YAMNet.

As seen in figure 7.7, we drop the final layer after utilising MobileNet for classification, and attach our fully connected dense network of long-short-long

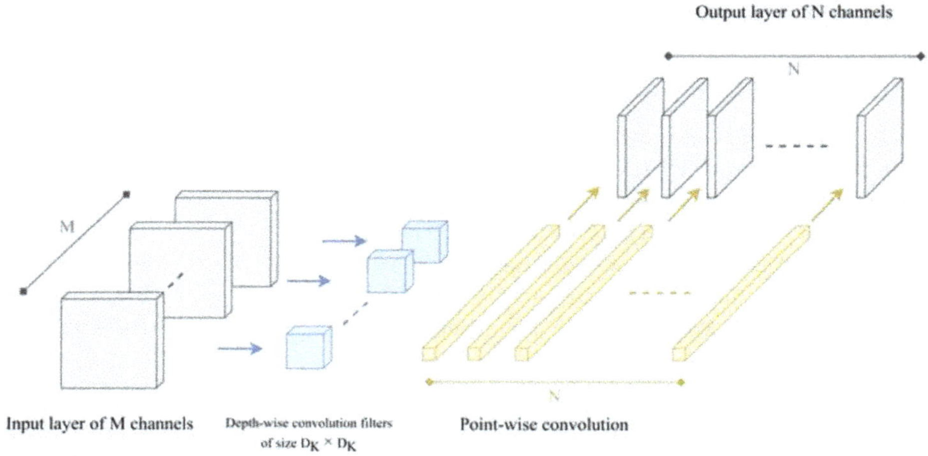

Figure 7.6. The YAMNet architecture.

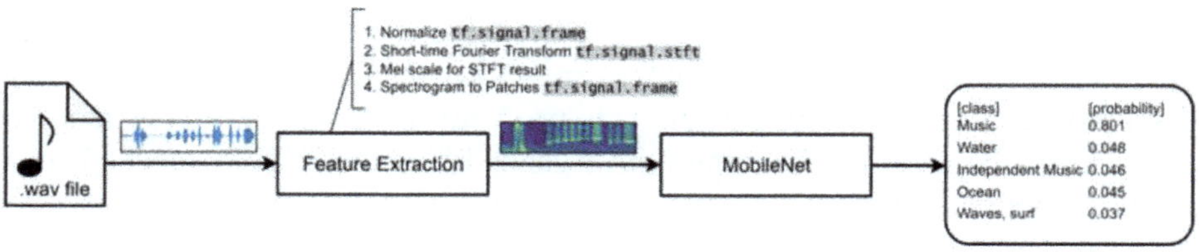

Figure 7.7. The overall working principle of YAMNet.

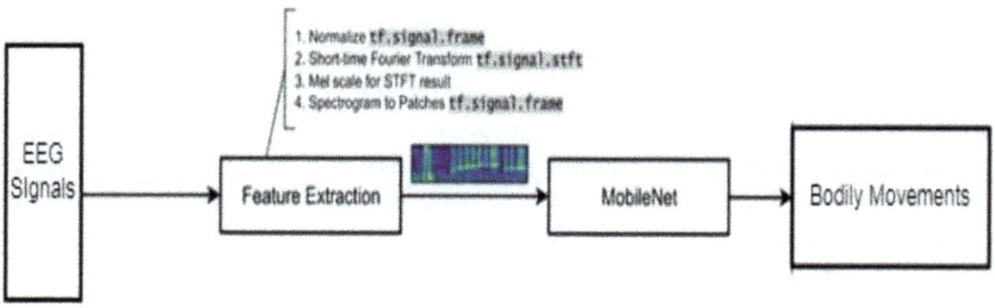

Figure 7.8. Our modified YAMNet architecture for EEG classification.

chains. As a last step, then, we secure the categorical values to classify bodily movements. Figure 7.8 shows this modified layer of our YAMNet model.

Our modified YAMNet transfer-learning architecture consists of a total of 19 845 256 hyperparameters.

We next compare these three strategies to evaluate which is the best at mapping bodily movements. The results are shown in the next section.

7.4 Results

This section includes a comparative analysis of the three different strategies outlined in our proposed system. It also contains pictorial representations of the various parameters associated with our other networks. We validated the hardware amplification circuit by mimicking sample signals using a simulated millivolt generator via the Multisim software. Further, we utilised four standard datasets that are openly available to the research community. In each dataset, we used 70% of the samples for training and the remaining partition for testing. A detailed description of the utilised datasets is first given in section 7.4.1.

7.4.1 Summary of the utilised datasets

Our proposed system consists of mimicking EEG signals extracted from 64 channels placed around the brain, similar to the mounting of an EEG cap in a real-world scenario. The required mimicking is done via the Neurosity operating system, installed on a virtual machine. The EEG signals are collected separately under the custom dataset D04 (Custom Motor Imagery Dataset). We have also used some standard existing datasets, D01 (Left Right-Hand motor Imagery Dataset), D02 (Motor Movement Dataset), and D03 (The most extensive SCP data of Motor-Imagery) to efficiently compare our networks. Table 7.4 gives a brief overview of our datasets.

Table 7.4. The datasets used in our proposed system.

Dataset type	Dataset code	Dataset name	Description
Motor imagery	**D01**	Left Right-Hand motor Imagery Dataset	A total of 52 subjects are present in this dataset, out of which there are 38 valid subjects. Further, the dataset contains results of different questionnaires corresponding to physiology and psychology.
	D02	Motor Movement Dataset	This dataset is composed of 109 different volunteers, two baseline tasks (eyes open and eyes closed), and 64 electrode signals corresponding to fists and feet movement.
	D03	The most extensive SCP data of Motor-Imagery	This dataset consists of 60 hr of EEG brain–computer interface recordings across 75 odd session recordings connected to 13 variable participants.
	D04	Custom Motor Imagery Dataset	This dataset includes 42 mimicked subjects distributed across 64 channels for different bodily movements.

7.4.2 Comparison of different hyperparameters

As mentioned earlier, each of our proposed system strategies includes a set of parameters. The higher the number of hyperparameters, the more time the system requires for computation. Table 7.5 gives a summary of the hyperparameters used for our system.

As we can see from table 4.2, the transformer architecture surpassed all the alternatives by a considerable factor, followed by the transfer-learning approach and then the LSTM model.

7.4.3 Statistical parameter comparison of different datasets

To prove the ability of our model and analyse its effectiveness, we set some standard parameters, namely, precision, accuracy, sensitivity, specificity, and F1 score. We performed the analysis on all four datasets.

7.4.3.1 Analysis of the long short-term memory system

We utilised all four datasets from table 7.4; the achieved results are shown in table 7.6, which shows the statistical parameters of our LSTM-based neural network. For each sample, we supplied 64 input features corresponding to 64 different electrode signals.

Table 7.5. The number of hyperparameters used in our system.

Strategy type	Network used	Number of hyperparameters	Rank
Strategy 1	LSTM	5 400 567 123	III
Strategy 2	**Transformer**	**5 798 123**	**I***
Strategy 3	Transfer learning	19 845 256	II

Table 7.6. Statistical analysis parameters used for strategy 1.

Evaluation metrics		Dataset type			
		D01	D02	D03	D04
No. of samples	TP↑	4445	**4540***	4425	4370
	TN↓	246	**163***	268	313
	FP↑	9136	**9213***	9118	9013
	FN↓	206	**163***	268	313
Percentage	Precision (%) ↑	**33%**	**33%***	**33%**	**33%**
	Recall (%) ↑	**95%**	**97%***	**94%**	**93%**
	Specificity (%) ↓	**3%**	**2%***	**3%**	**3%**
	F1 Score (%) ↑	**49%**	**49%***	**49%**	**48%**

Figure 7.9 portrays a visualised interpretation of the results displayed in table 7.6.

From figure 7.9, it can be inferred that the average precision rate of the LSTM system is fixed at 33%. The system's recall ability has bypassed all expectations, including specificity and F1 score. Such poor precision is due to environmental factors not considered during training.

7.4.3.2 Analysis of the transformer-based system

We implemented the above four datasets from table 7.4; the achieved results are shown in table 7.7, which shows the statistical parameters of our transformer-based architecture. For each sample, we supplied 64 input features corresponding to 64 different electrode signals.

Figure 7.10 portrays a visualised interpretation of the results displayed in table 7.7.

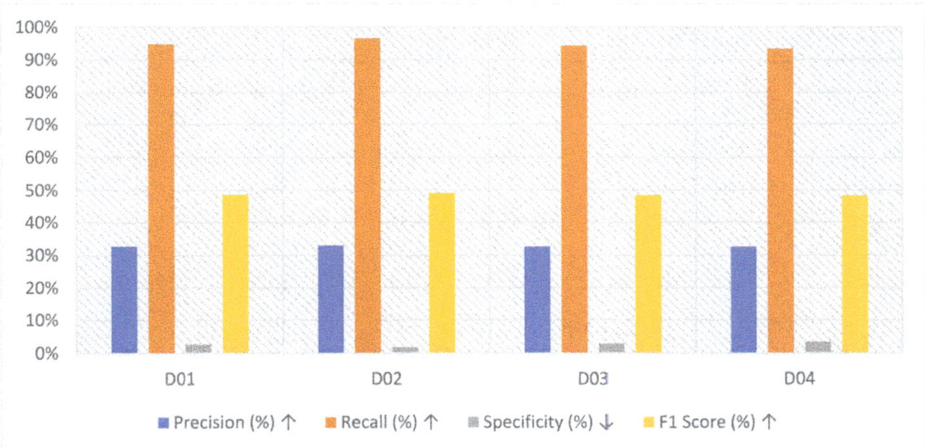

Figure 7.9. Bar chart depicting the analysis of statistical parameters presented in table 7.6.

Table 7.7. Statistical analysis parameters used for strategy 2.

Evaluation metrics		Dataset type			
		D01	D02	D03	D04
No. of samples	TP↑	5445	**5540***	5425	5370
	TN↓	346	**263***	368	413
	FP↑	9236	**9313***	9218	9313
	FN↓	306	**263***	368	413
Percentage	Precision (%) ↑	37%	**37%***	37%	37%
	Recall (%) ↑	94%	**95%***	94%	93%
	Specificity (%) ↓	4%	**3%***	4%	4%
	F1 Score (%) ↑	53%	**54%***	53%	52%

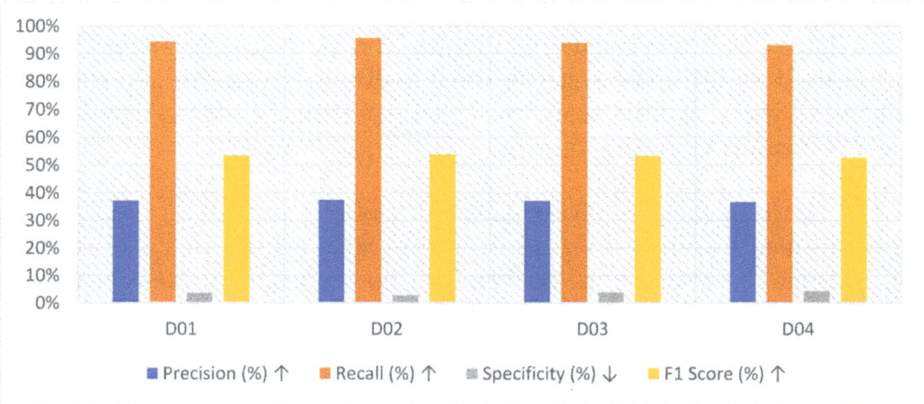

Figure 7.10. Bar chart depicting the analysis of statistical parameters presented in table 7.7.

Table 7.8. Statistical analysis parameters used for strategy 2.

Evaluation Metrics		Dataset Type			
		D01	D02	D03	D04
No. of samples	TP↑	3421	**3520***	3254	3564
	TN↓	243	**164***	168	235
	FP↑	8321	**7256***	7254	8254
	FN↓	205	**153***	152	235
Percentage	Precision (%) ↑	29%	**33%***	31%	30%
	Recall (%) ↑	93%	**96%***	95%	94%
	Specificity (%) ↓	3%	**2%***	2%	3%
	F1 Score (%) ↑	44%	**49%***	47%	46%

From figure 4.2, it is evident that there is a slight increase in the precision ability when using transformers. The main reason behind this effect is the multiple attention layers paying attention to different waves in the EEG pattern.

7.4.3.3 Analysis of the transfer-learning-based system

We then implemented the same four motor-imagery datasets from table 7.4; the achieved results are shown in table 7.8, which shows the statistical parameters of our transfer-learning-based architecture. For each sample, we supplied 64 input features corresponding to 64 different electrode signals.

Figure 7.11 portrays a visualised interpretation of the results displayed in table 7.8

Figure 7.11 shows clear evidence that the precision value gradually drops. This fall is solely due to the strategy's indifference to the time domain, in which the system takes the sequence as a whole and performs classification. Overall, the system

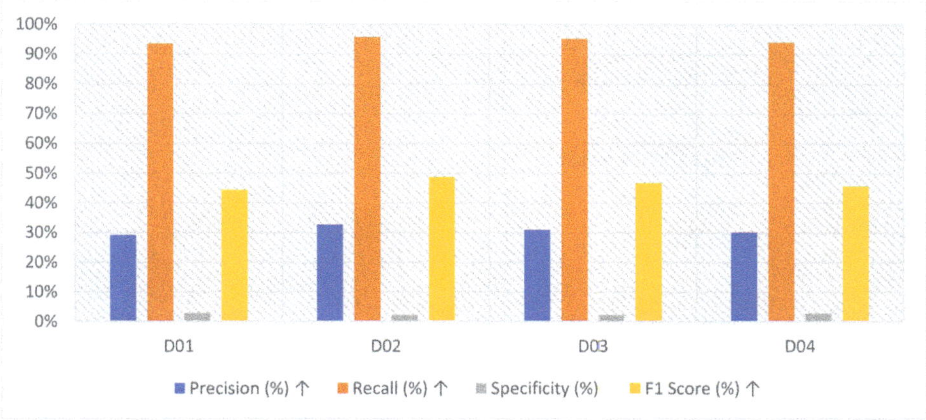

Figure 7.11. Bar chart depicting the analysis of statistical parameters presented in table 7.8.

Table 7.9. The individual accuracies of the different brain waves for each tested strategy.

Strategy vs. classification	Strategy 1 (LSTM)↑	Strategy 2 (transformer)↑	Strategy 3 (YAMNet)↑
Alpha waves	64	**68***	63
Beta waves	33	**47***	40
Theta waves	12	**12***	8
Delta waves	26	**28***	12
Overall accuracy	33	**38***	31

has a clear difference in these terms too. Table 7.9 compares the accuracies of the different techniques.

From table 7.9, it is evident that the transformer system outperforms the other systems. This is due to the multiple attention layers in the neural network. It can also be seen that our system performs best in the recognition of alpha waves. The main reason for this is that our sensor was chiefly designed to be capable of accurately mapping alpha waves via an EEG cap, and body movements are predominantly associated with alpha waves. Figure 7.12 portrays a graphical representation of the different accuracies of the different wave bands.

7.4.4 Comparative analysis

Apart from the abovementioned techniques, we also evaluated our classifier models with other state-of-art techniques. Table 7.10 depicts the ability of these others models in the same field. The parameters chosen were the classifiers used and their predicted accuracy.

The comparison in table 7.10 reveals that our proposed system outperforms other state-of-art techniques. This is due to the involvement of multiple-sequence

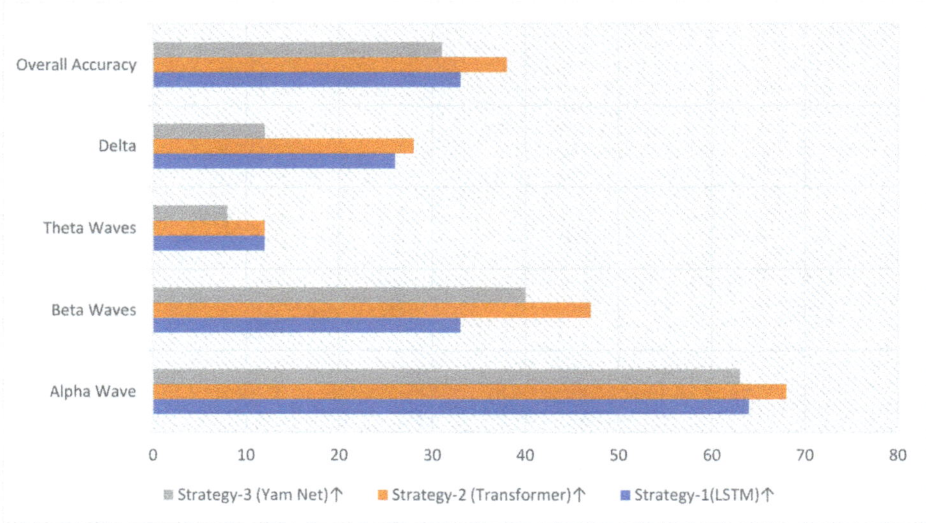

Figure 7.12. The accuracies attained for the different wave bands.

Table 7.10. Comparison of our work with existing research.

Authors	Model used	Classification type	Accuracy ↑
Zhou *et al* [25]	LSTM	Binary classification	65%
Zhnag *et al* [26]	Transfer learning	Three-class classification	63%
Xie *et al* [27]	Transformer architecture	Three-class classification	64%
Proposed system	**Modified transformer**	**Five-class classification**	**68%**

motor-imagery samples for five-class classification, thereby making movement recognition easier with higher accuracies.

7.5 Conclusion

In our proposed system, collected EEG signals are classified into alpha (8–13 Hz), beta (13–30 Hz), theta (4–8 Hz), and delta (<4 Hz) wave sequences based on the range of their frequencies. Various brain activities and bodily movements corresponding to motor imagery are recognised, and multiple categorisations are inferred by incorporating three key chosen strategies: LSTM, transformer-based, and YAMNet transfer-learning-based neural models. Depending on the subjects considered, the transformer-based approach outperforms the other techniques and yields better performance, with an overall recall rate of 90%. A brief comparative analysis, given in table 7.9, clearly indicates that the transformer technique outperforms LSTM and YAMNet neural network models by achieving a significant accuracy of 68% for alpha-wave, 47% for beta-wave, 28% for theta-wave, and 36% for delta-wave sequences.

7.6 Limitations and future work

Our proposed system has successfully achieved the required outcomes as per the outlined requirements. However, in connection to the broader scope of the work, the proposed method has the following limitations.

1. Lack of high-quality sensors that could avoid noise and increase the efficiency of signal identification.
2. Utilisation of above-average training time while handling abruptly varying sequences.
3. Insufficient samples for training patterns of additional body movement recognition.

Considering these limitations, in future the proposed system can be improved by incorporating a platinum-based hybrid transformer architecture to map a vast range of bodily movements. Further, mapping of delta and theta waves would be combined for mapping of thought patterns in the medical field. Also, the utilisation of neural network correction to help patients with epilepsy and dysplasia needs to be addressed. Finally, much effort on improving the proposed system's performance should be directed at using more robust hybrid neural models.

References

[1] Bucci P and Galderisi S 2011 Physiologic basis of the EEG signal *Standard Electroencephalography in Clinical Psychiatry: A Practical Handbook* ed N Boutros, S Galderisi, O Pogarell and S Riggio (New York: Wiley) ch 2 pp 7–12

[2] Venkata Phanikrishna B, Pławiak P and Jaya Prakash A 2021 A brief review on EEG signal pre-processing techniques for real-time brain–computer interface applications https://doi.org/10.36227/techrxiv.16691605.v1 techRxiv:16691605.v1

[3] López-Hernández J L, González-Carrasco I, López-Cuadrado J L and Ruiz-Mezcua B 2021 Framework for the classification of emotions in people with visual disabilities through brain signals *Front. Neuroinform.* **15** 642766

[4] Tandle A L, Joshi M S, Dharmadhikari A S and Jaiswal S V 2018 Mental state and emotion detection from musically stimulated EEG *Brain Inform.* **5** 1–13

[5] Hallett M *et al* 2021 Evaluation of movement and brain activity *Clin. Neurophysiol.* **132** 2608–38

[6] Abtahi M *et al* 2020 Merging fNIRS-EEG brain monitoring and body motion capture to distinguish Parkinsons disease *IEEE Trans. Neural Syst. Rehabil. Eng.* **28** 1246–53

[7] Moreira J, Moreira M, Pombo N, Silva B M C and Garcia N M 2020 Identification of real and imaginary movements in EEG using machine learning models ed A Badnjevic, R Škrbić and L Gurbeta Pokvić *CMBEBIH 2019. IFMBE Proc.* vol 73 (Cham: Springer)

[8] Suhaimi N S, Mountstephens J and Teo J 2020 EEG-based emotion recognition: a state-of-the-art review of current trends and opportunities *Comput. Intell. Neurosci.* **2020** 8875426

[9] Jeon B I, Byung J K, Cho H C and Kim J 2019 Motion recognition and an accuracy comparison of left and right arms by EEG signal analysis *Appl. Sci.* **9** 4885

[10] Zhang G, Davoodnia V, Sepas-Moghaddam A, Zhang Y and Etemad A 2020 Classification of hand movements from EEG using a deep attention-based LSTM network *IEEE Sens. J.* **20** 3113–22

[11] Leon-Urbano C and Ugarte W 2020 End-to-end electroencephalogram (EEG) motor imagery classification with long short-term *2020 IEEE Symp. Series on Computational Intelligence (SSCI)* pp 2814–20

[12] Sun J, Xie J and Zhou H 2021 EEG classification with transformer-based models *2021 IEEE 3rd Global Conf. on Life Sciences and Technologies (LifeTech)* pp 92–3

[13] Lee Y E and Lee S H 2022 EEG-transformer: self-attention from transformer architecture for decoding eeg of imagined speech *2022 10th Int. Winter Conf. on Brain–Computer Interface (BCI)(February 2022) (Piscataway, NJ)* (IEEE) pp 1–4

[14] Tao Y *et al* 2021 Gated transformer for decoding human brain EEG signals *Annual Int. Conf. of the IEEE Engineering in Medicine and Biology Society. IEEE Engineering in Medicine and Biology Society. Annual Int. Conf., 2021* 125–30 pp

[15] Williams J M 2017 Deep learning and transfer learning in the classification of EEG signals *PhD Thesis* University of Nebraska - Lincoln http://digitalcommons.unl.edu/computerscidiss/134

[16] Wang X, Yang R and Huang M 2022 An unsupervised deep-transfer-learning-based motor imagery EEG classification scheme for brain–computer interface *Sensors* **22** 2241

[17] Zheng X *et al* 2020 Task transfer learning for EEG classification in motor imagery-based BCI system *Comput. Math. Methods Med.* **2020** 6056383

[18] Graña M, Aguilar-Moreno M, De Lope Asiain J, Araquistain I B and Garmendia X 2020 Improved activity recognition combining inertial motion sensors and electroencephalogram signals *Int. J. Neural Syst.* **30** 2050053

[19] Kumar S, Sharma A and Tsunoda T 2019 Brain wave classification using long short-term memory network based optical predictor *Sci. Rep.* **9** 9153

[20] Liu L and Zhang P 2021 A novel recommendation algorithm with knowledge graph *J. Phys. Conf. Ser.* **1812** 012035

[21] Türk Ö and Özerdem M S 2019 Epilepsy detection by using scalogram based convolutional neural network from EEG signals *Brain Sci.* **9** 115

[22] Michielli N, Acharya U R and Molinari F 2019 Cascaded LSTM recurrent neural network for automated sleep stage classification using single-channel EEG signals *Comput. Biol. Med.* **106** 71–81

[23] Yuan Y and Lin L 2020 Self-supervised pretraining of transformers for satellite image time series classification *IEEE J. Sel. Top. Appl. Earth Obs. Remote Sens.* **14** 474–87

[24] Sannidhan M S, Prabhu G A, Chaitra K M and Mohanty J R 2021 Performance enhancement of generative adversarial network for photograph–sketch identification *Soft Comput.* **27** 435–52

[25] Zhou J, Meng M, Gao Y, Ma Y and Zhang Q 2018 Classification of motor imagery EEG using wavelet envelope analysis and LSTM networks *2018 Chinese Control and Decision Conf. (CCDC) (Piscataway, NJ, June 2018)* (IEEE) pp 5600–5

[26] Zhang K, Robinson N, Lee S W and Guan C 2021 Adaptive transfer learning for EEG motor imagery classification with deep convolutional neural network *Neural Netw.* **136** 1–10

[27] Xie J *et al* 2022 A transformer-based approach combining deep learning network and spatial-temporal information for raw EEG classification *IEEE Trans. Neural Syst. Rehabil. Eng.* **30** 2126–36

IOP Publishing

Affective Computing in Healthcare
Applications based on biosignals and artif cial intelligence
M Murugappan

Chapter 8

Voice-enabled real-time affective framework for negative emotion monitoring

Parker Wilmoth and Prabha Sundaravadivel

Stress, anxiety, and depression are common problems for many people and can make life difficult if they become chronic. Knowing what someone is dealing with is an essential first step in fixing the problem. Our goal is to provide a device that can detect negative emotions in real time and attempt to alleviate them. In order to detect negative emotions in real time, we train a neural network to recognise emotions from uttered phrases. When negative emotions are chronic, we employ cognitive behavioural therapy (CBT) to train the user's brain to think more positively. Over time, the user will learn lasting coping skills to improve their emotional state. We have found that emotional state can be ascertained from phrases uttered over a user's day. Our prediction network can accurately predict the emotion of a phrase in real time. We intend to use this prediction framework to employ CBT at critical times when it is most effective. Positive psychology has proven effective for many people, but can take a long time to become second nature to those attempting to adopt it. With our device, this process can be reinforced and employed effectively in such a way that this process is faster and more permanent. We have demonstrated emotion detection at an accuracy of 98% with minimal training. This is accomplished using MATLAB's mel-frequency cepstral coefficients extractor and a convolutional neural network. Different voice types and parameters were varied, and their effects were noted to achieve this accuracy. Our model can be easily integrated into wearables-based real-time emotion monitoring and interventions.

8.1 Introduction

Stress, anxiety, and depression have become very common in our day-to-day lives [1]. Much of the time, we can handle occasional such symptoms and cope on our own. However, everyone is different, and these symptoms can become a chronic

doi:10.1088/978-0-7503-5182-9ch8

problem. These symptoms become a problem when they get in the way of someone having a successful life because they do not know how to cope. Coping mechanisms can be taught to people who suffer from many mental afflictions. Treating people in this way is called *cognitive behavioural therapy (CBT)*. This is where patients are taught to challenge how they view their feelings and view the world in a more positive light. One problem with CBT is that it can only help if the afflicted remember what to do now. Therapy should progress much faster if the person can be reminded of good coping mechanisms and positive thought processes when feeling anxious. This is different than just training the brain in moments of no negative input, which would likely take longer to be effective. The patient will become better at recognising negative emotions and behaviour and will be able to counter it faster. Our device aims to provide this therapy in a real-time manner to expedite the user's treatment and recovery.

8.1.1 Wearables for emotion monitoring

There exist many wearables that detect the emotional state of the wearer using a plethora of different methods. These devices keep track of the user's mood throughout the day and use this information in various ways. Some present this data to the user or their supporting physicians/therapists after a long period of use. Others, like the ones discussed below, are built to detect stress minute-by-minute. In each case, sensing hardware is constructed into a wearable band that collects heart rate, blood pressure, body temperature, motion, orientation, voice, and so on, and either stores or analyses it.

8.1.2 Real-time stress detection

Active devices need to analyse their data immediately to act on their conclusions. Passive devices can also analyse in real time or process it at a later point in time. Most of these devices are Internet-of-Things capable and can upload their data to the Internet, where it can be processed and compressed. Active devices can also use this connection to notify the user of their findings and encourage them when needed. By moving from passive to active real-time detection, problems can be addressed when they appear, and forms of intervention can be employed. This vastly improves the device's usefulness: rather than just detecting the user is in distress and documenting it, the device can do something about it.

8.1.3 Cognitive behavioural therapy

Using CBT training for positive affects has been deployed by many researchers in different scenarios. How and when it is employed is an ongoing field of study and research. The goal of CBT is to rewire the way a patient's brain reacts to negative stimuli in positive ways. When humans employ positivity and gratitude in the way they think, they are happier and can cope with adverse situations better [9]. This positive feeling of gratitude is an evolutionary adaptation that CBT utilises as a coping mechanism [10]. When patients practice this positive psychology, they are presented with different situations and are advised on how to approach them. When negative stimuli are received, patients are taught to challenge how to overcome negative emotions and focus on the good things. They better themselves through difficult situations and learn to 'look at the bright side'. The hope is that by practicing this way of thinking when times are easy, patients' brains will fall back on it when times are difficult. The world is subjective, and those who think positively will live a happier life. This can be used as a treatment for many mental health afflictions such as stress, anxiety, depression, addiction, post-traumatic stress disorder (PTSD), etc.

The first thing that may come to mind is a weekly visit to a therapist; however, there are several other ways CBT can be administered. An online therapy programme was provided to college students in 2018 [4]. Students logged on to an online session in their own time, where they learned to employ the principles of CBT. This programme was effective in decreasing negative emotions in those that participated. This solution would work well with our wearable due to the flexible nature of online services. When the device detects stress, the user can be prompted to view reinforcing therapy in real time. This will be a more effective way to employ CBT during stressful times in the user's day rather than when they are comfy at home on the couch.

There have been many attempts at designing devices that can intervene when they detect stress in the user. One extreme example of stress intervention is in use for those who suffer from suicidal ideation [6]. When stress is detected, the device can intervene appropriately in real time. Other intervention devices use a much simpler, passive approach to curb stress. One such device [7] uses calming music, good news, and so on, to help the user cope with stressful situations. CBT has been employed similarly for those suffering from drug addictions and PTSD [8]. The device in these cases could detect the user's upset and provide simple, reassuring, empathetic messages. We aim to take notes from these existing devices and use a much more active form of real-time CBT to help our users with stress.

8.1.4 Privacy in health-monitoring systems

Keeping patient data privacy is very important if that data can be used maliciously in the wrong hands. This is the case with the emotional state of a user; if that is made available to a criminal, it could potentially be used to take advantage of them. A user's current emotional state and emotional history are not thus public and must be encrypted when sent over the air. Each user's data should be kept private. The great thing about the emotional data we intend to collect is that it is easy to make anonymous. It is difficult to associate any specific person with an emotional history. This means that once a user's name is taken off their data, it is inherently anonymous and cannot be tracked back to them. This is important for our use case because every user's data are analysed. Another way to encapsulate user data that provides protection is to have the device only post a user's response to a specific CBT stimulus rather than their emotional state throughout the stimulus. The device can assess how successful a CBT stimulus was and hide precisely how the user felt through the time administered. Its effectiveness lies in what is sent to the database for analysis. The effectiveness of this stimulus is more anonymous than even raw emotional data, which provides further protection to the user.

8.2 Methods

There are two parts to our method. First, we must develop an emotion-detection framework that can detect emotions in the user's voice in real time. Second, we must employ CBT to improve the user's emotions. Figure 8.1 shows a flowchart for developing a neural network with emotion-tagged data.

8.2.1 Real-time emotion detection

Emotion detection through voice has been done before using the same valence–arousal approach. We used a convolutional neural network (CNN) in MATLAB to detect emotions in uttered phrases. The CNN was trained using MATLAB's audio feature extractor and CNN tool. Using the Toronto Emotional Speech Set (TESS) [5], we trained the CNN to recognise different emotions and map them to different valence–arousal values. For each emotion category (neutral, happy, sad, angry) we used 360 training phrases and 40 validation phrases. MATLAB's audio feature extractor enabled the network to recognise different characteristics in each phrase. Mel-frequency cepstral coefficients, pitch, harmonic ratio, bark spectrum, etc., were pulled from each audio clip and passed as inputs to the network.

The program flow for training the network is shown below.

emotions to recognise ***emotions*** = categorical([‘neutral’,‘happy’,‘sad’, … ‘angry’]);

each audio file is extracted and passed into network

afe = audioFeature- Extractor (… ‘SampleRate’,fs, … ‘FFTLength’, FFTLength,
… ‘Window’,hann(frameSamples,‘periodic’), … ‘OverlapLength’, overlapSamples, … ‘mfcc’,true, … ‘barkSpectrum’,true);

features = extract(afe,xPadded);

the neural network is trained and saved

trainedNet = trainNetwork(XTrain,YTrain,layers,options);

The layers of the CNN are shown below. All the bands of voice data are passed into CNN, 50 bands at length 150. At the convolution layers, filters are applied to each recognise specific patterns in the data passed. Max-pooling layers condense the data to make it run faster on the machine, but also minimise the information lost. At the end, an emotion is predicted. By using this network and the audio feature extractor, real-time audio clips can be passed into the trained network and the emotion predicted.

Another addition is made to correct for times where the user is not speaking, so that portions of audio clips where voices are not detected do not predict emotions. This was also very easy via MATLAB, as it has objects which detect portions of a clip where the user is speaking. One final feature which can be implemented is voice recognition that also discards phrases not uttered by the user. The user would train

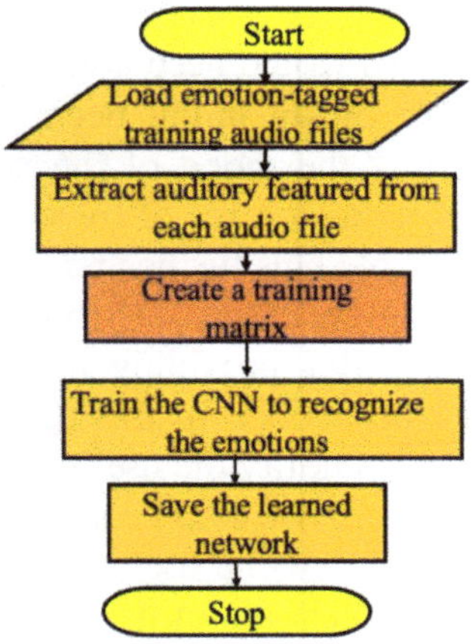

Figure 8.1. Program flowchart used for training the network.

the device to recognise their voice, and so others around them would not influence its emotion detection. This real-time prediction software can be ported into C and loaded onto hardware with an attached microphone. This can be used as a wearable with a microphone. The program can also be loaded onto a smartphone or smart speaker, in which case no additional hardware is required. However, this may pose added security hurdles, and would drain smartphone batteries by continuously running in the background. Thus, we intend to add it to a wearable in future work in order to test it in the ways explained in the next section. The program flow for real-time emotion detection is shown below.

8.2.2 Use of cognitive behavioural therapy in real time

The following describes how our device is designed to employ CBT in real time based on input from our emotion-detection software.

(1) **Determining when to intervene:** The emotion-detection software categorises the emotion of the user on a second-by-second basis. This poses problems for acting on input, as a person can exhibit many different emotions in a short period. One sentence may be exciting, and the next may be nervous, the next could be scared, etc. If our device prompted the user each instant that it detected they were stressed, it would very quickly become annoying and not helpful. Not only that, but the device will also be incorrect some of the time, and the user may be confused as to why the device is telling them they are depressed or stressed when they are not. Rather than acting on each detection, the device will keep track of recent emotions, and look for patterns and frequently detected emotions [21, 22]. By looking at these, the device can improve its accuracy and will be able to provide better help for each different type of situation. The device will be able to tell the difference between a person who is stressed and angry versus someone who just stubbed their toe. The severity of different emotions can be ascertained from the data, as well. Short but frequent periods of sadness can be addressed at

the end of the day when the user has time, but constant sadness and hopelessness in every word would need addressing in the moment. Not only can the device act once on an initial negative detection, but it can also provide encouragement if the mood of the person improves. By congratulating the user if they take control of their mood, it empowers them and makes them feel in control. This further reinforces positive psychology and will make the user feel even better [11] (building self-esteem). The device also needs to know if, after providing initial guidance, the user is not improving or even getting worse. In this case, the device should act with follow-up guidance or even notify the user's therapist, in which case the user could talk with them. The device could contact the user's significant other or good friend and tell them that the user is feeling stressed or sad, in which case they could talk with them about it. Talking about how one feels is yet another form of CBT. Figure 8.2 shows the network architecture for the trained data, and figure 8.3 shows the steps involved in training the network to recognise emotion.

(2) **Use of artificial intelligence (AI):** It is difficult to program a device to know what to do in each and every circumstance using reasoning alone. This is where AI can be used to detect patterns automatically. In our previous research, we integrated machine-learning algorithms in analysing affects for various scenarios [12–18]. Firstly, AI could detect specific times of the day or places where specific emotions are common. This would run all the time, tailoring to each user individually, for as long as the device is used. Secondly, it can be used during clinical trials to determine the most effective point in which to intervene and which forms of CBT work the best for all people. The longer the device is used and the more people that use it, the better it will become at helping them.

(3) **Integration of data in CBT training:** CBT typically uses hypothetical examples of things a person may face. With our detection framework, we intend to use actual events that happened to the user. This will further help

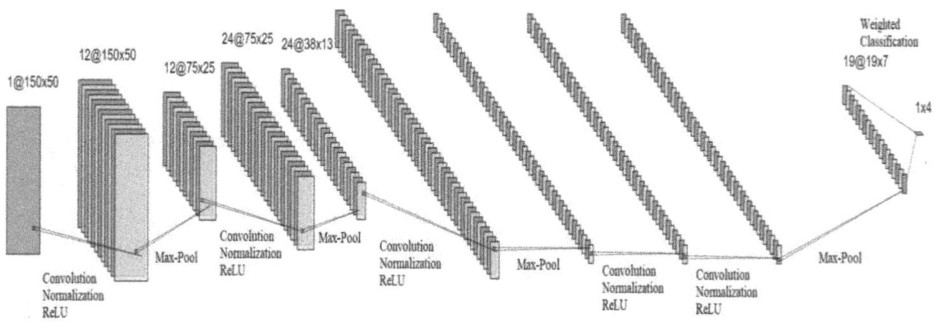

Figure 8.2. Our custom-built neural network architecture used for emotion-recognition training generated using neural network scalable vector graphics (NN-SVG) [23].

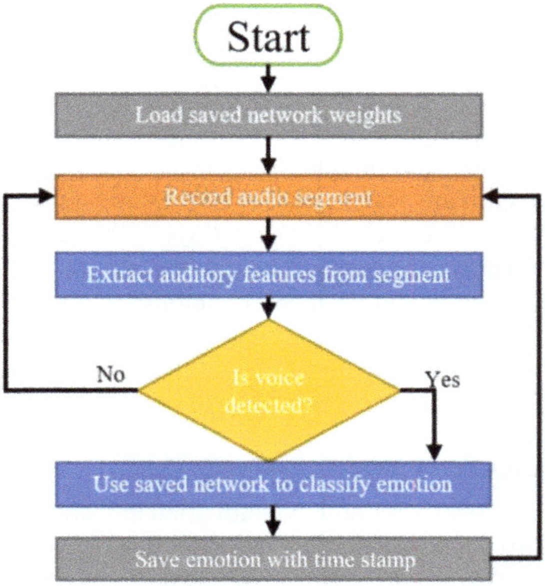

Figure 8.3. Program flow used for recognising emotion.

them to cope with their specific problems. For example, if the device detected the person was sad previously that day, it could ask the user to explain what they were feeling during those times. It can then ask them how they could make the situation better and keep track of what the user suggests as their coping mechanism. If on the next day the user is sad again, the device can suggest they try their coping mechanism. By building the device and online therapy framework so that they work together, CBT can be employed in a more effective manner. Some forms of CBT work better for one person but not another, and by using the data the device collects our solution will show improvements quickly where generic CBT may take longer.

8.3 Experimental results

8.3.1 Emotion-detection accuracy

Our emotion-detection software framework has shown similar results to those found in the literature [2, 3]. Our network shows about 98% accuracy, which falls on the higher end of the range of other's work (70%–99%). These results are from using only the TESS dataset, as proof of concept. This accuracy is only obtained after substantial training data is obtained for an individual user. The prediction accuracy for a new user with minimal training is about 70%, which falls on the lower end of the spectrum. Given more users, the accuracy will fall between these values, which are good enough to use CBT with.

8.3.2 False positives and audio sample size

It was the case that the CNN was more likely to produce false positives for known emotions, which must be considered when using real-time detection software. Table 8.1 shows a comparison of the accuracy of our algorithm with other examples in the field of emotion recognition and prediction.

Given these audio clips are very short (2–4 s), the sample size of a given emotion is small. This problem could be solved in two ways, either by ignoring brief single-emotion flags or by taking the average of groups of flags. The argument against simply increasing the sample duration for an emotion is that emotions can change quickly in a phrase, and potentially get lost inside of a larger frame. Decreasing the frame would have the opposite effect in that emotions may not be clearly extracted in such a short clip.

8.3.3 Voice types and unknown users

One problem with the CNN was that it was not good at recognising a new voice. The TESS dataset has two voice actors, one male and one female. One way to test the CNN on a new user was to only train it with one actor and validate it using the other. The table below shows the accuracy of the CNN given different combinations. The accuracy is near perfect when the system only encounters a single recognised user. Table 8.2 gives the validation of our results for both male and female datasets.

However, when it tried to recognise the emotions of a new user, it was about 50% less accurate. To further test the accuracy of the CNN when a new user was introduced, 15 recordings similar to the TESS 'Say the word (blank)' format were

Table 8.1. Best-case prediction accuracy comparison of our algorithm and others.

Author	Accuracy	Algorithm
Lika *et al* [3]	74%	ANFC and SOM
Bustamante *et al* [2]	95%	Std. CNN
Md. Sahidullah *et al* [19]	92%	MFLE
Vishwanathan *et al* [20]	86%	NFN
Our algorithm	**98%**	**Std. CNN**

The bold text indicates the best and highest accuracy achieved by our proposed methodology, which is also higher than the state-of-the-art methods.

Table 8.2. Prediction accuracy using male/female data for training and validation.

		Training	
Validation		Male	Female
	Male	100%	57%
	Female	49%	98%

collected for each emotion from a new user. Ten of each set of recordings were used for training and five for validation. Table 8.3 and the confusion matrices in figure 8.4 show the accuracy given in four scenarios.

The first scenario (48%) is when the TESS data were used to train the network and new users' data alone were used to validate it. This shows a very similar result to that of when an unrecognised TESS voice actor was validated on the other's training. This had the worst result because the CNN had never heard the new user before and could not predict their emotion well. The second scenario (72%) represents when the new user's data are added to the TESS data for training but only the new user validates the predictions. This increased the accuracy by 66%, which suggests that more data, even from different voices, does improve the accuracy of emotion detection. It also suggests that there may be information available in a recording of any type of voice that the CNN started to use, which could categorise emotion for any user (universal valence and arousal). Note there is no category for the new user's

Table 8.3. Prediction accuracy given different data used for training and validation.

		Training	
Validation		TESS	TESS and new user
	New user	48%	72%
	TESS and new user	94%	98%

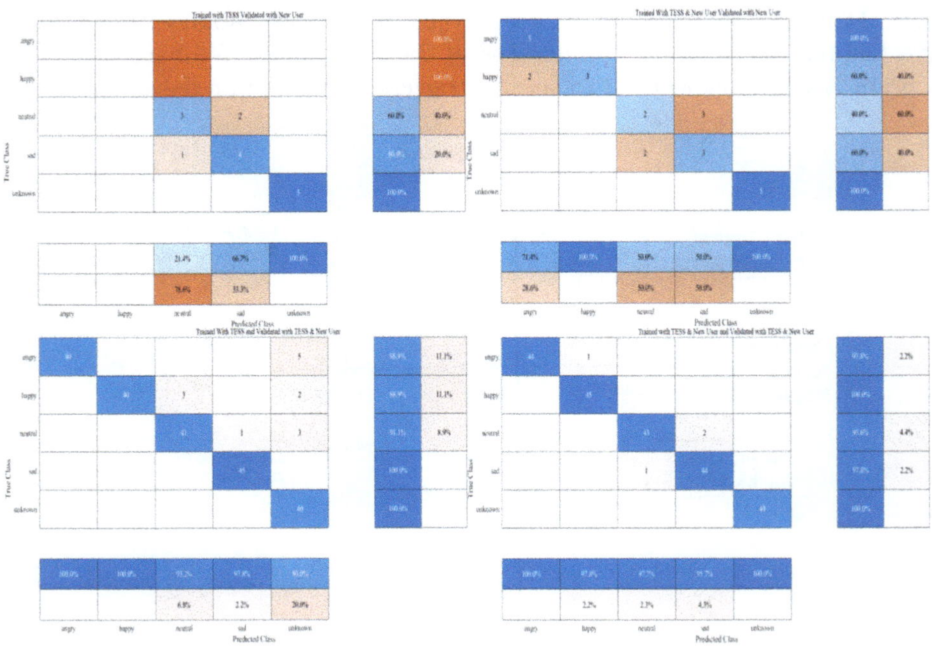

Figure 8.4. Confusion matrices of CNN accuracy given different data used for training and validation.

data alone to be used in training. This is done specifically because the end goal for the CNN is to make it work well for all new users with minimal training effort on their part. Given the use of 10 recordings for each emotion, the CNN would be very bad at predicting new phrases with the small amount of training data. The third and fourth scenarios demonstrate that the accuracy of the system is best when the most data are used. The CNN is the best for every individual user when all user data are used in training.

8.3.4 Error patterns

In the times that the CNN was incorrect, there were patterns in the predictions. The angry and happy emotions were often mixed up. However, the CNN was best at detecting sadness. This suggests that it was better at differentiating negative versus positive arousal than negative versus positive valence. Figure 8.5 shows our implementation of Russel's circumplex model of affect for emotions. Note the vertical axis is arousal and the horizontal axis is valence; also note that the neutral emotion is in the centre of the diagram. This happy/angry error may be because sadness is the only emotion in the negative arousal area that it was trained to recognise. Neutral emotions were occasionally miscategorized, as well, but less often than anger and happiness were. It was equally likely to be mixed up with the other three emotions, which makes sense as it is an equal distance from each on the model.

8.3.5 Employing cognitive behavioural therapy

Due to restrictions from the COVID-19 pandemic, clinical trials are not currently an option, but we intend to employ our software in trials in future work. By studying how CBT is employed and the situations where positive psychology can be used, we have tailored our software to intervene at the right times. We have developed a program flow of how to react to specific triggers from emotion detection.

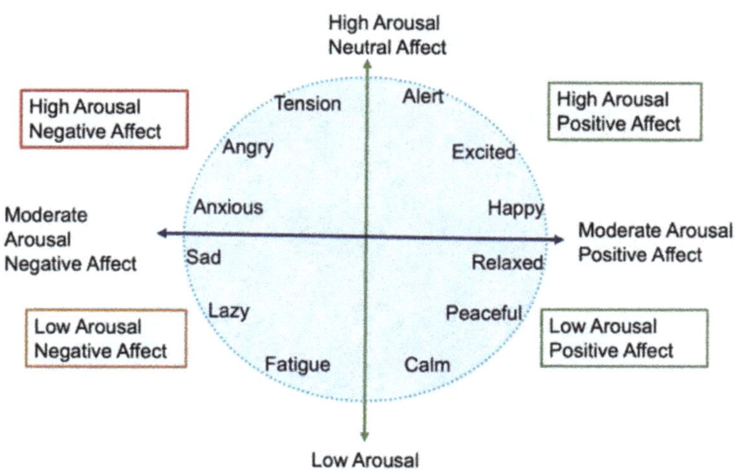

Figure 8.5. Valence–arousal model of affects. © 2020, IEEE. Adapted from [18].

8.3.6 Conclusion for deployment

Given the 72% accuracy from when a new user adds minimal training to the CNN, and that the accuracy improves the more voices are added to the network, this software is in a state which can be deployed for use with CBT. Before new users begin to use the software, they should record a few phrases in order to 'introduce' the CNN to them. The software can be expected to predict their emotion in real time with a high level of accuracy. The software is best at detecting sadness and, as a result, will be better when used with those with anxiety or depression than those with stress.

8.4 Conclusion

One big problem the device will encounter is when a user feels pressure to conceal their emotions and does not speak how they feel. In social settings, people tend to conceal their anger or sadness from others with whom they are not close. Unless the user can speak how they really feel, the device will not be able to detect their emotion and guide them to improve it. Users will be encouraged to verbally reflect on how they feel constantly throughout their day in order to maximise the detection of their emotions. This is not possible for every individual, but for those who it is, it can be used effectively. Voice detection can easily be paired with other emotion-sensing devices, which each contribute to the overall accuracy of real-time emotion detection. Further, life can be very tough and cause people to suffer from severe depression or anxiety that CBT alone cannot fix; for example, when someone loses a loved one. They could become depressed for weeks to months, and no amount of CBT would make their situation much less painful. This is especially true if the emotion is extreme, as in this case, and people in certain situations do not want to seek help. CBT should be used when the user actively wants to put the work in to recover and change how they think. Negative emotions are a part of life: they make us human. It is okay to not be okay all the time, and negative emotion can be a good thing.

References

[1] Karthikeyan P, Murugappan M and Yaacob S 2011 A review on stress inducement stimuli for assessing human stress using physiological signals *Proc. IEEE 7th Int. Coll. on Signal Processing and Its Applications (Penang, Malaysia)* pp 420–5

[2] Bustamante P, Celani N, Perez M and Montoya O 2015 Recognition, and rationalization of emotions in the arousal-valence plane *Proc. 37th Annual Int. Conf. of the IEEE Engineering in Medicine and Biology Society (EMBC) (August 2015)* pp 6042–6045

[3] Lika R, Seldon H and Kiong L 2014 Feature analysis of speech emotion data on arousal-valence dimension using an adaptive neuro-fuzzy classifier *Proc. Int. Conf. on Industrial Automation, Information, and Communications Technology (August 2014)* pp 104–10

[4] Palacios J, Richards D, Palmer R, Coudray C, Hofmann S, Palmieri P and Frazier P 2018 Supported Internet-delivered cognitive behavioral therapy programs for depression, anxiety, and stress in university students: open, non-randomised trial of acceptability, effectiveness, and satisfaction *JMIR Ment. Health* **5** e11467

[5] Pichora-Fuller M and Dupuis K 2020 Toronto emotional speech set (TESS) (Scholars Portal Dataverse, 2020) (https://doi.org/10.5683/SP2/E8H2MF)
[6] Sundaravadivel P, Salvatore P and Indic P 2020 M-SID: an IoT-based edge-intelligent framework for suicidal ideation detection *Proc. 2020 IEEE 6th World Forum on Internet of Things (WF-IoT) (New Orleans, USA, June 2020)* pp 1–6
[7] Akmandor A and Jha N 2017 Keep the stress away with SoDA: stress detection and alleviation system *IEEE Trans. Multi-Scale Comput. Syst.* **3** 269–82
[8] Fletcher R, Tam S, Omojola O, Redemske R, Fedor S and Moshoka J 2011 Mobile application and wearable sensors for use in cognitive behavioral therapy for drug addiction and PTSD *Proc. 2011 5th Int. Conf. on Pervasive Computing Technologies for Healthcare (Pervasive-Health) and Workshops* pp 202–3
[9] Emmons R and Shelton C 2002 *Gratitude and the Science of Positive Psychology* (Oxford: Oxford University Press)
[10] Nowak M and Roch S 2006 Upstream reciprocity and the evolution of gratitude *Proc. R. Soc.* B **274** 605–10
[11] Mruk C 2008 The psychology of self-esteem: a potential common ground for humanistic positive psychology *Humanist. Psychol.* **36** 143–58
[12] Sundaravadivel P, Tumwesigye C, Mohanty S P and Kougianos E 2020 iMED-Tour: an IoT-based privacy-assured framework for medical services in smart tourism *Proc. IEEE Int. Conf. on Consumer Electronics (ICCE)* pp 1–5
[13] Sundaravadivel P, Fitzgerald A and Indic P 2019 i-SAD: an edge-intelligent IoT-based wearable for substance abuse detection *Proc. IEEE Int. Symp. on Smart Electronic Systems (iSES) (Formerly iNiS) (Rourkela, India)* pp 117–22
[14] Sundaravadivel P, Wilmoth P and Fitzgerald A 2021 SolicitudeSavvy: an IoT-based edge intelligent framework for monitoring anxiety in real-time *Proc. 22nd Int. Symp. on Quality Electronic Design (ISQED) (Santa Clara, CA, USA)* pp 576–80
[15] Wilmoth P and Sundaravadivel P 2021 An interactive IoT-based framework for resource management in assisted living during pandemic *Proc. 22nd Int. Symp. on Quality Electronic Design (ISQED) (Santa Clara, CA, USA)* pp 571–5
[16] Sallah A and Sundaravadivel P 2020 Tot-Mon: a real-time Internet of Things based affective framework for monitoring infants *Proc. IEEE Computer Society Annual Symp. on VLSI (ISLVSI)* pp 600–1
[17] Yadav G, Sundaravadivel P and Kesavan L 2020 Affect-learn: an IoT-based affective learning framework for special education *Proc. IEEE 6th World Forum on Internet of Things (WF-IoT)* pp 1–5
[18] Sundaravadivel P, Goyal V and Tamil L 2020 i-RISE: an IoT-based semi-immersive affective monitoring framework for anxiety disorders *Proc. IEEE Int. Conf. on Consumer Electronics (ICCE)* pp 1–5
[19] Sahidullah M and Saha. G 2012 Design, analysis and experimental evaluation of block-based transformation in MFCC computation for speech recognition *Speech Commun.* **54** 543–65
[20] Viswanathan M, Zhang Z, Tian X and Lim. J S 2012 Emotional-speech recognition using the neuro-fuzzy network *Proc. 6th Int. Conf. on Ubiquitous Information Management and Communication (ICUIMC'12) (New York)* (Association for Computing Machinery) pp 1–5
[21] Maithri M, Raghavendra U, Gudigar A, Samanth J, Datta Barua P, Murugappan M, Chakole Y and Rajendra Acharya U 2022 Automated emotion recognition: current trends and future perspectives *Comput. Methods Programs Biomed.* **215** 106646

[22] Murugappan M, Baharuddin N Q I and Jerritta S 2012 DWT and MFCC based human emotional speech classification using LDA *2012 Int. Conf. on Biomedical Engineering (ICoBE) (Penang, Malaysia)* pp 203–6
[23] Lenail A 2019 NN-SVG tool (version 1.0) GitHub https://github.com/alexlenail/NN-SVG

IOP Publishing

Affective Computing in Healthcare
Applications based on biosignals and artificial intelligence
M Murugappan

Chapter 9

Differential diagnosis tool in healthcare application using respiratory sounds and convolutional neural network

Rajkumar Palaniappan, Kenneth Sundaraj, Fizza Ghulam Nabi and Vikneswaran Vijean

Affective computing is a field of research in which human emotions are recognised using physiological signals. In recent years, human breath-sound signal analysis has provided significant results in recognition of emotions and stress. Studying breath sounds can be of use in the development of low-cost devices for emotion recognition. This chapter focuses on the classification of respiratory pathology using breath-sound signals. The development of a computerised breath-sound analysis system could improve the standard of living of people affected by respiratory-related disease and further also be used as a differential diagnosis tool in affective computing. Accordingly, in this chapter, respiratory sounds recorded according to the Computerised Respiratory Sound Acquisition standard were obtained from subjects with respiratory sounds belonging to five different respiratory pathologies, namely, normal, wheezes, rhonchi, fine crackles, and coarse crackles. The breath sounds were filtered first and then segmented into respective breath cycles using an adaptive neuro-fuzzy inference system. Then, the breath cycles were reconstructed and fed into a classification model. Two different input types were extracted from the breath sounds and inputted into a convolutional neural network (CNN): (i) a spectrogram of the segmented breath cycles was provided as the input to the CNN for training (method I), and (ii) the segmented breath cycle itself was provided as an input to the classification model (method II). Once the training was completed, the network model was tested using a new dataset. The maximum classification accuracies obtained while testing the system using methods I and II were 94.46% and 83.32%, respectively. The sensitivity and specificity for method I while attaining maximum classification accuracy with 13 convolution layers were 90.67% and 95.32%, respectively. Similarly, the sensitivity and specificity for method II while attaining

doi:10.1088/978-0-7503-5182-9ch9

maximum classification accuracy with 16 convolution layers were 83.53% and 83.68%, respectively. The experimental results show that both proposed network models perform effectively, although the classification accuracy of the model based on the spectrogram-based data was better than that of the model obtained using the normal image plot as the input. Similarly, the time needed to train the model using spectrogram images was less than that required to train the model with an image plot as input. In the future, the proposed network will be trained with more samples to increase its effectiveness and ability to classify more pathological conditions. This research can be further adapted to discriminate human emotions using respiratory sounds.

9.1 Introduction

Affective computing has gained extensive focus in recent years. This field deals with emotion recognition using physiological signals [1]. Many types of physiological signal have come to the attention of researchers while investigating the topic of emotion recognition, such as electroencephalography signals, photoplethysmography signals, and so on [2]. Recently, researchers have opted for analysis of respiratory signals in recognising emotion [3]. Apart from emotion recognition using respiratory signals, heart sounds have also been used in classifying human emotions [4]. These results, taken together, demonstrate that breath-sound signals can act as prominent markers in discriminating human emotions. Computerised respiratory sound analysis is a non-invasive technique that can be used in respiratory pathology classification, and also further extended to classification of human emotions as per research studies [5]. Hence, analysing these breath sounds and classifying the breath-sound signals may be helpful in the development of low-cost devices to detect respiratory pathologies and, in the field of affective computing, in recognising human emotions. The analysis of respiratory sounds and the classification of respiratory pathology have received much interest in recent years [6]. In the early 1980s, researchers started to become interested in developing computer-based diagnostic methods for the classification of respiratory pathology, and these methods have gained importance in the 2000s [7]. In a report of the World Health Organization (WHO), respiratory-related disorders such as pneumonia, pulmonary fibrosis, asthma, chronic obstructive pulmonary disease (COPD), and other respiratory-related illnesses are ranked as the third most common cause of fatalities globally. Specifically, the WHO reported 3 million deaths caused due to COPD in the year 2012 [8], and indicated that millions of people were suffering from asthma in 2011 [9]. In a report regarding pneumonia cases, 1 million deaths were reported by WHO in the year 2013 [10]. The major causes of respiratory-related diseases are air pollution, continued exposure to certain toxic agents, smoking, and hereditary factors [11]. In addition, many patients do not consult their physician at the initial stages of these pathologies and only seek medical attention after their respiratory system is badly affected, at which point the damage might be irreversible [12].

Thus, early-stage diagnosis and action can substantially reduce loss of life and improve healthy standards of living. In addition, a major causes of mortality is due to the lack of available treatment services and physicians in rural areas [13]. The methods used for the diagnosis of respiratory disease include but are not limited to radiography techniques, auscultation, and analysis of pulmonary function, and these are very costly and time-consuming, requiring medical facilities and trained practitioners. Furthermore, the use of radiography techniques, such as computer tomography scans and X-rays, for a prolonged duration can have serious side effects on the human body [14], and some obstructive pathologies cannot be easily diagnosed using these radiography techniques. Although the pulmonary function test provides extra information, such as the estimated respiratory flow, lung volume, and the severity level of the respiratory condition [15], as well as not involving any serious side effects, it is nevertheless time-consuming and expensive and can also be considered an invasive procedure because patients need to make extra exertion in some tests, such as in spirometry [16].

To overcome these downsides, different methodologies for respiratory sound analysis need to be developed in order to recognise different respiratory conditions [17]. The benefits of using breath-sound analysis using computer technology include the non-invasive nature of such approaches, the ability to obtain a rapid diagnosis, their low cost, and the increased accuracy of the method. This approach can also aid as a differential diagnosis tool for the physicians. Differential diagnosis is the process whereby a practitioner either identifies a patient's specific disease or condition or otherwise eliminates the possibility of certain diseases or conditions [18]. Further, these kinds of respiratory sound analysis and classification will lead to further investigate the emotional pattern using respiratory sounds.

9.1.1 Literature review

Research into breath-sound-based diagnosis of respiratory pathologies began in the early '80s [12]. Initially, the field focused on the implementation of signal-processing algorithms to aid visual inspection because the diagnosis of a respiratory pathology through visual inspection alone was challenging [17]. Advancements in the field of signal processing led to the implementation of algorithms for the detection of prominent features in respiratory sounds, which subsequently have been used as inputs for artificial intelligence algorithms or classification approaches [13].

Sengupta *et al* [19] performed lung sound classification using mel-frequency cepstral features and an artificial neural network (ANN). However, the number of subjects used for this study was only 30, and thus a higher number of subjects is needed to ensure the reliability of the system. The number of classification classes was three, namely, normal sounds, wheezes, and crackles, and no sub-classes of respiratory sounds were used. The overall classification accuracy was approximately 99.70%.

In 2017, Khodabakhshi *et al* [20] proposed a recurrent fuzzy wavelet network for the classification of lung sounds, which achieved a classification accuracy of 95%. In their study, respiratory sounds were recorded from 40 normal and 40 abnormal subjects and classified through the extraction of chaotic features. In the same year, Liu *et al* [21] obtained respiratory sounds with an electronic stethoscope and classified these sounds using a Gaussian mixture model. In total, respiratory data from 60 subjects were recorded; the cepstral features from the data were used to train the model. The overall classification accuracy of the obtained model was 98.4%. The same researchers proposed the use of a Hilbert–Huang transform and multi-layer perceptron for the classification of respiratory sounds [22], and obtained an overall accuracy of 95.84% using data from the RALE database.

Islam *et al* [23] compared an ANN and a support vector machine (SVM) in terms of the classification of respiratory sounds using spectral sub-band features. In the study, respiratory sounds from 60 subjects with normal and abnormal sounds were recorded using a four-channel data-acquisition system, and the mean classification accuracy obtained with the SVM-based classifier was 93.3%. In a different study using the same data, the same researchers [24] proposed the use of statistical features and an ANN for the classification of lung sounds, and the overall classification accuracy performance was 60%. In the same year, Serbes *et al* [25] proposed a SVM-based classifier for classifying respiratory sounds into four different classes. The dataset used in their work included various types of noises, and the researchers obtained a classification accuracy of 49.86% using non-linear novel spectral features.

Ulukaya *et al* [26] developed an algorithm to classify polyphonic and monophonic wheezes. Using a rational dilation wavelet transform, energy features were extracted; for classification, a SVM, a *k*-nearest neighbours(K-NN) classifier, and an extreme learning machine were used. The SVM classifier performed best, with a 86% classification accuracy.

In 2020, Meng *et al* [27] collected respiratory sounds from 130 patients. A total of 705 respiratory sound recordings were used in their study to classify normal, rhonchi, and wheeze respiratory sounds, in which 205 recordings were normal respiratory sounds, 260 were rhonchi respiratory sounds, and 240 were wheeze sounds. Wavelet energy and wavelet entropy were used as a feature vector to train and test an ANN model. The model's performance was evaluated using a fivefold cross-validation scheme, and the developed model achieved an accuracy of 85.43%. In the same year, Yadav *et al* [28] developed a SVM-based model for classifying normal and abnormal respiratory sounds. A wavelet packet transform was used in the extraction of features, and a SVM model was used to classify the respiratory sounds. The accuracy obtained in classifying the respiratory sounds was found to be 92.30%.

Jaber *et al* [29] performed classification of normal, coarse crackles, fine crackles, monophonic wheezes, polyphonic wheezes, stridor, and squawk respiratory sounds. The recordings used in their work were obtained from the RALE database, of which only 15 recordings were used in their work. Mel-frequency cepstral coefficients and wavelet-based features were extracted from the respiratory sound signals and three different classifiers, namely, an improved random forest, AdaBoost, and a gradient boosting classifier, were used to classify the respiratory sounds. It was found that the improved random forest performed better than the other two classifiers, obtaining a classification accuracy of 99.04%.

In 2021, Mukherjee *et al* [30] proposed a random-forest-based classification of breath sounds. The ICBHI dataset was used to evaluate the performance of the classifier. Filter-band energy-based features were extracted from the breath-sound signals for classification. The performance of the proposed method was satisfactory in distinguishing crackle and wheeze breath-sound signals.

Apart from conventional machine-learning algorithms, few researchers have implemented deep-learning approach in classifying respiratory sounds. The work of Petmezas *et al* [31] performed classification of respiratory sounds using a hybrid convolutional neural network (CNN). The ICBHI 2017 Respiratory Sound Database was used in their research. Short-time Fourier transform spectrograms were fed as input to their model. The data were split into conventional (60/40), 10-fold cross-validation, and leave-one-out cross-validation. The reported accuracy for the conventional, leave-one-out cross-validation, and 10-fold cross-validation were 73.69%, 76.39%, and 74.57%, respectively.

The classification models used in these previous studies show that the results are dependent on the dataset used, and that the implementation of deep-learning neural networks with bigger samples of data would aid the easier and faster analysis of respiratory pathology. The present study focuses on the implementation of a CNN for the classification of respiratory pathologies. In the present study it is further proposed to segment the respiratory cycles before inputting them to the CNN model, unlike approaches that provide the whole signal or features extracted from the signals themselves to the model.

9.2 Methodology

The data used in the study conducted previously by Palaniappan *et al* [32] were also used in the present study. The breath sounds were collected using a digital stethoscope from both normal and abnormal patients with respiratory-related conditions. The breath sounds were segmented into breath cycles, and the cycles with wheezes, rhonchi, fine crackles, coarse crackles, and normal sounds were separated using an adaptive neuro-fuzzy inference system (ANFIS) algorithm proposed by Palaniappan *et al* [32]. After the segmentation and identification of the respective breath cycles, the segments were reconstructed to form a complete breath cycle. After the cycles were separated, two methods were used before the data were inputted into the CNN. In the second method, the data were plotted and the image plots of the respiratory cycles were then inputted into the CNN. In contrast, in method I, the spectrogram of the breath cycles was obtained and used as the input for the CNN In contrast, in method I, the spectrogram of the breath cycles was obtained and used as the input for the CNN.

9.2.1 Dataset

The breath sounds used in this chapter's study were recorded and verified at Kempegowda Institute of Medical Sciences (KIMS) in Bengaluru, Karnataka, India. The research proposal was approved by the KIMS Institutional Ethics Committee, and KIMS permitted the researchers to perform the data collection at the department of pulmonary medicine. The dataset was obtained from 40 normal individuals, 40 individuals with continuous breath sounds, and 40 individuals with discontinuous breath sounds. The 40 continuous breath sounds were further subdivided into 20 individuals with wheeze sounds and 20 individuals with rhonchi. Similarly, the 40 discontinuous breath sounds were subdivided into 20 fine crackles and 20 coarse crackles. The breath sounds were recorded using an electronic stethoscope developed by WISE. The breath-sound recordings were obtained from three different locations, namely, the trachea and the left and right lung bases, according to the Computerised Respiratory Sound Acquisition (CORSA) standard [33]. The breath sounds were recorded for a duration of 20 s in the three abovementioned locations, and five trials were performed. The breath sounds were segmented into respective breath cycles using the ANFIS, and the first five complete cycles from each recording were segmented and labelled. The verification and labelling of the segments were also carried out at KIMS by two experts in pulmonary medicine. After segmentation, 3000 normal respiratory cycles, 1500 wheeze cycles, 1500 rhonchi cycles, 1500 fine crackle cycles, and 1500 coarse crackle cycles were subjected to further analysis. To ensure an equal distribution of sample size, only 1500 samples of normal respiratory cycles were considered in this study, and thus a total of 7500 samples were used to train the CNN.

9.2.2 Pre-processing

In the pre-processing step, the breath sounds are filtered to remove heart sounds and other noise that affects the quality of the signal. This is followed by segmentation of the breath cycles from the breath sounds using the ANFIS. Finally, the breath segments are reconstructed to form a complete breath cycle.

9.2.2.1 Filtering

The filtering process is carried out on the breath sounds specifically to eliminate noises related to heart sounds and other physiological signal interference in the breath-sound signals. The original sampling rate of the breath-sound signal recordings obtained using an electronic stethoscope was 10 000 Hz. The sampling rate was downsampled to 8 kHz as per the proposed CORSA standard [34]. After down-sampling, the breath sounds were filtered using a high-pass filter at 7.5 Hz (1st-order Butterworth filter) to eradicate the DC offset and a low-pass filter at 2500 Hz (8th-order Butterworth filter) to evade aliasing. The breath sounds were then filtered using a 4th-order Butterworth bandpass filter (150–2 kHz) to eliminate the heart sounds and any other unwanted noise that may affect the signal. The breath sounds thus collected using the electronic stethoscope are free from periodical power-line interference noise because the stethoscope is driven by a direct current. The filters applied to the breath-sound signals and the order of the filters were all obtained from the CORSA standard specifications [35].

9.2.2.2 Cycle segmentation

The breath sounds are segmented into breath phases and reconstructed to form separate breath cycles. Segmenting the breath cycle and classifying the breath sounds, as compared to segmenting a signal based on samples and classifying the breath sounds, has been demonstrated to provide an improved performance in the model. In the breath cycle segmentation part, the input given to the ANFIS is the power spectral density of the breath-sound signal, which is segmented to obtain 1024 samples per segment, and the output of the ANFIS is the equivalent cycle of each segment. The ANFIS outputs whether the segment is part of an inspiratory phase or expiratory phase, or a pause of the breath cycle. The segments of each cycle are reconstructed using a previously proposed algorithm [32]. The proposed method was also matched with another strategy using a fuzzy inference system (FIS) that was described in another work [36]. However, the prior results showed that ANFIS performs better than the FIS-based method. The proposed ANFIS model for breath cycle segmentation was also validated by two medical professionals at KIMS. As aforementioned, in method I, the plotted images of the segmented breath cycles are fed directly into the CNN as the input; in method II, spectrogram images of the breath cycles are obtained and provided as input to the CNN.

9.2.3 Classification using deep-learning algorithms

In recent years, deep-learning algorithms have had a great impact in biomedical signal processing [37]. A CNN is a type of deep-learning algorithm inspired by multi-layer feed-forward neural networks that resembles a back-propagation algorithm [38]. The CNN has two main layers, namely, a hidden layer, which is also known as the feature-extraction stage, and a classification layer [39]. The hidden layer (feature-extraction stage) comprises at least one convolutional layer with rectification linear units and pooling layers [40]. The classification layer comprises a fully connected layer similar to that used in a multi-layer perceptron neural network. The convolutional layer includes a convolution filter followed by a rectification linear unit, which is again followed by max pooling. The number of convolutional layers can be increased or decreased and the parameters of each layer can be varied. The input to the CNN is often two-dimensional (2D) images or any other 2D signal, such as speech signals and respiratory sound signals [41]. In the CNN, the 2D signals are converted into translation-invariant features using the pooling layer, which results in a more effective classification. The rectification linear units act as an activation function for the convolution layer, and a softmax activation function is used in the final layer. The softmax function is otherwise known as a normalised exponential function, and is used generally in multi-class classification problems. It assigns decimal values to the different classes to be classified. A typical CNN model shows improved learning through more in-depth training. Another important advantage of using a CNN is that notably fewer parameters need to be used to train the neural network compared to those needed to train other neural network models. A CNN possesses the capability of combining both feature-extraction and classification processes into one process [42]. With its feasibility and aforementioned advantages, the proposed method will thus implement CNN models in classifying respiratory pathologies from respiratory cycles rather than considering the whole signal.

9.2.3.1 Convolutional neural network architecture

The architectures proposed in this work are given in figures 9.1 and 9.2; the only difference between them is the input, where *n* is the total number of convolution layers, which was varied to obtain the best possible outcome from both the proposed models. As shown in figure 9.1, the input in the first architecture is a plot of the

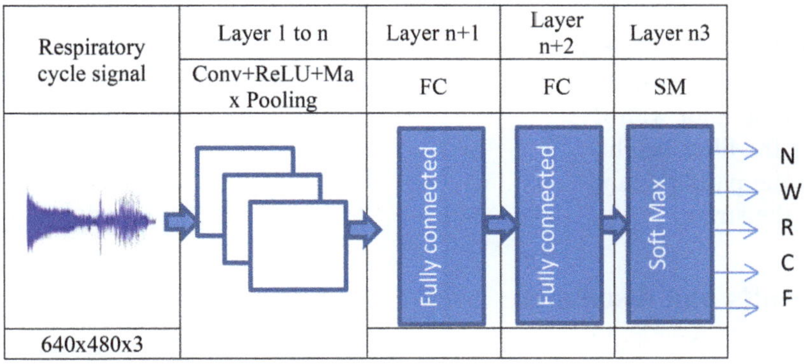

Figure 9.1. CNN architecture (method I).

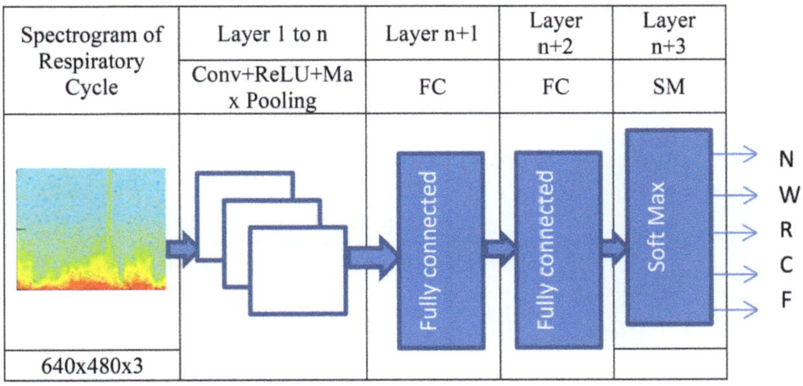

Figure 9.2. CNN architecture (method II).

respiratory cycle. In contrast, in the architecture shown in figure 9.2, the input is a spectrogram plot of the respiratory cycle, wherein the respiratory cycle is transformed into an equivalent image and inputted to the neural network. The proposed architecture was finalised after repetitive analysis and training using different configuration for the architecture. The output width and output height in the proposed network were calculated using equations 9.1 and 9.2. The proposed configuration provided better results than other configurations. In addition, the computation time required with the proposed configuration was considerably decreased when compared with that needed with the other configurations; the results for various configurations are provided. The proposed method was evaluated using a 10-fold cross-validation scheme:

$$\text{Output width} = \frac{W - F_{\text{w}} + 2P}{S} + 1, \tag{9.1}$$

$$\text{Output height} = \frac{H - F_{\text{h}} + 2P}{S} + 1, \tag{9.2}$$

where
W is the width of the input,
H is the height of the input,
F_w is the filter width,
F_h is the filter height,
P is the padding, and
S is the stride.

9.3 Results and discussion

The proposed CNN architectures were implemented and the classification accuracy was obtained using a 10-fold cross-validation scheme. The results for methods I and II are summarised in tables 9.1 and 9.2, respectively. For both network architectures, the number of convolutional layers, the classification accuracy, sensitivity, and specificity while testing the network are reported. The classification accuracy, sensitivity, and specificity are calculated based on equations (9.3), (9.4), and (9.5), respectively:

$$\text{Sensitivity} = \frac{\text{True Positive}}{(\text{True Positive} + \text{False Negative})}, \tag{9.3}$$

$$\text{Specificity} = \frac{\text{True Negative}}{(\text{True Negative} + \text{False Positive})}, \tag{9.4}$$

$$\text{Classification Accuracy} = \frac{(\text{True Positive} + \text{True Negative})}{(\text{False Negative} + \text{False Positive} + \text{True Positive} + \text{True Negative})}. \tag{9.5}$$

The maximum classification accuracies obtained while training the system using methods I and II were 83.32% and 94.46%, respectively. The times required to train and test the system using methods I and II to achieve the maximum classification accuracy were 324 and 457 s, respectively. This shows that the time taken for

Table 9.1. Results for method I.

No. of convolutional layers	Sensitivity (%)	Specificity (%)	Accuracy (%)
7	80.33	64.12	83.67
6	81.62	86.81	84.66
8	82.11	87.22	84.71
9	84.09	88.52	86.59
10	85.75	89.62	87.90
11	87.11	91.74	89.61
12	88.42	92.18	92.53
13	90.67	95.32	94.46

Table 9.2. Results for method II.

No. of convolutional layers	Sensitivity (%)	Specificity (%)	Accuracy (%)
9	74.18	76.82	75.88
10	75.32	77.27	76.13
11	77.53	78.31	76.22
12	78.62	79.00	77.74
13	79.93	80.03	78.33
14	81.05	81.67	80.63
15	82.74	83.15	82.81
16	83.53	83.68	83.32

training and testing method II is greater compared to method I. Different numbers of convolution layers were implemented and tested. The table for method I clearly shows that the maximum classification accuracy was obtained with 13 convolution layers, whereas for method II it was 16 convolution layers. Further increases in the number of convolutional layers resulted in no further improvements in the classification accuracy. The sensitivity and specificity for method I while attaining maximum classification accuracy with 13 convolution layers was 90.67% and 95.32%, respectively. Similarly, the sensitivity and specificity for method II while attaining maximum classification accuracy with 16 convolution layers was 83.53% and 83.68%, respectively. This shows that the sensitivity and specificity of method I is better compared to method II.

Tables 9.3 and 9.4 show confusion matrices for methods I and II, respectively, in which the matrices display the numbers of missed classifications with both methods. The results shown in the tables indicate that the number of missed classifications with method II was lower than that obtained with method I.

The results obtained show that the use of spectrogram images as input to the network model resulted in improved performance to that obtained using normal signal plot images as input. Satisfactory results were obtained using a decreased amount of data to train the model. In addition, the results can be further improved by using images obtained in the time–frequency domain. For example, the use of images obtained with an S-transform matrix can further improve the classification accuracy of the proposed system.

A comparison of the results of the proposed method with those obtained using the methods described in the literature reveals that some techniques mentioned in the literature show better performance than the method proposed in this study. For example, Sengupta *et al* [19] used data from 30 subjects to evaluate the performance of various classifiers and reported an overall accuracy of approximately 97%. Although this classification accuracy is higher than that obtained in the present work, the number of subjects included and the number of tested samples were notably lower compared with those used in the present study. In addition, the training time used in the previous study was substantially higher compared with that

Table 9.3. Confusion matrix for method I.

Confusion matrix		Predicted					
		N	W	R	FC	CC	Total
Actual	N	2885	34	26	36	19	3000
	W	38	1356	28	43	35	1500
	R	35	52	1338	30	45	1500
	FC	26	34	46	1365	29	1500
	CC	41	18	35	28	1378	1500
Total		3000	1500	1500	1500	1500	

Note: *N—Normal, W—Wheeze, R—Rhonchi, FC—Fine crackles, CC—Coarse crackles.

Table 9.4. Confusion matrix for method II.

Confusion matrix		Predicted					
		N	W	R	FC	CC	Total
Actual	N	2765	64	53	61	57	3000
	W	47	1272	56	37	88	1500
	R	55	49	1285	58	53	1500
	FC	87	68	60	1251	34	1500
	CC	46	47	46	93	1268	1500
Total		3000	1500	1500	1500	1500	

Note: *N—Normal, W—Wheeze, R—Rhonchi, FC—Fine crackles, CC—Coarse crackles.

used in this study. Lui *et al* [22] used the RALE database, which includes only 70–100 recordings from subjects with a wide range of ages, to classify the respiratory sounds. In another study [21], the researchers collected data from 60 subjects and obtained a classification accuracy of 98.4%. However, the classification step only considered wheezes, crackles, and normal sounds, and rhonchi and further classification of crackles (fine and coarse crackles) were not considered. Similarly, Khodabakhshi *et al* [20] obtained an accuracy of 95% with their developed system for classifying lung sounds using data from 80 subjects (40 normal subjects and 40 patients). The 40 patients included both COPD and asthma patients, but the researchers did not consider rhonchi, fine crackles, or coarse crackles in their classification of lung sounds. In the work of Rizal *et al* [43], only 99 recordings were used to classif, with an obtained accuracy of 98.88%. The 99 recordings were collected from various sources and the age groups of the subjects varied. In this study, 7500 samples were considered to train the CNN, and thus the number of samples used for training was considerably higher compared with the number of samples used in the previous studies detailed in the literature. In the work of Petmezas *et al* [31], the ICBHI 2017 Respiratory Sound Database was used, with which an almost 75% classification accuracy was reported using various validation methods such as conventional validation and 10-fold cross-validation. In addition, the diversity of the classifications performed in this study was greater compared with the diversity of the classification categories considered in previous studies. Similarly, the time required to train the CNN was less that the reported times needed to train some of the previously established models.

The results clearly show that improved results can likely be obtained by training the network model with more data, which is essential for all deep-learning networks. Furthermore, there is a possibility that the accuracy can further be improved when the input image resolution to the CNN model is increased. Currently, the resolution of the input used in this work is 640 × 480 × 3; however, improving this resolution could further improve the results. In the future, the number of data points in the dataset will be further increased, and other signal-processing techniques will be implemented. Further, the results show that the proposed method can be adapted to recognition of human emotions using respiratory sound analysis. This technique can be used in the development of low-cost devices in the field of affective computing in recognising human emotions using breath-sound signals.

9.4 Conclusions

In this study, a CNN network was implemented for the classification of respiratory conditions. Two different CNN models were developed, and the accuracies of the classification of different respiratory pathologies were compared. The breath cycles were segmented from the breath-sound signals using an ANFIS, and the cycles were labelled with the corresponding respiratory pathologies, validated by two physicians. The two inputs given to the CNN model were time-domain signal plot images and spectrograms of the images, and the classification results from the two models with these inputs were obtained. The achieved classification accuracy of the model using time-domain plot images as input (method II) was 83.32%, and the classification accuracy achieved by the model using frequency-domain spectrogram images as input (method I) was 94.46%. The sensitivity and specificity for method I while attaining maximum classification accuracy with 13 convolution layers was 90.67% and 95.32% respectively. Similarly, the sensitivity and specificity for method II while attaining maximum classification accuracy with 16 convolution layers was 83.53% and 83.68%, respectively. The results reveal that the classification model obtained using spectrogram images as the input showed better performance than the model obtained using time signal plot images. These findings show that signals exhibit more significant differences between pathologies in the frequency domain than in the time domain, and it is possible that the classification accuracy in the time–frequency domain can be further improved. These findings also show that the adapted method is effective in classifying respiratory sounds and that this methodology can further be used in respiratory-sound-based human emotion recognition in the near future. In specific, this tool would be highly helpful in developing a multimodal system to detect emotional impairment in patients with neurological disorders [44–48]. The findings also reflect the possibility of this kind of methodology being implemented in the classification of human emotions using breath-sound signals.

Authors' contributions

R.P. and K.S. implemented the algorithms and performed the analysis. F.G.N. and V.V drafted the manuscript and participated in the design of the study. R.P. and K. S. helped with the data validation and the study coordination.

Conflict of interest

The authors of this article declare that they have no conflicts of interest.

Acknowledgements

The authors of this research study thank the management and staff of KIMS for providing the ethical clearance for this study, allowing us to collect the data at their institution and providing valuable insights in the field of respiratory sound analysis.

Ethical approval

This research complies with the principles laid down in the Declaration of Helsinki. The respiratory sounds used in this research study were recorded at Kempegowda Institute of Medical Sciences (KIMS) in Bangalore, India, and this research was approved by the Institutional Ethics Committee at KIMS.

References

[1] Rushambwa M C, Gezimati M, Palaniappan G P, Vijean R and Nabi FG V 2021 Cloud based analysis and classification of EEG signals to detect epileptic seizures *2021 7th Int. Conf. on Bio Signals, Images, and Instrumentation (ICBSII) (March 2021)* pp 25–7

[2] Filippini C, Di Crosta A, Palumbo R, Perpetuini D, Cardone D and Ceccato I *et al* 2022 Automated affective computing based on bio-signals analysis and deep learning approach *Sensors* **22** 1789

[3] Deshpande G, Batliner A and Schuller B W 2022 AI-based human audio processing for COVID-19: a comprehensive overview *Pattern Recognit.* **122** 108289

[4] Xiefeng C, Wang Y, Dai S, Zhao P and Liu Q 2019 Heart sound signals can be used for emotion recognition *Sci. Rep.* **9** 6486

[5] Zulfiqar R, Majeed F, Irfan R, Rauf H T, Benkhelifa E and Belkacem A N 2021 Abnormal respiratory sounds classification using deep CNN through artificial noise addition *Front. Med. (Lausanne)* **8** 714811

[6] Andrès E, Gass R, Charloux A, Brandt C and Hentzler A 2018 Respiratory sound analysis in the era of evidence-based medicine and the world of medicine 2.0 *J. Med. Life* **11** 89–106 (PMID: 30140315)

[7] Kim Y, Hyon Y, Jung S S, Lee S, Yoo G and Chung C *et al* 2021 Respiratory sound classification for crackles, wheezes, and rhonchi in the clinical field using deep learning *Sci. Rep.* **11** 17186

[8] WHO 2012 Chronic obstructive pulmonary disease (COPD) (Accessed: 11/03/2015) http://who.int/mediacentre/factsheets/fs315/en/

[9] WHO 2013 Asthma (Accessed: 11/03/2018) http://who.int/mediacentre/factsheets/fs307/en/
[10] WHO 2013 Pneumonia (Accessed: 11/03/2018) http://who.int/mediacentre/factsheets/fs331/en/
[11] Ghulam Nabi F, Sundaraj K, Iqbal M S, Shafiq M and Palaniappan R 2022 A telemedicine software application for asthma severity levels identification using wheeze sounds classification *Biocybern. Biomed. Eng.* **42** 1236–47
[12] Nabi F G, Sundaraj K, Lam C K and Palaniappan R 2020 Analysis of wheeze sounds during tidal breathing according to severity levels in asthma patients *J. Asthma* **57** 353–65
[13] Nabi F G, Sundaraj K, Lam C K and Palaniappan R 2019 Characterization and classification of asthmatic wheeze sounds according to severity level using spectral integrated features *Comput. Biol. Med.* **104** 52–61
[14] Kandaswamy A, Kumar C S, Ramanathan R P, Jayaraman S and Malmurugan N 2004 Neural classification of lung sounds using wavelet coefficients *Comput. Biol. Med.* **34** 523–37
[15] Shephard R J and Turner M E 1959 On the probability of correct diagnosis by pulmonary function tests *Thorax* **14** 300–4
[16] Palaniappan R, Sundaraj K, Sundaraj S, Huliraj N and Revadi S S 2015 A telemedicine tool to detect pulmonary pathology using computerized pulmonary acoustic signal analysis *Appl. Soft Comput.* **37** 952–9
[17] Nabi F G, Sundaraj K and Palaniappan R 2020 Identification of asthma severity using wavelet transform and K-nearest-neighbour classifier *2020 Int. Conf. on Data Analytics for Business and Industry: Way Towards a Sustainable Economy (ICDABI) (Sakheer, Bahrain, October 2020)* pp 1–4
[18] Fan G 2022 Differential diagnosis of respiratory system diseases *Atlas of Differential Diagnosis: MRI* ed G Fan (Singapore: Springer) pp 271–84
[19] Sengupta N, Sahidullah M and Saha G 2016 Lung sound classification using cepstral-based statistical features *Comput. Biol. Med.* **75** 118–29
[20] Khodabakhshi B M, Moradi, Hassana M, Sanat and Momayezb Z *et al* 2017 Lung sound decomposition using recurrent fuzzy wavelet network *J. Intell. Fuzzy Syst.* **33** 2497–508
[21] Liu Y, Lin Y, Zhang X, Wang Z, Gao Y and Chen G *et al* 2017 Classifying respiratory sounds using electronic stethoscope *2017 IEEE SmartWorld, Ubiquitous Intelligence and Computing, Advanced and Trusted Computed, Scalable Computing and Communications, Cloud and Big Data Computing, Internet of People and Smart City Innovation (SmartWorld/SCALCOM/UIC/ATC/CBDCom/IOP/SCI) (August 2017)* pp 4–8
[22] Liu Y, Yang Y and Chen Y 2017 Lung sound classification based on Hilbert–Huang transform features and multilayer perceptron network *2017 Asia-Pacific Signal and Information Processing Association Annual Summit and Conf. (APSIPA ASC) (December 2017)* pp 12–5
[23] Islam M A, Bandyopadhyaya I, Bhattacharyya P and Saha G 2018 Multichannel lung sound analysis for asthma detection *Comput. Methods Programs Biomed.* **159** 111–23
[24] Islam M A, Bandyopadhyaya I, Bhattacharyya P and Saha G 2018 Classification of normal, asthma and COPD subjects using multichannel lung sound signals *2018 Int. Conf. on Communication and Signal Processing (ICCSP) (Chennai, India, April 2018)* pp 3–5
[25] Serbes G, Ulukaya S and Kahya Y P (ed) 2018 An automated lung sound preprocessing and classification system based on spectral analysis methods *Precision Medicine Powered by pHealth and Connected Health IFMBE Proceedings* vol 65 (Singapore: Springer)
[26] Ulukaya S, Serbes G and Kahya Y P 2019 Wheeze type classification using non-dyadic wavelet transform based optimal energy ratio technique *Comput. Biol. Med.* **104** 175–82

[27] Meng F, Shi Y, Wang N, Cai M and Luo Z 2020 Detection of respiratory sounds based on wavelet coefficients and machine learning *IEEE Access* **8** 155710–20

[28] Yadav A, Dutta M K and Prinosil J 2020 Machine learning based automatic classification of respiratory signals using wavelet transform *2020 43rd Int. Conf. on Telecommunications and Signal Processing (TSP) (Milan, Italy, July 2020)* pp 7–9

[29] Jaber M M, Abd S K, Shakeel P M, Burhanuddin M A, Mohammed M A and Yussof S 2020 A telemedicine tool framework for lung sounds classification using ensemble classifier algorithms *Measurement* **162** 107883

[30] Mukherjee H, Salam H and Santosh K C 2021 Lung health analysis: adventitious respiratory sound classification using filterbank energies *Int. J. Pattern Recognit. Artif. Intell.* **35** 2157008

[31] Petmezas G, Cheimariotis G-A, Stefanopoulos L, Rocha B, Paiva R P and Katsaggelos A K *et al* 2022 Automated lung sound classification using a hybrid CNN-LSTM network and focal loss function *Sensors* **22** 1232

[32] Palaniappan R, Sundaraj K and Sundaraj S 2017 Adaptive neuro-fuzzy inference system for breath phase detection and breath cycle segmentation *Comput. Methods Programs Biomed.* **145** 67–72

[33] Palaniappan R, Sundaraj K and Sundaraj S 2014 Artificial intelligence techniques used in respiratory sound analysis – a systematic review *Biomed. Tech./Biomed. Eng.* **59** 7–18

[34] Laitinen T, Sovijärvi A, Malmberg P, Turjanmaa V and Hartiala J 2022 The birth and development of clinical physiology in Finland *Clin. Physiol. Funct. Imaging* **42** 151–80

[35] Khodaie M, Nafisi V R and Moghadam F F 2021 Design and implementation of an apparatus for respiratory parameters estimation based on acoustic methods *2021 28th National and 6th Int. Iranian Conf. on Biomedical Engineering (ICBME) (Tehran, Iran, November 2021)* pp 15–21

[36] Palaniappan R, Sundaraj K, Sundaraj S, Huliraj N and Revadi S S 2016 A novel approach to detect respiratory phases from pulmonary acoustic signals using normalised power spectral density and fuzzy inference system *Clin. Respir. J.* **10** 486–94

[37] Patel V and Shah A K 2021 Machine learning for biomedical signal processing *Machine Learning and the Internet of Medical Things in Healthcare* ed K K Singh, M Elhoseny, A Singh and A A Elngar (New York: Academic) ch 3 pp 47–66

[38] Zhu Y, Li G, Tang S, Wang R, Su H and Wang C 2022 Acoustic signal-based fault detection of hydraulic piston pump using a particle swarm optimization enhancement CNN *Appl. Acoust.* **192** 108718

[39] Ciompi F, de Hoop B, van Riel S J, Chung K, Scholten E T and Oudkerk M *et al* 2015 Automatic classification of pulmonary peri-fissural nodules in computed tomography using an ensemble of 2D views and a convolutional neural network out-of-the-box *Med. Image Anal.* **26** 195–202

[40] Aslan M F, Sabanci K, Durdu A and Unlersen M F 2022 COVID-19 diagnosis using state-of-the-art CNN architecture features and Bayesian optimization *Comput. Biol. Med.* **142** 105244

[41] Prasoon A, Petersen K, Igel C, Lauze F, Dam E and Nielsen M 2013 Deep feature learning for knee cartilage segmentation using a triplanar convolutional neural network *Medical Image Computing and Computer-Assisted Intervention—MICCAI 2013* vol 8150 ed K Mori, I Sakuma and Y Sato *et al* (Berlin: Springer)

[42] Li Z, Wang F, Cui L and Liu J 2022 Dual mixture model based CNN for image denoising *IEEE Trans. Image Process.* **31** 3618–29

[43] Rizal A, Hidayat R and Nugroho H A 2019 Lung sound classification using Hjorth descriptor measurement on wavelet sub-bands *J. Inf. Process. Syst.* **15** 1068–81

[44] Choong W Y *et al* 2022 Investigation of the brain activation pattern of stroke patients and healthy individuals during happiness and sadness ed M Murugappan and Y Rajamanickam *Biomedical Signals Based Computer-Aided Diagnosis for Neurological Disorders* (Cham: Springer)

[45] Chawla P, Rana S B and Kaur H *et al* 2023 A decision support system for automated diagnosis of Parkinson's disease from EEG using FAWT and entropy features, biomedical signal processing and control *Biomed. Signal Process. Control* **79** 104116

[46] Dar M N and Akram M U *et al* 2022 EEG-based emotion charting for Parkinson's disease patients using convolutional recurrent neural networks and cross dataset learning *Comput. Biol. Med.* **144** 105327

[47] Murugappan M, Zheng B S and Khairunizam W 2021 Recurrent quantification analysis-based emotion classification in stroke using electroencephalogram signals *Arab. J. Sci. Eng.* **46** 9573–88

[48] Choong W Y and Khairunizam W *et al* 1997 Correlation analysis of emotional EEG in alpha, beta and gamma frequency bands *J. Phys.: Conf. Ser.* **1** 2021

Chapter 10

Virtual reality and augmented reality based affective computing applications in healthcare, challenges, and its future direction

Suma Dawn

In the digital world, virtual reality (VR) and augmented reality (AR) are the buzzwords of the moment. Most of these applications can be found on gaming platforms and on utilities like Google Maps. However, in recent years, these cutting-edge technologies have also made remarkable strides in the healthcare industry. Different applications have benefitted from technological advancements in terms of device configurations and processing hardware. Of these, affective computing (AC) is a related interdisciplinary branch of computer science that studies, processes, and simulates emotions. This chapter presents current research in the field of AC with AR and VR in the healthcare and medical fields. There are many uses of AR and VR in healthcare, not just in medical training, teaching, and education, but also in patient education and communication, among others. AC has been utilised in many forms of rehabilitation, mental health, adjunctive and physical therapies, fitness programmes, in the managing and controlling of addiction and phobias, etc. Any newly developed interactive interfaces based on AR can make collaboration between practitioners, patients, and wider stakeholders more engaging and useful. Professional practitioners and students of various medical disciplines can use AR/VR systems to help increase their competence before performing actual treatments on patients, thereby decreasing the risk of patient injury or death. In recent years, AR/VR have become increasingly popular in medical studies. Accordingly, several types of AR/VR system development platforms for clinical applications are also discussed in this chapter. A few commercially available softwares and related hardware are also discussed, as well as some emerging challenges associated with such systems. Although explicit pedagogical and theoretical frameworks are still in their infancy, AR/VR are quickly becoming accepted in the medical field.

doi:10.1088/978-0-7503-5182-9ch10

10.1 Introduction

The continued increase of computing power has made the dreams of yesterday into the reality of today. Recent technological advancements have made higher computational budgets an attainable reality in other domains, especially the medical domain, where interventions need to be timely, effective, and cost efficient to be widely accepted by population. Affective computing (AC), first pioneered by Rosalind Picard in 1997, relates to and is capable of deliberately influencing human emotions. It is as an interdisciplinary field that can help investigate and understand human emotional health, and assist with many medical applications. Further, social cues can be gathered by using multiple sensors, such as in wearable cameras and audio devices, and so-called affective intelligence platforms can be used in many ways, such as by analysing consumer engagement with products, content, or services in general with respect to human emotions, as well as in biometric sensors. Some current examples include Affectiva[1], DeepAffex[2], MyPinWheel[3], Emotibot[4], NVISO[5], among others, which assist in the fields of medical and healthcare, automotive, finance, product engagement, and so on. A parallel thread of investigation is the usage of augmented reality (AR) and virtual reality (VR) in the domains of medical and healthcare. VR aims at stimulating human senses to the largest extent, in which multi-sensory stimuli create a sense of presence so that a user can interact with a simulated virtual environment. The simulation of this real-life-like experience is especially important. AR, by contrast, allows a user to interact with simulated virtual objects in conjunction with the real-world. Figure 10.1 shows a virtual continuum of these technologies amalgamation with the real world. As can be seen, AR (or mixed reality) integrates with structures from the real-world by

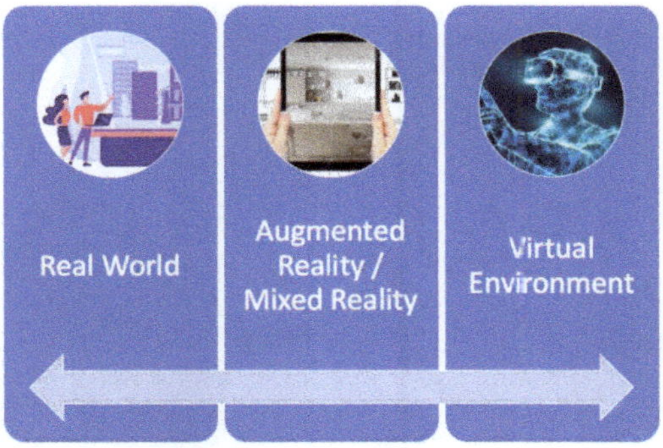

Figure 10.1. Virtual continuum of AR/VR technologies.

[1] www.affectiva.com
[2] www.deepaffex.ai
[3] www.mypinwheel.com
[4] www.emotibot.com
[5] www.nviso.ai

adding virtual objects, while in VR the whole environment is simulated multi-sensorily through virtual objects.

Various kinds of events can trigger different types of emotions in humans. To this end, different features and functionalities can be used in the design and development of VR applications, some elements of which can elicit emotions unconsciously too. Immersive experiences, enhanced by technological advances in mutual interaction, can enhance this emotional design space. Mapping and understanding of user behaviour can be accomplished by using in-built sensors, such as eye-tracking and movement sensors in VR/AR hardware devices [1]. Instead of exposing a target population or users to general situations that may not be controllable, it is easier as well as more reliable to control the stimuli presented to an immersed user. These stimuli can be designed so as not to be random, but rather with specific purposes and intentions, such as the evocation of certain presences, physical experiences, or emotional experiences for the user. These instigations may be explicit or implicit. Explicit methods or subjective methods may require users to actively express their own experiences such as during an interview, questionnaires, etc [2]. However, a user's behaviour in response to certain stimuli can also be analysed in terms of implicit evaluation methods. These behaviours include direct observation of the user's responses including facial expression, using audio/voice inputs to record physiological data such as endodermal activity, electroencephalogram (EEG) and electrocardiogram (ECG) signal-acquisition devices, etc [3–5]. Data from gyroscopes and accelerometers can also be used in conjunction to provide movement data. Figure 10.2 showcases some generic forms of interaction in an affective intelligence engine with AR/VR application.

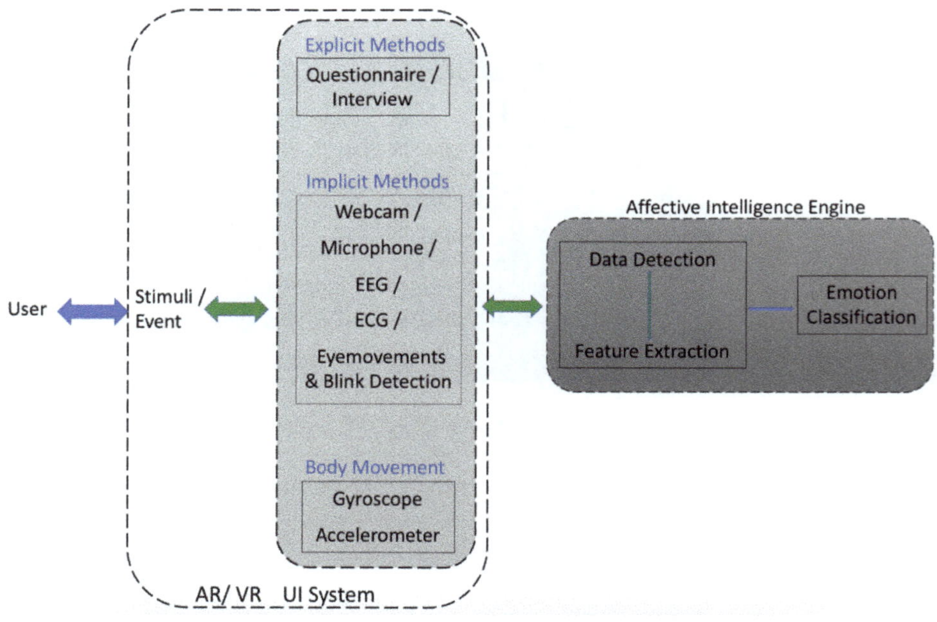

Figure 10.2. Generic forms of interaction in an affective intelligence engine with AR/VR application.

The responses and emotions elicited by an event are extremely important in the healthcare and medical domain. They are integral to many applications, particularly so when the disorder is due to psychological or neuropsychological irregularities rather than being purely physical in nature. The emotions experienced by an individual in response to event may vary in intensity. In addition, for any given particular event, one person may react mildly whereas the same event may trigger an intense reaction in another. Such differences in experiences can be due to many reasons. Hence, while designing an AR/VR system, care must be taken with regards to the mental states of the users, too, as it involves playing with immersion, presence, and multi-sensory stimuli.

10.2 Generic applications of augmented reality/virtual reality

There exist a wide range of applications for AR/VR. Their main areas of use include travel, navigation and maintenance, the automobile industry, real-estate, architecture and interior designing, manufacturing, aerospace and flight stimulation, advertising, gaming, marketing, retail, defence, occupational safety, communication, education, sports, fitness and well-being, social engagements, entertainment, art and design, the fashion industry, conferences and meetings, etc [6–8]. Taking the generic field of healthcare itself as an example, AR/VR have proven their utility in a huge number of possible applications. Applications created for ensuring a healthy lifestyle, such as in fitness instruction, dieting and healthy eating, as well as forms of physical therapy can make use of interactive environments to present novel and interesting artificial-reality-based solutions [1, 9, 10]. The teaching and learning of human anatomy, virtualization of surgery, management of patient insights, conducting of rehabilitation programmes, medical training, the practice of nursing, doctor training, operating theatre set-up, and various other such requirements can all be augmented with specialised AR/VR applications. As such, the usage of physical specimens can be reduced, and virtual objects can be used instead in practice sessions. The handling of emergency situations, epidemic outbreaks, health education, and telemedicine too can make use of the extensive reach of artificial reality, in a manner that encourages community-based understanding and cost-effective outreach to locales [11, 12]. Further, domains of medical device handling such as device operation training, their maintenance, marketing pitches, etc, can use AR-based media to greater advantage, in which any potential users such as buyers, doctors, and healthcare workers can get a 360° view of objects and elements.

In the treatment of patients, many VR applications have had a profound impact. They can be useful in planning complex operations, neurosurgical procedures, and other sensitive aspects of healthcare. Various multi-modal images such as inputs from X-rays, CT scans, MRIs, ultrasound scans, etc, can be complemented by haptic devices, and VR can aid in the reconstruction of actual body parts [13, 14]. Surgical robots that use robotic arms, controlled by surgeons at a console, can use tactile and sensory feedback provided by VR devices. Many patients suffering from mental health disorders (MHDs), most commonly phobias, post-traumatic stress disorders, and others, may be recommended to use event-triggering stimulations in

AR/VR application to help face situations [7]. Pain management, rehabilitation, and physiotherapy sessions can be augmented with haptic devices and VR applications to realise the practical benefits of on-site coaching sessions.

10.3 Design of affective augmented reality/virtual reality applications for the medical domain

As can be seen, the creation of appropriate VR/AR experiences can be of immense use. Further study must be undertaken to determine the cases wherein these technologies would be useful. However, rampant (over)use of virtual or augmented systems may have some detrimental effects on users too. Physically, they may be required to make use of their hands or other body parts in AR applications. Mentally, when users are asked to concentrate on such applications, apart from their short-term and long-term memory being engaged[5], their emotions too get entangled. Many such applications can be designed that present cognitive and epistemic experiences, i.e., awareness and intuition, to users. Applications can also be designed to invoke emotional experiences apart from these purely sensory or instrumental experiences. These aspects of UI/UX/XR designs are, nowadays, being incorporated into applications that are designed for particular medical requirements [8, 15].

Another such contributing factor is the user's sense of presence. This sense of presence is generated by the user characteristics, system characteristics, and task characteristics. The user characteristics include disability condition, age, gender, immersive tendencies, and prior experience. VR system characteristics include factors of representation, dimensionality, multi-modality, encumbrance, etc. VR task characteristics incorporate factors of realism, meaningfulness, types of interaction, and others. In applications that use AR/VR solutions, the users of such solutions are physically as well as mentally involved in the events showcased in these applications, thereby being totally engrossed within them. With such technology, users can interact with objects in the virtual world that are simulated by computer graphics. These interactions can help users in observing the simulated environment, in exploring the types of possible interactions and their effects on other objects, to learn new possible movements, and to understand the repercussions of actions and their associated emotional impacts. Such interactions can even influence neural systems to a great extent. Mirroring of behaviour is a pattern that humans perform after observing the same or similar actions by others. Such mirroring events can trigger neurons to be distributed in different regions of the brain, thereby activating perceptions of actions. This principle is useful in VR therapy and rehabilitation.

The creation of appropriate VR/AR experiences can have multitude of applications, many of which may have very common requirements. Figure 10.3 presents the usual requirements of a VR application. In this, there are three main stakeholders: a client, an administrator, and a database. The client-side design includes the VR visualisation module that in turn incorporates physics simulation and artificial intelligence (AI)-based interactions, with most virtual objects modelled on the patient data; alternatively, these may be rendered based on certain specifications

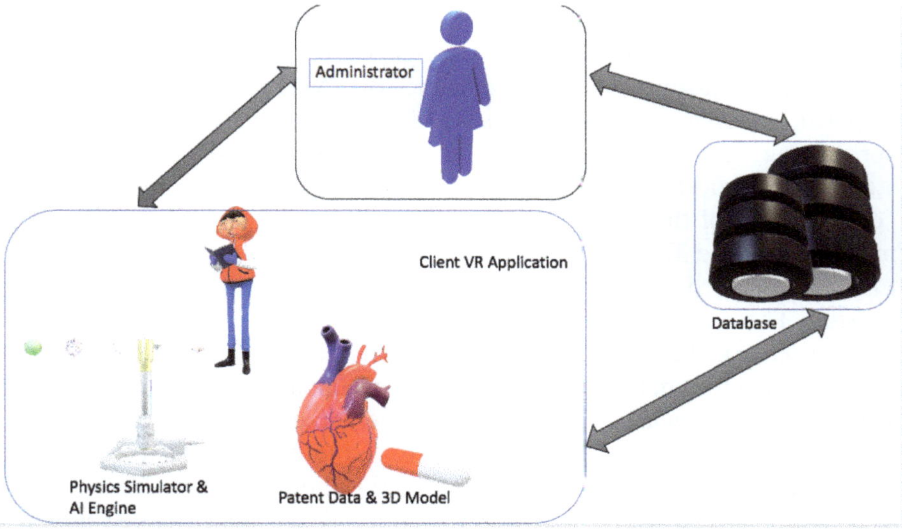

Figure 10.3. Common requirements of a VR application.

into the scenario simulation system. The initial database can include three-dimensional (3D) models and assets, user data, and various scenes. The same is extendable to most AR applications, too.

There exist a few known companies and organisations that have made a name for themselves in designing AR/VR applications for the medical domain. These include Fundamental VR, Karuna Labs, OxfordVR, Augmedics, Surgical Theatre, EchoPixel, Medivis, Health Scholars, Vicarious Surgical, Touch Surgery, Proprio Vision, Immersive Touch, OSSO VR, Senti AR, Holo Anatomy, XR Health, and Mind Maze [16, 17]. These companies are undertaking groundbreaking work in designing relevant applications for clinics, hospitals, and schools of medicine so that the AR/VR content experience is clinically accurate as well as meaningful. Many of their applications incorporate 5G technology as well as AI and machine learning to present appropriate two-dimensional (2D) and 3D representations through screens and holographic display devices [17].

Effective interactive interface elements such as framing and use of texts, colours, graphics, and sound can help in creating a good immersive environment for users, providing sufficient auditory and visual inputs, as well as other sensory contributions. Several types of games are used in rehabilitation services, such as 2D, 3D, VR and AR games, and other widely available consumer-console-based user interfaces such as Wii, PlayStation, Wii Balance, Xbox, and Kinect. Peripherals and gear such as Samsung Gear VR glasses, Oculus headsets, Vuforia, etc., are useful in tracking user movement when rotating in the three axes. Devices such as the Samsung Galaxy S6, S7, Galaxy Tab S2, and Nexus are known to offer comprehensive augmentation features. Additional hardware, such as Leap Motion controllers, may be used to process spatial information in three dimensions and to detect and understand hand movement and distance variation [18]. Some development frameworks that are in common use include Apple's AR Kit, Google's AR Core, Wikitude AR, Vuforia, Easy AR, the open-source augmented framework ARToolKit, and others [19].

Application development is composed of five basic stages: (i) data acquisition and pre-processing; (ii) data streaming P of transferring real-word data and information into the virtual world or AR environment; (iii) network and security requirements; (iv) development of the application framework using SDKs and a coding environment to incorporate 3D model creation, defining of functionality, and environment features; and (v) designing of a user interface for effective interaction and immersion. These are shown in figure 10.4.

Interactions can be made meaningful only if the interface and the objects and events in the environment have a symbiotic and timely communication. The three cornerstones of VR technology, immersion, interactivity, and imagination, must be in sync with the user requirements to achieve an affective application. Developmental platforms such as the Unity 3D graphics engine have been found to be compatible with many AR/VR software development kits [20]. Software such as 3D Max and Blender can be used to make virtual medical kits and scenes too. Viewing formats in AR environments, VR environments, and web-based environments must also be considered for aggregation with the design of the application. These must be considered in conjunction with the now generic model for implementation of a web service on cloud platforms using various integrations of database interactions, servers, and plugins [21]. Figure 10.5 presents the various layers of

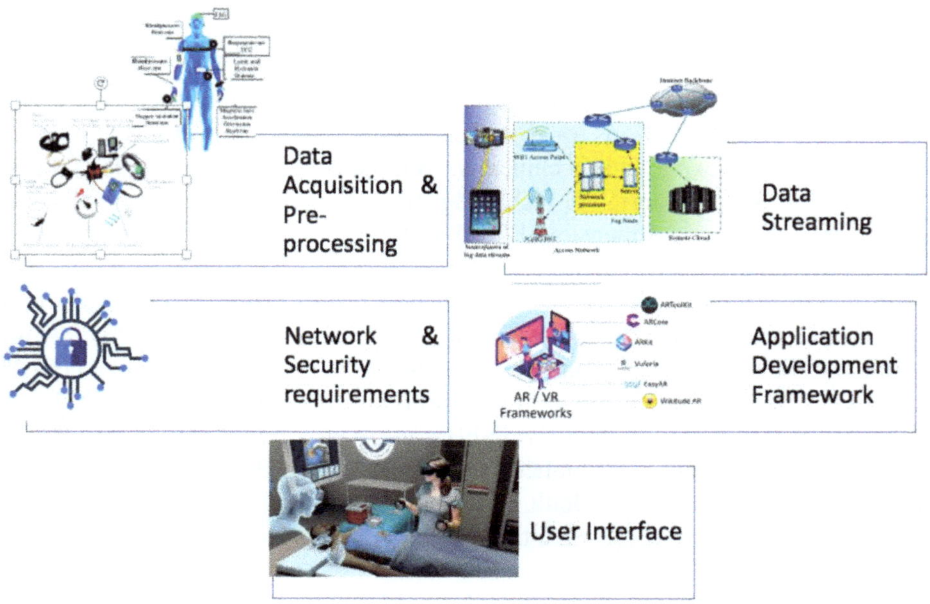

Figure 10.4. The five phases of augmented healthcare application development.

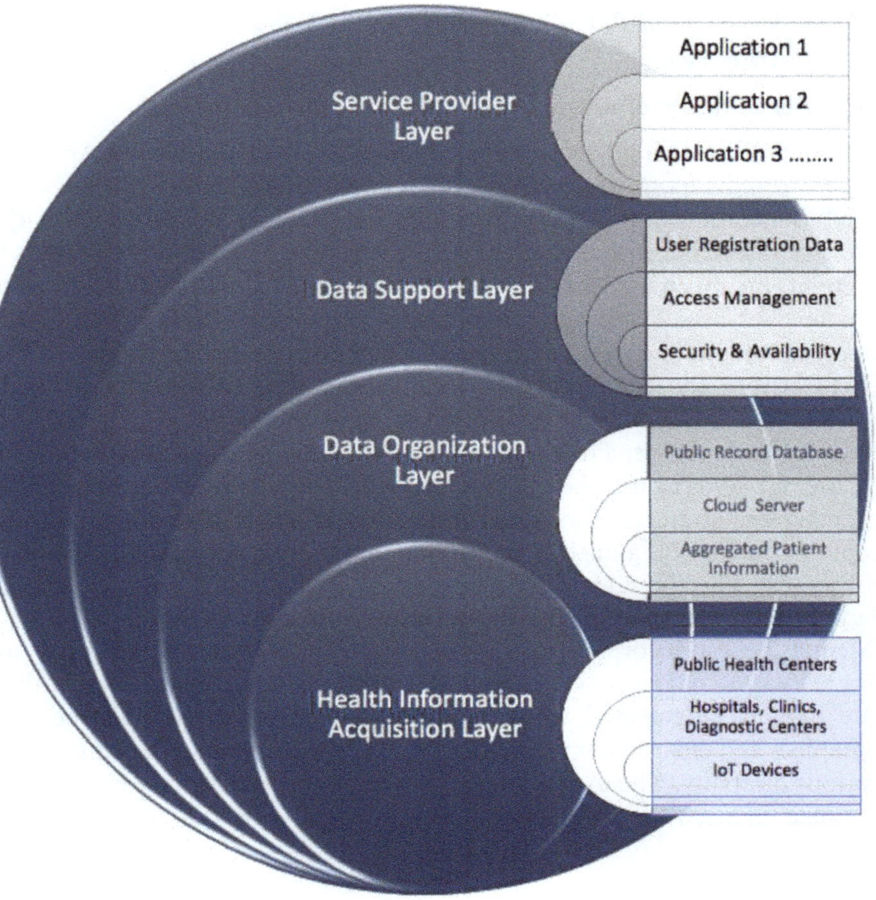

Figure 10.5. Various layers of association between stakeholders for creation of a comprehensive affective application using AR/VR technology.

association between stakeholders for creation of a comprehensive affective application using AR/VR technology.

The physiological signals that are commonly used in VR applications include ECGs to measure heart rate, heart rate variability, blood volume pulse through photoplethysmograms, and blood pressure sensors; skin conductance level and skin potential response through electrodermal activity sensors, galvanic skin response sensors, and skin temperature; respiration rate, tidal volume, and O_2 consumption to acquire information about breathing activity; the strength of contraction of skeletal muscles using electromyogram devices, and eye movements and pupil properties using cameras; and the electrical activity of the brain via the scalp through EEG devices. All such devices are very commonly used. Haptic devices have also found usage in these applications.

10.4 Affective augmented reality/virtual reality applications in healthcare

10.4.1 Mental health disorders

MHDs have been found to be very common all over the world. Among health burdens, in India alone nearly about 200 million people require care for conditions related to mental health [22]. Further, approximately 50 million people suffer with depressive disorders, with a similar count for people with anxiety disorders [2, 23]. The counts are much higher worldwide. Following the global COVID-19 pandemic, this count has been significantly increased. Diagnosis of MHDs, though not very tedious, is still a taboo in many societies. Such diseases can be diagnosed based on medical history and lab reports, physical examination of the patients, and, most importantly, a psychological evaluation to note and evaluate patients' thoughts, behaviour, and feelings. Treatment of MHDs should be given very high priority as they are no longer just the burden of rich. Their treatments need to involve comprehensive strategies for the dissemination of knowledge about MHDs, their acceptance in society, and their prevention, apart from the tasks of treatment and recovery [23]. This should apply not only at the personal level, but also at the level of policy for total inclusion in government healthcare systems (figure 10.6).

Mental health incorporates individual attributes that include, but are not restricted to, managing one's behaviour, emotions, and interactions with others. These may be augmented with a number of socioeconomic, genetic, political, geographic, and environmental factors. Neuropsychiatric disorders may even result in serious disability. The losses due to these are known to be very high [24]. MHDs can range in severity, from minor incidents and episodes to becoming major

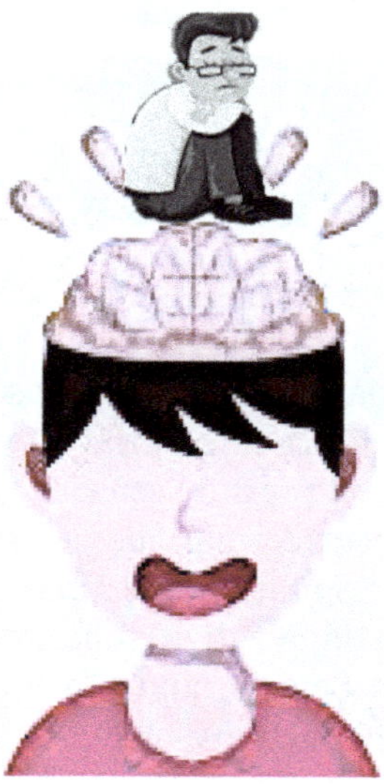

Figure 10.6. MHDs are usually viewed with less empathy but they actually have a huge impact in overall well-being.

disruptions to a person's life and well-being, as shown in Figure 10.6. While occasional outbursts, impulsiveness, defiance, and losing of temper is not considered a problem, their continuous occurrences can hinder an individual in leading a healthy, normal life. Furthermore, such disorders can also manifest themselves either as internalised disorders or externalised behaviours [25–28].

The various forms of MHDs include the following:

- Anxiety disorders, panic disorders, obsessive-compulsive disorders, and phobias.
- Depression, bipolar disorders, and mood disorders.
- Post-traumatic stress disorder (PTSD).
- Psychotic disorders such as schizophrenia.
- Eating disorders.
- Disruptive behaviour, dissocial disorders, defiance disorder, and conduct disorder.
- Attention deficit hyperactive disorder.
- Developmental problems such as speech/language delay and intellectual disability.
- Neuro-developmental and neurodegenerative disorders.
- Personality disorders.

Such disorders can occur at any stage of life. Many tend to occur in later childhood and may be difficult to recognise early by parents or caregivers, while many others are known to occur in the senior population. Treatment of MHDs depends on the disorder and its seriousness. Proper and timely medication, counselling, group discussions, and activities with mental health professionals and other patients have been known to be highly effective.

Identification, treatment, and management of MHDs in primary-care settings are cost effective as they are more acceptable to the patient and their caregivers so as to avoid any social stigma. Some of these are shown in Figure 10.7. Further, the environment of the treatment setup itself should be amenable to the patients, such as its locality or familiarity, etc. If appropriate care can be provided in familiar settings, the patients are known to respond in a more positive manner efficiently and effectively (figure 10.7).

However, geographic location, unavailability of appropriate treatment facilities, pandemic-like situations, and many such issues can lead to incomplete or non-ideal situations for treatment. With the advancements in the fields of AR and VR, including devices, computing capability, networks, and so on, there is now a possibility of putting such technologies to use [7, 8]. These systems may be web-based or app-based and may work with or without internet service depending on their usability and design structures [29]. Further, psychological, cognitive, and behavioural interventions through the use of AR and VR have been demonstrated to have particular advantages too. These advantages include the ability to control the stimuli, events, and environments to which the patients may be exposed to check and compare their adaptability. These are especially advantageous as control in real-world situations may be difficult to achieve. In addition, it has been found through

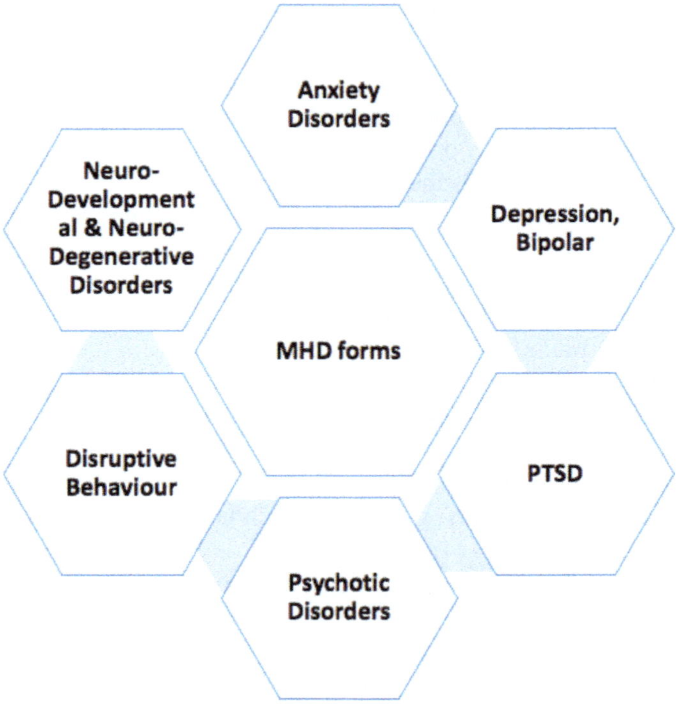

Figure 10.7. Some of the various forms of disease related to MHDs.

deliberations that patients' subjective performance when making use of the presence and immersion of AR/VR is better in cognitive-neuropsychological tests as compared to their performance in lab environments. In many such cases, AR- and VR-based evaluations are more comfortable for neurologically affected patients. Further, such applications can also be used as empathic tools for doctors, in which the actual simulation of events can help doctors to relate with patients' problems in a more engaging and understanding manner.

Many of the common symptoms of anxiety disorders, depression, PTSD, behavioural and developmental problems, personality disorders, and other such related mental health problems are mostly related to how the patient is feeling. These include symptoms such as hopelessness, feeling sad, loss of interest in normal day-to-day activities, feelings of frustration, anxiousness, suicidal tendencies, guilt, appetite disorder, etc. Symptoms may occur as isolated episodes or as multiple events that may be triggered suddenly or due to a particular factor. Another type of disorder, seasonal affective disorder, affects patients who may suffer from clinical depression due to changes in seasons or weather. Though depression may be triggered due to the effect of certain chemicals in the body, it may also be psychologically triggered. The psychological aspect of the afflictions may be reduced with the use of proper VR environments.

VR-based applications for MHDs also use other sensors to understand the feelings and emotions displayed in humans. Emotions in humans may be classified into discrete categories or understood as dimensional models. The various forms of dimensional models include the circumplex model, the vector model, positive activation–negative activation model, Plutchk's model, and the pleasure–arousal–dominance model. Six basic emotions of anger, fear, disgust, joy, surprise, and sadness are accounted for in the discrete categorisation model; other emotions are said to be a combination of these basic emotions. On the other hand, dimensional models conceptualise emotions as per their spatial location in two or three dimensions such as in valence–arousal or intensity graphs. When medical VR applications are augmented using other sensory devices such as EEG or ECG signal-acquisition devices, these emotion models can give an indication of a person's emotional state. The analysis presented by these models can complement direct clinical observations as multi-source feedback and help caregivers and medical personnel in charting the course of treatments [12]. A recent work by Srivastava and Agnihotri [23] relates studies wherein Google Glass AR innovation was used to assist youngsters with MHDs to decipher their emotions and feelings. The Autism Glass Project from Stanford University also deals with such work. In a study by Sharma *et al* [13], the authors compiled works on how VR-based applications can be designed to help people cope with depression.

The design of an affective AR/VR application would need affective input too. These inputs would help in triggering responses from patients. The relationship between affective input, immersion and presence, and affective response is depicted below in figure 10.8.

Affective and emotional content must be created to enhance the user's feelings of presence and immersion. This can then lead to increased affective and emotional responses. These responses in turn can be read and analysed by relevant experts to expedite treatment. In [19], the authors presented similar design paradigms. They further proposed that an understanding of the reactions and responses of patients in earlier sessions be compared to present sessions to help as a feedback mechanism to generate better future events. They also emphasised the use of a definite emotional space (i.e., valence, arousal, dominance, emotion typology and intensity) in the design of AR/VR applications. A narration of the events triggered at a particular response or time interval would be helpful in shaping the experiences too.

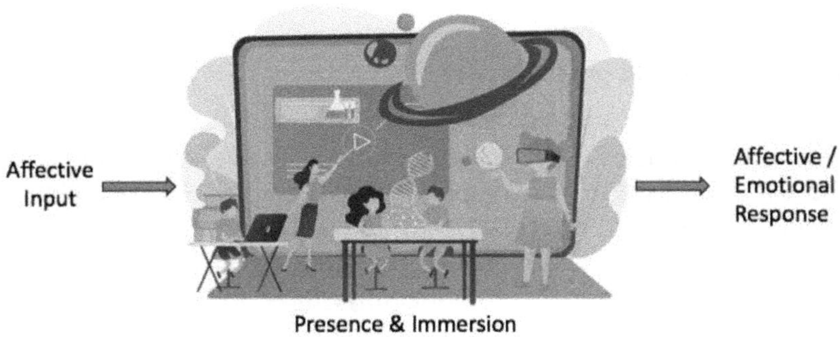

Figure 10.8. Figure showing the relationship between affective input, feeling of presence and immersion by user, and their affective response to the events.

10.4.2 Rehabilitation related to traumatic brain injuries

Traumatic brain injuries (TBIs) are often referred to as a silent epidemic. Such injuries can occur due to neurodegenerative diseases, brain strokes, or accidents, etc. As a conseqeunce of these injuries, a patient's understanding of mental imagery may show a deterioration. The so-called mental-rotation paradigm is a well-known psychological study [30] that has long established that there is a relation between the time it takes for the human brain to distinguish between an image and its mirror image or a rotated figure. The Shepard and Metzler test discusses the perception of physical rotation of a real object by considering it as a representation of visual information [30]. Related studies by Tomasino and Rumiati in [30] and Rose *et al* in [10] showcase the possibilities of using computers for the generation, maintenance, scanning, and manipulation of images that can be used as mental images to be used in this mental-rotation paradigm for TBI-affected populations. Two-dimensional as well as 3D user interfaces were also developed. This form of brain rehabilitation can be further enhanced in virtual-environment-assisted applications, wherein patients can practice multiple times in their own time and space without strict and multiple supervision of doctors. This research can further be augmented by utilising other medical devices to record which portions of the brain are involved in solving mental-rotation-related tasks.

In their work, Marusan *et al* [31] presented details of using VR for various mental-rotation-related tasks to improve visuospatial ability. The various stakeholders in this model were the administrators, doctors, and patients. Each had its role defined within the application. The patients are allowed access to a test schedule and the tests themselves only. Doctors and healthcare practitioners are granted a wider access, i.e., to the patient results too, along with test-related actions. Administrators were required to manage the doctor and patient accounts and records. Three-dimensional objects can be designed, and their rotation enabled in various directions. These include not only regular geometric shapes, but virtual objects such as sofas, tables, lamps, and so on. The main intended purpose of the application was to engage users (i.e., patients) in finding the differences between image models and their mirror images or rotated forms. Implementing this application as a VR application allowed the patients to perform these tasks repeatedly as well as to make the experience more attractive (i.e., more present and immersive). Some examples of the UI designed in [11] is shown in figure 10.9.

10.4.3 Rehabilitation and physiotherapy

VR and AR have been commonly used in the gaming industry, for example in the games *Ingress* and *Zombies, Run!*. In addition to this, these applications have shown the potential to be utilised to increase physical activity in players, thereby improving cardiovascular health [32]. According to the authors (Heng *et al* [14]), these applications can motivate adolescents to perform certain health-related exercises. To combat obesity and related physiotherapy, these may be used to entice the younger, game-oriented population to engage in physical activities. In a related case, the treatment of phantom-limb pain involves the rehabilitation of a patient with phantom appendages [13]. Using an AR application, patients will see a virtual arm

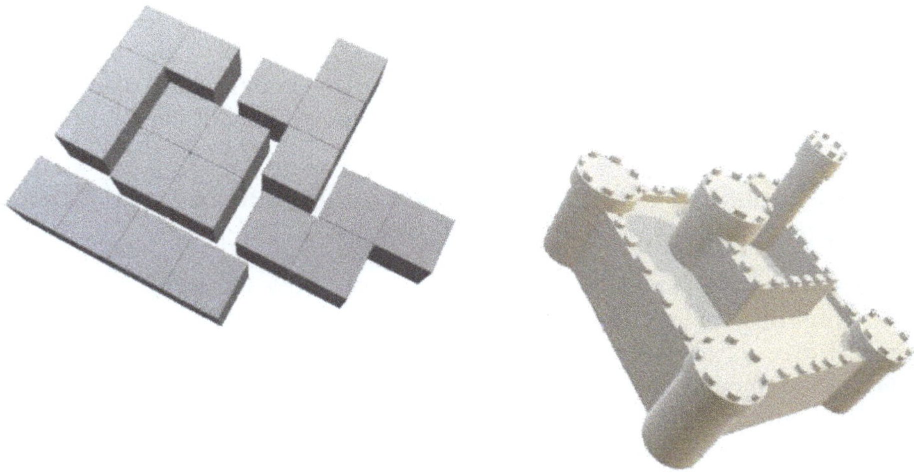

Figure 10.9. Examples of mental images used in VR-based mental-rotation tasks.

or limb appear on the screen during the treatment plan. As a result, this can provide a restorative effect.

In [32], authors Mubin *et al* presented information about the usage of AR/VR and the above related concept of gamification for stroke patients' rehabilitation through robot-assisted therapy. They studied the various manners in which technologies and practices of AR/VR or gamification are adaptable for the rehabilitation of post-stroke patients by assessing the effectiveness of exoskeleton robotics. They studied MEDLINE, EMBASE, Science Direct, and the Cochrane Library databases. They also found participation in VR/AR-based games, either as exercises or through interactions, was much more efficient and effective for repeated sessions. Haptic devices have previously been used in conjunction with AR experiments for the rehabilitation of patients with restricted limb movements such as hand stiffness. A good example of such an application is Physio@Home, which helps in exploring visual guidance and feedback techniques for physiotherapy exercises [33].

Gamification based on immersion and interaction can also be used to manage acute and chronic pain through psychological simulations. Apart from physiotherapy, other fields of therapy and rehabilitation where many AR/VR applications have been utilised are exposure therapy, addiction therapy, and relaxation therapy [21]. Other common applications of AR/VR in the healthcare sector have been in the teaching and learning of human anatomy, nursing, medical equipment training, simulating surgery procedures [34] including pre-surgery planning and post-surgery necessities, implantology, radiology, gynaecologist, obstetrics, medical social skills learning, patient education and communication, telemedicine, medical or emergency case simulations, raising awareness in the community, as well as for other end-to-end healthcare requirements [2, 13, 35]. Existing applications such as AR Human Anatomy [18], 4D APP, and others can be installed on handheld mobile devices along with appropriate head-mounted display devices to engage in self-learning. There are many more applications such as eye disease diagnosis, cardiac treatment, cancer detection, brain tumour detection, and monitoring guidelines wherein AR-based healthcare applications find relevance [24]. The use of such applications is fuelled by the demand for quality healthcare services, the need for a reduction in healthcare costs, and the increased role of connected sensory devices.

10.5 Assessment of affective responses in augmented reality/virtual reality applications

The effectiveness of an application can be determined while it is being developed and can be confirmed by the response of users. Typically, AR/VR applications are designed for medical professionals, such as physicians, therapists, etc., as well as patients. Even though most applications are designed with the patients' needs in mind, it is imperative to also consider the views of healthcare professionals, especially for critical applications where the doctor's input or empathy is necessary to assess the progress of MHD patients. It is necessary for virtual agents acting as mentors in such applications to adapt their behaviour in accordance with the mood, feelings, and personalities of their patients. Furthermore, while most assessments are subjective in nature, some may be based on real-time mapping using additional sensors such as EEG devices.

According to a study by Alimardani *et al* [36], estimating the patient's personality traits can also improve human–agent interaction and therefore a given application's immersive quality. Their findings were based on the use of EEGs measuring responses from generic study participants. The authors aimed to enhance participants' interaction with the virtual agent by using the EEG as a real-time physiological measure of affective empathy. Using Kruskall–Wallis tests, they tested between different experimental phases for each brain area (frontal and central) and frequency bands of delta, theta, alpha, beta, and gamma waves. Most of their analysis was based on regression analysis.

10.6 Design challenges of affective applications using augmented reality/virtual reality technology in healthcare

The accessibility of VR/AR applications to end users is a continuous challenge. Further, the designed user interface must be intuitive so that familiarity with the application may be established quickly and efficiently. There are times when users need to be given instructions or shown movements at the right time and place for them to become familiar with the application; it is not enough to use the application only once. In addition, the experience should be enticing enough to hold the attention of the participant for multiple sessions. Figure 10.10 illustrates a number of these design challenges. It is also imperative to consider how 'real' the objects appear. This is conditional on the requirements of the application, its budget, and the level of experience of the VR object designers. There are several factors that influence the overall cost of designing a successful application, including the number of 3D objects, their interaction, the level of immersion, and the number of man-hours required for their development. Enhancing motivation in users, especially

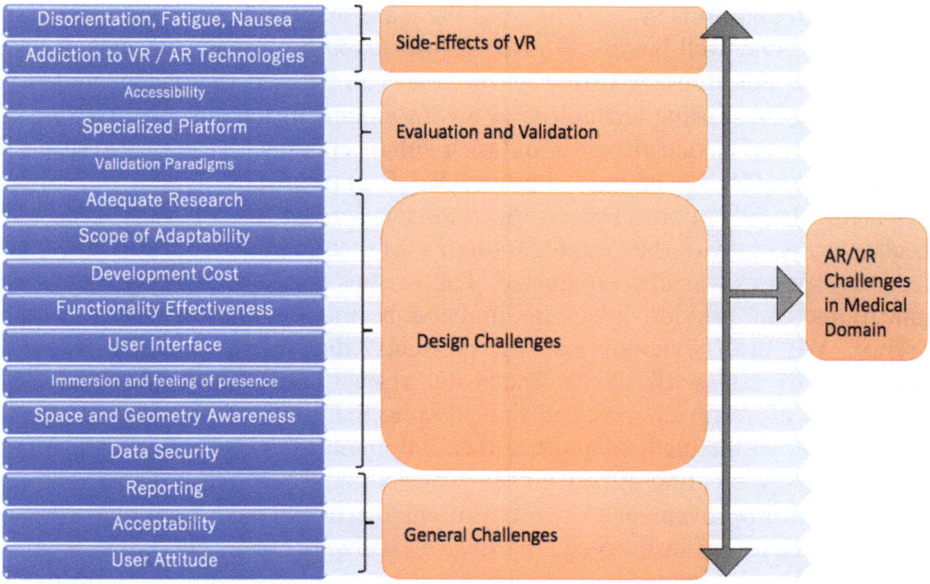

Figure 10.10. Challenges in the design of affective AR/VR applications in the medical domain.

patients, through audiovisual cues is difficult and varies from user to user according to their requirements, and even their moods.

When designing applications, consideration should be given to featuring social context (i.e., multiplayer versus single player), motion types (that is, single muscle versus multiple muscles), and cognitive challenges (easy, medium, difficult, or level 0 to higher). The aim of group therapy sessions is to motivate patients through collaboration or competition. The design of an application that incorporates this level of interaction and realism is challenging. In addition, patients may also feel overwhelmed or isolated when using these advanced technologies. In addition, a suitable and appropriate reporting format should be created for doctors, therapists, and healthcare workers.

Several factors, such as immersion, freedom of movement, navigation, camera control, etc., need to be catered to and improved upon in future. Other common challenges include the use of non-standard equipment and user interfaces, as well as side-effects of disorientation, fatigue, and nausea. Even though these are common side-effects of VR technology, they can have an adverse effect on the usability of applications designed in this manner. Last but not least, there is the massive issue of data and network security for AR platforms [37]. Concerns include the collaboration of data, scalability, confidentiality, integrity, resilience, availability, privacy, network issues, protocols, and standards, among others.

10.7 Conclusion

Humans are complex beings with many capabilities and emotions. As a result of our capabilities, we can reach the pinnacle of our potential. There is no denying the importance of emotions in our lives, and there are many subtle ways in which they can affect us. Our well-being can also be threatened by imbalances and disorders that affect our emotions. A variety of methods can be used to enhance and enrich quality of life by utilising technological advancements in the fields of AR and VR, via the creation of virtual elements and their enhancement with real-world scenarios. A variety of MHDs can be treated using AR/VR applications, as well as a range of other medical applications. These various applications of AR/VR were discussed in this chapter. A study of the design paradigms for creating adequate systems to elicit affective responses was also conducted. The various stages of development of such applications can provide adequate immersion and enhance a user's sense of presence. We also reviewed existing products and frameworks. It is equally challenging to assess all of the medically relevant AR/VR applications. This chapter's literature review revealed that, despite the multitude of AR/VR applications available in the medical and healthcare domain, they are still in their infancy when it comes to creating affective-response-eliciting applications. There remains a huge scope for improvement. A few recent enhancements have been made possible due to advances in technology, hardware, software, and networks, with the possibility of undertaking new developments. A rigorous assessment protocol is also necessary, as these advances are directly related to human health and well-being. This chapter further discussed some of the challenges that exist in the field. These challenges include human nature's reluctance to accept unknown applications, as well as their accessibility to the public. The challenges of the AR/VR technology itself are not the only ones. There are also challenges in the design, evaluation, and validation of new products. Several of these challenges may persist so long as there are no standards or protocols in place.

References

[1] Massetti T, Da Silva T D, Crocetta T B, Guarnieri R, De Freitas B L, Bianchi Lopes P and de Mello Monteiro C B 2018 The clinical utility of virtual reality in neurorehabilitation: a systematic review *J. Cent. Nerv. Syst. Dis.* **10** 1179573518813541

[2] Müller-Wittig W 2011 Virtual reality in medicine ed R Kramme, K P Hoffmann and R S Pozos *Springer Handbook of Medical Technology. Springer Handbooks* (Berlin: Springer)

[3] Murugappan M 2015 Frequency band localization on multiple physiological signals for human emotion classification using DWT *Emotion Recognition: A Pattern Analysis* ed A Konar and A Chakraborty (New York: Wiley) ch 12 pp 293–313

[4] Maruthapillai V and Murugappan M 2016 Optimal geometrical set for automated marker placement to virtualized real-time facial emotions *PLoS One* **11** e0149003

[5] Murugappan M, Nagarajan R and Yaacob S 2015 KNN and LDA based discrete human emotions classification using electroencephalogram (EEG) *Softw. Technol. Eng.* **2009** 322–7

[6] She W J *et al* 2022 Investigation of a Web-based explainable AI screening for prolonged grief disorder *IEEE Access* **10** 41164–85

[7] Tabbaa L, Ang C S, Siriaraya P, She W J and Prigerson H G 2021 A reflection on virtual reality design for psychological, cognitive and behavioral interventions: design needs, opportunities and challenges *Int. J. Hum.–Comput. Interact.* **37** 851–66

[8] 2020 Usability and UX in mobile and XR applications https://bimprove-h2020.eu/usability-and-ux-in-mobile-and-xr-applications/ (Accessed: 18/10/22)

[9] Riva G, Mancuso V, Cavedoni S and Stramba-Badiale C 2020 Virtual reality in neurorehabilitation: a review of its effects on multiple cognitive domains *Expert Rev. Med. Devices* **17** 1035–61

[10] Rose F D, Brooks B M and Rizzo A A 2005 Virtual reality in brain damage rehabilitation *Cyberpsychol. Behav.* **8** 241–62

[11] Boeldt D, McMahon E, McFaul M and Greenleaf W 2019 Using virtual reality exposure therapy to enhance treatment of anxiety disorders: identifying areas of clinical adoption and potential obstacles *Front. Psychiatry* **10** 773

[12] Srivastava S and Agnihotri R B 2019 Augmented reality and its implementation in health care sector *2019 Int. Conf. on Intelligent Computing and Control Systems (ICCS)(May 2019) (Piscataway, NJ)* (IEEE) pp 1391–6

[13] Sharma N, Kolekar M H and Chandra S 2012 Synthetic perception: new era of virtual reality in mental health care *CSI Commun.* **33** 413

[14] Heng P A, Cheng C Y, Wong T T, Xu Y, Chui Y P, Chan K M and Tso S K 2004 A virtual-reality training system for knee arthroscopic surgery *IEEE Trans. Inf. Technol. Biomed.* **8** 217–27

[15] Shepard R N and Metzler J 1971 Mental rotation of three-dimensional objects *Science* **171** 701–3

[16] 2023 AR VR in Healthcare Startups https://tracxn.com/explore/Top-AR-VR-in-Healthcare-Startups (Accessed: 18/10/22)

[17] 2020 Healthcare Augmented Reality and Virtual Reality Companies https://hitconsultant.net/2020/06/29/augmented-reality-and-virtual-reality-companies-to-watch/ (Accessed: 18/10/22)

[18] Ara J, Karim F B, Alsubaie M S A, Bhuiyan Y A, Bhuiyan M I, Bhyan S B and Bhuiyan H 2021 Comprehensive analysis of augmented reality technology in modern healthcare system *Int. J. Adv. Comput. Sci. Appl.* **12** 840–9.

[19] Marcolin F, Scurati G W, Ulrich L, Nonis F, Vezzetti E, Dozio N and Ferrise F 2021 Affective virtual reality: how to design artificial experiences impacting human emotions *IEEE Comput. Graph. Appl.* **41** 171–84

[20] Cong X and Li T 2020 Design and development of virtual medical system interface based on VR–AR hybrid technology *Comput. Math. Methods Med.* **2020** 7108147

[21] Halbig A and Latoschik M E 2021 A systematic review of physiological measurements, factors, methods, and applications in virtual reality *Front. Virtual Real.* **2** 694567

[22] Chauhan V S and Chauhan S 2022 Mental Health in India: A Perspective https://indianexpress.com/article/lifestyle/health/mental-health-in-india-a-perspective-anxiety-depression-stress-7764309/#:~:text=In%202017%2C%20an%20estimation%20of,million%20people%20with%20anxiety%20disorders (Accessed: 18/10/22)

[23] 2023 Mental Health https://who.int/india/health-topics/mental-health (Accessed: 18/10/22)

[24] 2023 National Mental Health Programme (NMHP) https://nhm.gov.in/index1.php?lang=1&level=2&sublinkid=1043&lid=359 (Accessed: 18/10/22)

[25] Bong S Z and Khairunizam W K *et al* 2017 Implementation of wavelet packet transform and non-linear analysis for emotion classification in stroke patient using brain signals *Biomed. Signal Process. Control* **36** 102–12

[26] Yuvaraj R, Murugappan M and Sundaraj K 2012 Methods and approaches on emotions recognition in neurodegenerative disorders: a review *2012 IEEE Symp. on Industrial Electronics and Applications (Bandung, Indonesia, 2012)* pp 287–92

[27] Dar M N and Akram M U *et al* 2022 EEG-based emotion charting for Parkinson's disease patients using convolutional recurrent neural networks and cross dataset learning *Comput. Biol. Med.* **144** 105327

[28] Anandhi B and Jerritta S *et al* 2020 Performance analysis of wavelet transform in the removal of baseline wandering from ECG signals in children with autism spectrum disorder (ASD) *Advances in Electrical and Computer Technologies. Lecture Notes in Electrical Engineering* vol 672 (Singapore: Springer)

[29] Tabbaa L, Searle R, Mirzaee S, Hossain M M, Intarasirisawat J, Glancy M and Ang C S 2021 VREED: virtual reality emotion recognition dataset using eye tracking and physiological measures *Proc. ACM on Interactive, Mobile, Wearable and Ubiquitous Technologies* pp 1–20

[30] Tomasino B and Rumiati R I 2004 Effects of strategies on mental rotation and hemispheric lateralization: neuropsychological evidence *J. Cogn. Neurosci.* **16** 878–84

[31] Marusan M, Kulistak J and Zara J 2006 Virtual reality in neurorehabilitation: mental rotation *Proc. 3rd Central European Multimedia and Virtual Reality Conf. (November 2006)* pp 77–83

[32] Mubin O, Alnajjar F, Jishtu N, Alsinglawi B and Al Mahmud A 2019 Exoskeletons with virtual reality, augmented reality, and gamification for stroke patients' rehabilitation: systematic review *JMIR Rehabil. Assist. Technol.* **6** e12010

[33] Tang R, Yang X D, Bateman S, Jorge J and Tang A 2015 Physio@Home: exploring visual guidance and feedback techniques for physiotherapy exercises *Proc. 33rd Annual ACM Conf. on Human Factors in Computing Systems (Seoul, Republic of Korea, April 2015)* pp 4123–32

[34] González Izard S, Juanes Méndez J A, Ruisoto Palomera P and García-Peñalvo F J 2019 Applications of virtual and augmented reality in biomedical imaging *J. Med. Syst.* **43** 1–5

[35] Muñoz-Saavedra L, Miró-Amarante L and Domínguez-Morales M 2020 Augmented and virtual reality evolution and future tendency *Appl. Sci.* **10** 322

[36] Alimardani M, Hermans A and Tinga A M 2020 Assessment of empathy in an affective VR environment using EEG signals arXiv preprint arXiv:2003.10886

[37] Weiss P L, Kizony R, Feintuch U and Katz N 2014 Virtual reality in neurorehabilitation *Textbook of Neural Repair and Rehabilitation* ed M Selzer, S Clarke, L Cohen, G Kwakkel and Miller R (Cambridge: Cambridge University Press) pp 198–218

[38] Lopes D S, Medeiros D, Paulo S F, Borges P B, Nunes V, Mascarenhas V and Jorge J A 2018 Interaction techniques for immersive CT colonography: a professional assessment *Int. Conf. on Medical Image Computing and Computer-Assisted Intervention (Cham, September 2018)* pp 629–37

www.ingramcontent.com/pod-product-compliance
Ingram Content Group UK Ltd.
Pitfield, Milton Keynes, MK11 3LW, UK
UKHW051855100926
8556IPUK00005B/639

9 780750 351805